# Advances in Oral Diseases Diagnosis and Management: 2nd Edition

# Advances in Oral Diseases Diagnosis and Management: 2nd Edition

Guest Editors

**Dimitris Tatsis**
**Konstantinos Paraskevopoulos**

MDPI

Basel • Beijing • Wuhan • Barcelona • Belgrade • Novi Sad • Cluj • Manchester

*Guest Editors*
Dimitris Tatsis
Department of Oral and Maxillofacial Surgery
Aristotle University of Thessaloniki
Thessaloniki
Greece

Konstantinos Paraskevopoulos
Department of Oral and Maxillofacial Surgery
Aristotle University of Thessaloniki
Thessaloniki
Greece

*Editorial Office*
MDPI AG
Grosspeteranlage 5
4052 Basel, Switzerland

This is a reprint of the Special Issue, published open access by the journal *Diagnostics* (ISSN 2075-4418), freely accessible at: https://www.mdpi.com/journal/diagnostics/special_issues/LS00BP9ED8.

For citation purposes, cite each article independently as indicated on the article page online and as indicated below:

| Lastname, A.A.; Lastname, B.B. Article Title. *Journal Name* **Year**, *Volume Number*, Page Range. |
|---|

**ISBN 978-3-7258-4501-9 (Hbk)**
**ISBN 978-3-7258-4502-6 (PDF)**
**https://doi.org/10.3390/books978-3-7258-4502-6**

# Contents

# About the Editors

**Dimitris Tatsis**

Dimitris Tatsis is an oral and maxillofacial surgeon, serving as a consultant at the University Department of Oral and Maxillofacial Surgery, General Hospital G. Papanikolaou, Thessaloniki. He holds medical and dental degrees from Greece and is a Fellow of the European Board of Oro-Maxillo-Facial Surgery/Head and Neck Surgery (EBOMFS). With advanced training as a Post-CCT Senior Clinical Fellow in Head and Neck Surgery at the University College London Hospitals NHS Foundation Trust, United Kingdom, as well as microsurgery and flap reconstruction from prestigious institutions in London and Aachen, Dr. Tatsis' special interest lies in head and neck oncology, reconstructive surgery, and traumatology. He has contributed to numerous publications in high-impact journals, including *Diagnostics*, *Oral Maxillofacial Surgery*, and *European Journal of Surgical Oncology*, and is a frequent speaker at international conferences, such as the European Association for Cranio Maxillo Facial Surgery Congress, where he has been recognized with the John Lowry Scholarship. Dr. Tatsis actively participates in collaborative research, including the COVIDSurg Collaborative, and is dedicated to advancing patient care and education in oral and maxillofacial surgery.

**Konstantinos Paraskevopoulos**

Konstantinos Paraskevopoulos serves as an assistant professor at the Aristotle University of Thessaloniki, Greece and practices as an oral and maxillofacial surgeon at the University Department of Oral and Maxillofacial Surgery, General Hospital G. Papanikolaou, Thessaloniki. Holding both medical and dental degrees, he addresses the full scope of his specialty surgically, with a particular focus on oncology, facial reconstruction, traumatology, and research. He has earned a doctoral degree and conducted postdoctoral research, complemented by advanced training at European centers for oral and maxillofacial surgery. Dr. Paraskevopoulos has contributed to numerous research protocols, collaborating extensively with oncologists, pathologists, and biologists. A frequently invited speaker at international conferences, he maintains a prominent presence in the field and has authored multiple international publications in peer-reviewed journals, as well as books on oral and maxillofacial surgery and related medical topics. For many years, he has been deeply engaged in educating medical, dental, and Erasmus students, as well as oral and maxillofacial surgery residents

# Preface

The Special Issue "Advances in Oral Diseases Diagnosis and Management: 2nd Edition", published in *Diagnostics* (ISSN 2075-4418) under the section "Pathology and Molecular Diagnostics," presents a comprehensive collection of research advancing the diagnosis and management of oral diseases. Edited by Dr. Dimitris Tatsis and Dr. Konstantinos Paraskevopoulos from the Aristotle University of Thessaloniki, Greece, this issue addresses critical public health challenges posed by oral conditions, including oral potentially malignant disorders, oral cancer, autoimmune disorders, infections, temporomandibular joint disorders, osteomyelitis, and medication-related osteonecrosis of the jaws.

Featuring 15 peer-reviewed papers, this Special Issue encompasses a wide spectrum of head and neck pathologies. Key contributions explore innovative diagnostic tools such as mucoscopy, bioimpedance, and optical coherence tomography, alongside histopathological and clinical analyses of conditions like oral lichen planus, leukoplakia, and peri-implantitis. The research highlights interdisciplinary approaches, integrating molecular biology, genetics, and microbiology, emphasizing early detection, personalized treatment, and patient-centered care to improve oral and systemic health outcomes.

The Reprint of this Special Issue serves as a resource for researchers, clinicians, and policymakers, offering insights into diagnostic technologies and management strategies to reduce the global burden of oral diseases and enhance patient quality of life.

**Dimitris Tatsis and Konstantinos Paraskevopoulos**
*Guest Editors*

diagnostics

MDPI

Editorial

# Editorial for "Advances in Oral Diseases Diagnosis and Management: 2nd Edition"

**Dimitris Tatsis * and Konstantinos Paraskevopoulos**

Department of Oral & Maxillofacial Surgery, Aristotle University of Thessaloniki, Specialized Cancer Treatment and Reconstruction Centre, General Hospital of Thessaloniki "George Papanikolaou", 57010 Thessaloniki, Greece; kostparas@yahoo.gr

* Correspondence: dtatsis@outlook.com or dimitats@auth.gr

The field of oral disease diagnosis and management has undergone significant transformation in recent years, propelled by innovations in diagnostic technologies, molecular biology, and interdisciplinary clinical approaches. Oral diseases, ranging from periodontal disease to oral cancers, pose a major global health challenge due to their prevalence and impact on patients' quality of life [1]. The second edition of the Special Issue, titled "Advances in Oral Diseases Diagnosis and Management", published in *Diagnostics*, builds on the success of its predecessor by presenting innovative research that addresses critical gaps in the early detection, diagnosis, and treatment of these conditions.

Recent advancements in oral diagnostics have leveraged tools such as high-resolution imaging, biomarker profiling, and artificial intelligence-driven analytics to enable earlier and more precise detection of oral pathologies [2]. However, challenges remain, including the need for standardized diagnostic protocols across diverse populations, a deeper understanding of molecular mechanisms underlying disease progression, and the development of targeted therapies for complex conditions such as oral squamous cell carcinoma [1,3]. This Special Issue addresses these gaps by highlighting studies that integrate novel diagnostic methodologies, therapeutic strategies, and research into host–microbiome interactions to advance patient-centered care.

The contributions to this Special Issue highlight a range of innovative approaches. For instance, a retrospective study on pathological fractures of the mandible explored the challenges of managing compromised bone quality due to conditions like osteoradionecrosis and medication-related osteonecrosis, offering applied insights into multidisciplinary treatment strategies [4]. Another investigation utilized mucoscopy as a non-invasive tool to assess oral lichen planus, demonstrating its potential to differentiate inflammatory conditions and enhance diagnostic accuracy [5]. Additionally, the application of targeted optical coherence tomography (OCT) in oral cancer diagnosis has shown promise for evaluating tissue microstructure, paving the way for standardized protocols [6]. These works, alongside broader research on microbial dynamics and clinical interventions, underscore the importance of integrating advanced diagnostics with clinical practice [7,8].

Beyond the Special Issue, the recent literature has emphasized the interplay between oral and systemic health. Studies have explored the efficacy of interventions such as sodium hypochlorite mouthwash for periodontal disease management [8], as well as the association between oral health and broader disease outcomes [2]. These findings highlight the need for holistic diagnostic and management strategies that bridge oral and systemic health.

Looking to the future, several research priorities emerge. Standardizing diagnostic criteria across global populations is essential to ensure equitable access to early detection and treatment [1]. The integration of AI into clinical workflows requires robust, multicenter validation studies to confirm its reliability and applicability. Furthermore, personalized therapies informed by genetic and epigenetic profiling could transform the management of oral cancers and autoimmune disorders. Interdisciplinary collaboration across oral pathology, maxillofacial surgery, and molecular biology will be critical to translating these innovations into clinical practice.

This Special Issue serves as both a milestone in current research and a call to action for future exploration. We hope it will inspire researchers, clinicians, and policymakers to address the remaining challenges in oral disease diagnosis and management, ultimately improving patient outcomes on a broader scale.

We extend our gratitude to the authors, reviewers, and editorial team for their dedication to this Special Issue. We invite readers to engage with the research presented here and to contribute to the ongoing advancement of this vital field.

**Author Contributions:** Writing—original draft preparation, D.T.; writing—review and editing, K.P. All authors have read and agreed to the published version of the manuscript.

**Funding:** This research received no external funding.

**Conflicts of Interest:** The authors declare no conflicts of interest.

## References

1. Peres, M.A.; Macpherson, L.M.D.; Weyant, R.J.; Daly, B.; Venturelli, R.; Mathur, M.R.; Listl, S.; Celeste, R.K.; Guarnizo-Herreño, C.C.; Kearns, C.; et al. Oral diseases: A global public health challenge. *Lancet* **2019**, *394*, 249–260, Erratum in Lancet **2019**, *394*, 1010. [CrossRef] [PubMed]
2. Ilhan, B.; Lin, K.; Guneri, P.; Wilder-Smith, P. Improving Oral Cancer Outcomes with Imaging and Artificial Intelligence. *J. Dent. Res.* **2020**, *99*, 241–248. [CrossRef] [PubMed]
3. van der Ploeg, G.R.; Rosema, N.A.M.; Keijser, B.J.F.; Zaura, E.; van der Weijden, G.A.; Shemesh, H. Multi-way modelling of oral microbial dynamics and host-microbiome interactions during induced gingivitis. *NPJ Biofilms Microbiomes* **2024**, *10*, 89. [CrossRef] [PubMed]
4. Chatziantoniou, G.; Tatsis, D.; Politis, S.; Saramantos, A.; Koukolis, N.; Paraskevopoulos, K. Pathological Fractures of the Mandible: Our Department's 15-Year Experience. *Diagnostics* **2025**, *15*, 1216. [CrossRef] [PubMed]
5. Toader, M.P.; Hritcu, O.M.C.; Botoc, C.C.; Hutanu, A.E.; Munteanu, C.A.; Ciobanu, R.P.; Toader, S.V.; Colac, A.G.; Costan, V.V.; Andrese, E.P.; et al. Mucoscopic Features of Oral Lichen Planus: A Retrospective Comparative Study with Inflammatory Mimickers. *Diagnostics* **2025**, *15*, 1084. [CrossRef] [PubMed]
6. Panzarella, V.; Buttacavoli, F.; Rodolico, V.; Maniscalco, L.; Firenze, A.; De Caro, V.; Mauceri, R.; Rombo, S.E.; Campisi, G. Application of Targeted Optical Coherence Tomography in Oral Cancer: A Cross-Sectional Preliminary Study. *Diagnostics* **2024**, *14*, 2247. [CrossRef] [PubMed]
7. Hussain, A.M.; Khan, F.A.; Alsaif, S.S.; Alqahtani, N.; Alqahtani, A.; Alali, Y.; Alolayan, M.; Alghannam, A.; Alolayan, A. Effect of a sodium hypochlorite mouthwash on plaque and clinical parameters of periodontal disease—A systematic review. *Int. J. Dent. Hyg.* **2022**, *20*, 40–52. [CrossRef] [PubMed]
8. Cosgarea, R.; Pollmann, R.; Sharif, J.; Schmidt, T.; Stein, R.; Bodea, A.; Auschill, T.; Sculean, A.; Eming, R.; Greene, B.; et al. Photodynamic therapy in oral lichen planus: A prospective case-controlled pilot study. *Sci. Rep.* **2020**, *10*, 1667. [CrossRef] [PubMed]

*diagnostics*

MDPI

*Article*

# Pathological Fractures of the Mandible: Our Department's 15-Year Experience

**Georgios Chatziantoniou [1,*], Dimitris Tatsis [1,*], Solon Politis [2], Antonios Saramantos [1], Nikolaos Koukolis [3] and Konstantinos Paraskevopoulos [1]**

[1] Department of Oral & Maxillofacial Surgery, Aristotle University of Thessaloniki, Specialized Cancer Treatment and Reconstruction Center, General Hospital of Thessaloniki "George Papanikolaou", 57010 Thessaloniki, Greece; saramantosant@gmail.com (A.S.); kostparas@yahoo.gr (K.P.)

[2] Oral and Maxillofacial Surgery Clinic, 424 Military Hospital of Thessaloniki, 56429 Thessaloniki, Greece; solonpolitis88@gmail.com

[3] Private Practice, 57010 Thessaloniki, Greece; koukolisn@yahoo.gr

* Correspondence: ghatziadoniou@gmail.com (G.C.); dtatsis@outlook.com (D.T.)

**Abstract: Background/Objectives**: Pathological fractures of the mandible are uncommon and often result from underlying conditions such as osteoradionecrosis, malignancies, or medication-related osteonecrosis of the jaw (MRONJ). Their management is challenging due to compromised bone quality and complex patient comorbidities. This study presents a 15-year experience from a tertiary oral and maxillofacial surgery center, highlighting the clinical characteristics, etiologies, treatment approaches, and outcomes of these fractures. **Methods**: A retrospective review was conducted on patients diagnosed with pathological mandibular fractures between 2010 and 2024. Data collected included demographics, fracture etiology and location, diagnostic imaging, treatment modality, complications, and long-term outcomes. **Results**: Fifty patients met the inclusion criteria. The mean age was 66.4 years, with a predominance of male patients (78%). The most common etiology was osteoradionecrosis (48%), followed by primary malignancy (22%) and MRONJ (16%). In 82% of cases, surgical management was required, most frequently involving marginal or segmental mandibular resection (gnathectomy), with or without immediate reconstruction. Conservative treatment was reserved for select cases with high surgical risk. Complications occurred in 54% of patients, including persistent fistulas, pathological communication with the skin or oral cavity, and the need for revision surgery. Long-term follow-up revealed variable survival, with many patients experiencing reduced quality of life due to complex postoperative courses. **Conclusions**: Pathological fractures of the mandible present significant diagnostic and therapeutic challenges, particularly in patients with osteoradionecrosis or malignancies. Early diagnosis and individualized, multidisciplinary treatment planning are essential. This study underscores the need for a standardized classification system and treatment algorithm to guide management and improve outcomes in this complex patient population.

**Keywords:** pathological jaw fracture; MRONJ; ORN; spontaneous fracture; mandible

## 1. Introduction

Pathological fractures of the jaws, particularly the mandible, are a unique category of fractures, which are relatively rare, amounting to less than 1% [1]. Most of these data are documented in independent case series and reports. Nonetheless, although infrequent, pathological fractures present a significant clinical challenge because they negatively impact the quality of life for affected patients, as well as needing a possibly complex and patient personalized treatment planning.

Patients presenting with pathological fractures have both functional and aesthetic impairments and are psychologically affected as well. Functionally, these patients experience high levels of chronic pain [2], especially during the mastication process, due to the underlying fracture. In patients with underlying conditions, especially elderly ones, this further deteriorates their well-being [3]. Speech and overall oral hygiene may also be hindered [4,5]. Aesthetically, the facial contour may also be adversely affected, leading to a possible decline in self-esteem and increased anxiety about daily social interactions. Overall, these conditions may exacerbate social withdrawal and mental health issues [6–9].

Pathological fractures of the mandible occur due to weakened bone integrity from underlying systemic or localized conditions. Pathologic fractures, in general, are predominantly secondary to metastatic disease rather than primary bone malignancies or other conditions [10], with metastatic lesions from lung, breast, thyroid, renal, and prostate cancer being the most common contributors [10,11]. However, mandibular pathologic fractures and their etiology differ in that regard, as the most prominent underlying causal factors involve osteonecrosis of the jaws (osteoradionecrosis and medically related osteonecrosis of the jaws (MRONJ)), tumors, surgical procedures, and infections. Iatrogenic causes are eminent in the majority of the cases, with osteoradionecrosis representing the majority of cases, while exodontia is the main culprit for the otherwise healthy population [1,12–18]. Osteoradionecrosis is a severe complication following radiotherapy for head and neck cancer patients. While osteoradionecrosis's occurrence is on the decline, thanks to the use of Intensity-Modulated Radiation Therapy, it still lingers around 7% [19–23].

The diagnosis of pathological fractures of the mandible depends on both clinical examination and imaging. Pain, especially during mastication, difficulty in movement or structural deformation of the mandible, and changes to the patient's occlusion may be indicative of a pathological fracture [24]. Pathological fractures of the mandible occur during mastication most of the time [12]. The initial imaging of choice for mandibular pathological fractures is an orthopantomogram (OPG) as it is a cheap and readily available examination. CT allows for more thorough structural visualization and possible surgical planning. Furthermore, it can contribute diagnostically to cases of suspected malignancy.

Treatment choice is determined by the etiology, location, and severity of the fracture. The body of the mandible is the most frequent fracture site, followed by the angle [12,17,24,25]. As no consensus or clear guidelines exist, there are several different approaches and subsequent treatment algorithms. The most crucial point is whether surgical intervention would be the most appropriate treatment choice or non-surgical management should be considered first [1,12,16,17,24,26–31].

Non-surgical management consists of pain management protocols (NSAIDS, opioids, corticosteroids), the administration of bisphosphonates and denosumab in metastatic bone disease, and radiotherapy for local control of malignant cases. Surgical management includes prophylactic fixation (for severely compromised structures or fractures awaiting biomechanical assessment), resection, and possible reconstruction with free flaps and bone grafts and/or internal fixation [32].

Osteoradionecrosis and pathological fractures related to malignant tumors pose a significant challenge in the management of head and neck oncology, primarily due to compromised bone quality, delayed healing, and the intricate anatomical factors involved [33]. Existing treatment protocols are hindered by several limitations, notably high rates of postoperative complications and inconsistent reconstruction outcomes, which impede effective patient recovery. Non-surgical approaches, including hyperbaric oxygen therapy or bisphosphonates, are often insufficient for managing advanced osteoradionecrosis or fractures related to tumors and are unable to prevent progression in severe mandibular ORN, necessitating surgical intervention [34]. Furthermore, the efficacy of hyperbaric oxygen in revitalizing necrotic bone is questionable, resulting in authors advocating for surgical management in advanced cases [35]. Current treatment protocols often lack individualization, failing to consider patient-specific factors such as radiation dose, tumor biology, or bone integrity. The variability in outcomes of ORN reconstructions due to the neglect of these factors calls for tailored treatment strategies [36]. The lack of consensus on the ideal timing for surgery following radiation or chemotherapy further complicates outcomes, as optimal conditions for bone and soft tissue recovery are frequently overlooked.

The development of evidence-based protocols for ORN prevention and management is hindered by the scarcity of high-quality clinical trials, with much of the current data originating from retrospective studies. This limitation hinders the establishment of robust treatment guidelines [37]. Additionally, the 2024 ISOO-MASCC-ASCO guidelines, which stress the importance of multidisciplinary approaches, fall short in providing detailed strategies for implementation, reflecting ongoing gaps in the evidence base [38].

Postoperative complications are largely associated with both systemic and local factors, particularly infections in hard and soft tissues or failures of the surgical hardware [39]. Patients with malignant tumors often present additional comorbidities, such as malnutrition or immunosuppression resulting from chemotherapy, which further exacerbate the risk of complications. These systemic factors are significant contributors to infections and delayed wound healing in ORN patients, emphasizing the critical need for thorough preoperative optimization [40].

An early diagnosis, along with proper planning and timely therapeutic intervention, is of paramount importance as it can greatly enhance patient treatment outcomes [41–43]. This study aims to present a series of 50 patients with pathological fractures of the mandible, their subsequent management, and the clinical and demographic data of this particular yet extremely diversified group of patients.

## 2. Materials and Methods

A retrospective, analytical study was conducted at the Oral and Maxillofacial Surgery Department of Aristotle University of Thessaloniki, Greece, a specialized center in the General Hospital G. Papanikolaou for the surgical treatment and rehabilitation of patients with head and neck cancer. The medical records and management of all patients with pathological fractures of the mandible treated in our clinic between January 2010 and December 2024 were examined.

The patients' medical records were carefully examined by two of the researchers, who meticulously recorded the patient's medical records for the following variables: age, gender, fracture location, length of hospital stay (after surgical intervention and total), type of management (surgical or conservative), type of surgical intervention (when applicable) etiology, pre- and post-surgery imaging, survival, alcohol and tobacco consumption history, and major comorbidities. The follow-up of these patients was recorded in an effort to establish the long-term outcomes of the intervention provided. Medical records with missing data were excluded from this study. Also, patients with a history of drug abuse were excluded from the present study. Lastly, patients presenting with a pathological fracture that had undergone therapeutic interventions elsewhere were excluded as well.

This retrospective study was performed in accordance with the tenets of the Declaration of Helsinki and the Medical Research Involving Human Subjects Act (WMO).

Approval from the local Scientific Committee of the Hospital was obtained (Protocol No. 332/5-5-2025).

## 3. Results

### 3.1. Patient Characteristics

This study evaluated the medical records of 54 patients with pathological fractures of the mandible between January 2010 and December 2024. Four patients with a pathological fracture were excluded from the present study as they had significantly missing data.

The majority of the patients were male (78%, $n = 39$) and had an age > 60 years (58%, $n = 29$). The age range was 19–90 years. Tobacco (74%) and alcohol (60%) use was observed in most patients. Major comorbidities, such as cardiovascular disease, diabetes mellitus, history of malignancy, renal failure, COPD, etc., were also prevalent in this patient group (78%) (Table 1).

**Table 1.** Patient characteristics.

| | **Patient Characteristics** |
|---|---|
| **Variable** | **Number of Patients (%)** |
| Age | |
| <60 years | 21 (42%) |
| >60 years | 29 (58%) |
| Median Age | 66.4 years |
| Sex | |
| Male | 39 (78%) |
| Female | 11 (22%) |
| Major comorbidities | |
| Yes | 39 (78%) |
| No | 11 (22%) |
| Smokers | |
| Yes | 37 (74%) |
| No | 13 (26%) |
| Alcohol use | |
| Yes | 30 (60%) |
| No | 20 (40%) |

### 3.2. Fracture Characteristics

The most frequent cause of mandibular pathological fracture was osteoradionecrosis (48%), followed by malignancy (22%), MRONJ (16%), and atrophy (14%) (Figure 1). Single fractures of the body of the mandible were the most frequent (56%) among all categories. Single fractures in general consisted of 68% of the cases. Multiple fracture sites were observed in 16 of the 50 cases, amounting to 20% unilateral and 12% bilateral fractures. Lastly, angle fractures represented 12% of the cases, while the ramus as a possible fracture location was only present in the multiple fracture group in six cases (12%). Fistulae were observed in 56% of the patients, with 18% of them having both intra- and extraoral fistulae. Regarding initial diagnostic imaging, OPG was used in 37 cases, CT in 25, and both were used in 14 cases. Biopsy was not performed in 30% of the fractures, while malignancy occurred 36% of the time (Table 2).

**Table 2.** Fracture characteristics.

| | **Fracture Characteristics** |
|---|---|
| **Variable** | **Number of Patients (%)** |
| Etiology | |
| Medication-related osteonecrosis of the jaws | 8 (16%) |
| Osteoradionecrosis | 24 (48%) |
| Primary malignancy | 11 (22%) |
| Recurrence of malignancy | 7 (14%) |

**Table 2.** *Cont.*

| Variable | Fracture Characteristics<br>Number of Patients (%) |
|---|---|
| Benign tumours | 2 (4%) |
| Cysts | 1 (2%) |
| Osteoporosis | 1 (2%) |
| Mandibular atrophy | 7 (14%) |
| Osteomyelitis | 4 (8%) |
| Iatrogenic (after tooth extractions) | 1 (2%) |
| Fracture location | |
| Body only | 28 (56%) |
| Angle only | 6 (12%) |
| Ramus (as part of multiple locations) | 6 (12%) |
| Multiple (unilateral) | 10 (20%) |
| Multiple (bilateral) | 6 (12%) |
| Presence of fistula | |
| No | 22 (44%) |
| Yes, intraoral | 9 (18%) |
| Yes, extraoral | 10 (20%) |
| Yes, both | 9 (18%) |
| Imaging | |
| OPG | 37 (74%) |
| CT | 25 (50%) |
| Both | 14 (28%) |
| Biopsy | |
| No | 15 (30%) |
| Yes, inflammation | 17 (34%) |
| Yes, malignancy | 18 (36%) |

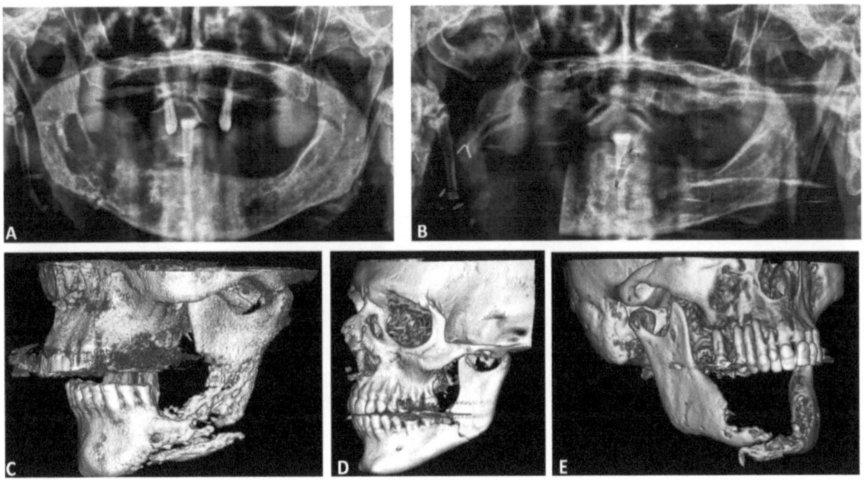


**Figure 1.** Imaging modalities of selected patients. (**A**) OPG of a female patient (78 years old) diagnosed with a mandibular pathological fracture of the right mandibular body due to MRONJ. (**B**) OPG of the same patient postoperatively, after right segmental mandibulectomy. (**C**) Three-dimensional anasynthesis of a CT scan of a male patient (83 years old) with a mandibular pathological fracture of the left angle due to osteoradionecrosis. (**D**) Three-dimensional anasynthesis of a CT scan of a male patient (50 years old) with a mandibular pathological fracture of the left angle after surgical extraction of a low-level-impacted third molar. (**E**) Three-dimensional anasynthesis of a CT scan of a female patient (64 years old) with an extended mandibular pathological fracture of the mandible due to malignancy.

### 3.3. *Intervention Characteristics*

In total, 41 patients underwent surgery (82%), of whom 25 underwent mandibular resection, 14 mandibular resection and immediate reconstruction of the mandible, and

2 MMF. Hyperbaric oxygen therapy (10%) and the administration of Pentoxifylline (4%) were adjunct therapies in patients with osteoradionecrosis. As for post-treatment imaging, OPG was used in most cases (72%), with CT scan use observed in 14 cases, while both exams were performed for 12% of the patients. The average postoperative hospital stay was 11.5 days (minimum stay = 2 days, maximum stay = 49 days) (Table 3).

**Table 3.** Intervention characteristics.

| Intervention Characteristics | |
|---|---|
| **Variable** | **Number of Patients (%)** |
| Surgical intervention | |
| Yes | 41 (82%) |
| No | 9 (18%) |
| Type of surgical intervention | |
| Mandibular resection | 25 (61%) |
| Mandibular resection and reconstruction | 14 (34%) |
| MMF | 2 (5%) |
| Adjunct Therapies | |
| Hyperbaric Oxygen Therapy | 5 (10%) |
| Pentoxifylline | 2 (4%) |
| Length of hospital stay (days) | 2–49 [median 11.5] |
| Postoperation imaging | |
| OPG | 36 (88%) |
| CT | 14 (34%) |
| Both | 6 (15%) |

### 3.4. Outcomes

Mean patient survival after treatment was 27.6 months, with the minimum value being 1 month and the highest being 106 months. Complications such as fixation luxation, the loss of flap tissue, the contamination of osteosynthesis materials, etc., were observed in 54% of the patients (Table 4).

**Table 4.** Outcomes.

| Outcomes | |
|---|---|
| **Variable** | **Number of Patients (%)** |
| Complications | |
| Yes | 27 (54%) |
| No | 23 (46%) |
| Overall survival (months) | 1–105 [median 27.6] |

## 4. Discussion

Pathological fractures of the mandible, although rare, can significantly worsen a patient's quality of life, having a negative impact on both psychological and physical welfare [2,44]. In the present study, most patients presenting with a pathological fracture were cancer patients, particularly head and neck cancer patients, who had undergone radiation therapy and subsequently developed osteoradionecrosis of the mandible. These findings are in line with the literature [1,12,13,16,17,25]. Recently, the occurrence of pathological fractures of the mandible associated with osteoradionecrosis has become increasingly frequent due to the wide use of adjuvant radiation therapy in head and neck cancer patients, in conjunction with better survival nowadays. Osteoradionecrosis of the jaws is considerably more common in continued tobacco users, in patients with diabetes mellitus, at the primary tumor site, with bony invasion of the primary tumor, and consequently in patients with pathological fractures. Ohori et al. (2023) [13] have determined the incidence of pathological fractures in patients with osteoradionecrosis to be 25.7%. As optimal treatment planning for osteoradionecrosis patients with mandibular pathological fractures is not standardized, surgical resection and free vascularized bone transfer have been proposed as the treatment of choice [26–28,30,31,41]. However, reconstructive surgery in patients with advanced-stage osteoradionecrosis is quite an endeavor since the quality of soft tissue healing is compromised due to both decreased blood supply and the loss of healthy tissues due to fistulae, occurring in more than 50% of this study's patients. The devastating effects of osteoradionecrosis in the mandible have been speculated to be affected by the devascularization of it during selective neck dissection, where part of the facial artery is typically ligated. In addition, age-related vascular compromise of the mandible further contributes to the effects of radiotherapy, leading to complications such as pathological fractures [45]. Also, the depleted neck due to the absence of cervical vessels may hinder microvascular reconstruction [46,47]. Without doubt, appropriate treatment planning should consider the patient's general health and nutritional status, as well as ruling out the possibility of recurrent cancer [25]. Cancer patients with osseous metastases who develop MRONJ have an increased survival rate, resulting in more patients developing pathological fractures due to MRONJ [48–51]. On the other hand, the incidence of osteomyelitis as a cause is not as frequent nowadays, probably due to the widespread use of and access to antibiotics. Fourteen percent of the pathological fractures had an underlying cause of atrophy of the mandible, which is in line with the early extraction of teeth being commonplace during the years of economic crisis in Greece. Bony lesions (cysts or benign tumors) can potentially lead to a pathological fracture, as they alter the adjacent bony structure, thus weakening the mandible and predisposing it to fractures.

Fractures resulting from cystic lesions are a rare occurrence [16]. There was only one pathological fracture due to iatrogenic reasons found in this retrospective study, clearly lower than other study findings [1,12,13,16,17,24]. This may be attributed to the fact that the institution of the authors mainly treats head and neck cancer patients. Furthermore, pathological fractures of the mandible following exodontia may be treated in the private sector more frequently than pathological fractures from other etiologies as they generally require shorter hospital stays and not particularly complex surgical procedures [14,18].

Diagnostic imaging plays an essential role in identifying pathological fractures of the mandible, guiding both diagnosis and treatment strategies. Conventional radiography, though commonly used, may not provide sufficient visibility of the underlying bone quality, structural integrity, or pathology present [52]. Instead, advanced imaging modalities such as CT provide detailed assessments of fracture patterns, enabling effective treatment planning. CT imaging is especially valuable in visualizing complex fractures associated with underlying pathologies and planning for reconstructive surgery [52,53]. Furthermore, high-quality CT imaging examinations are essential for presurgical treatment planning with the aid of 3D CAD/CAM technologies for the manufacturing of personalized surgical guides and/or internal fixation plates [54]. Thus, the integration of advanced imaging technologies in surgical planning is crucial, as it allows for a better understanding of the osseous anatomy, vascular supply, and existing lesions.

OPG and/or other types of radiographs of the visceral cranium, depending on the fracture site and type of surgical intervention, are the postoperative imaging of choice. CT is mainly performed when complications arise, or in future follow-ups when oncologic relapses are suspected.

Biopsy of the lesions of the pathological fracture is crucial, especially in cases of suspected malignancy, depending on the patient's anamnesis. In our study, 36% of the biopsies were positive for malignancy. This alters treatment and surgical planning significantly, as well as overall prognosis.

A fracture of the mandibular body is the most frequent in the present study, followed by the angle of the mandible. Fractures involving solely the mandibular ramus were not observed at all and were only found in the multiple fracture group. These findings are in line with the demographic data of this study as well as the literature [4,24]. Most patients are male (78%) in their 6–7th decade of life. Tobacco and alcohol use and abuse are more prominent in groups of males, while they also exhibit poorer oral hygiene, thus resulting in an even more unfavorable set of conditions for the already compromised state of oral hygiene of head and neck cancer patients who have undergone radiation therapy [4,5].

As aforementioned, more than half the patients presented with extraoral or intraoral fistulas, which are a hindering factor in the surgical management of this group of patients. Fistula formation compromises the surrounding soft tissue healing capacity and complicates the surgical planning with a subpar postoperative healing process. In fistula cases where bone reconstruction is considered, soft tissue coverage and/or regional flaps should be considered. Free tissue transfer remains the gold standard for soft and hard tissue reconstruction, but as expected, patients with pathological fractures may be frail and not fit for this surgical intervention. In patients unfit for surgery who are managed conservatively, fistulas further worsen the quality of life.

The treatment of pathological fractures of the mandible should be tailored to the individual, considering the fracture's causal factors, the fracture site, and the patient's overall health status. Therapeutic options range from conservative management, including medications for pain relief and infection control, to various surgical procedures.

Surgical interventions remain the cornerstone in treating pathological fractures of the mandible. Surgical treatment was performed in 82% of the patients in the present study. Antimicrobials were administered to all the patients perioperatively, along with low-molecular-weight heparin as per standard practice. The use of innovative techniques such as virtual surgical planning can significantly enhance outcomes, particularly in complex cases involving extensive bone loss, with the employment of free fibula flaps for reconstruction following the resection of pathologic lesions showing reliable results in restoring functionality and facial aesthetics [55]. When electing for a surgical procedure as the first treatment choice for a pathological fracture, many factors must be considered first. These include, but are not limited to, patient-specific prognosis, health status, major comorbidities, recurrence of malignancy, concurrent treatments, nutritional status, tobacco and alcohol use/abuse, gender, and patient compliance [4,49,50,56,57]. Most of the 50 patients of this study ($n$ = 39) had major comorbidities such as cardiovascular disease, diabetes mellitus, history of malignancy, renal failure, COPD, etc. These conditions further inhibit the patient's healing mechanisms and potential for an uneventful postoperative period. More often than not, conservative management was selected as the first-choice treatment due to the compromised fitness for surgery. Furthermore, surgical planning may be altered by electing for a more minimal treatment approach, not involving the reconstruction of the mandible, avoiding a free tissue transfer procedure.

Adjunct therapies used were hyperbaric oxygen therapy and administration of Pentoxifylline in patients diagnosed with osteoradionecrosis. While the current consensus for hyperbaric oxygen therapy is that it should not be used routinely for the treatment of osteoradionecrosis, it could be beneficial for a subgroup of patients where other treatment options have been fruitless [58–61]. On the other hand, the use of Pentoxifylline could potentially be more promising, although its use and dosage need to be standardized [62–64].

Half the patients presented complications in future follow-ups. This can be attributed to the compromised healing process, especially in cancer patients with major comorbidities. The past history of radiation therapy also hinders the healing process in the postoperative period. Patients should be followed closely to ensure that possible complications are diagnosed early, allowing for immediate intervention and treatment.

The median overall survival after therapeutic intervention (surgical or not) was 27.6 months, which can be attributed to the compromised health status of most individuals presenting with a pathological fracture in our study. As aforementioned, the majority of the patients treated were cancer patients, either head and neck cancer patients with osteoradionecrosis/primary malignancy/malignancy recurrence or patients with MRONJ for other types of malignancies. Also, 78% of the patients had major comorbidities too. In the case series reviewed, there was no mention of overall survival after intervention or diagnosis.

The potential limitations of the present study can be attributed to the inherent limitations of retrospective studies. Additionally, subgroup analysis could not be performed due to the heterogeneity of the data and the small number of patients in each subgroup. Furthermore, as mentioned in the etiology segment, there could be an underreporting of pathological fractures, especially those following exodontia, from the private sector. Also, as our department mainly treats head and neck cancer patients, center-specific bias cannot be excluded.

Lastly, there is a glaring gap in the present literature for a widely accepted classification system and a clear consensus for a cohesive algorithmic management for mandibular pathological fractures as opposed to other possible pathological fracture sites [10]. This issue must be addressed in order to enable more universally accepted treatment planning that leads to elevated therapeutic results for the patients treated.

## 5. Conclusions

This longitudinal retrospective analysis of patients presenting with pathological fractures of the mandible delineates the considerable clinical intricacies and therapeutic challenges inherent to this rare condition, predominantly encountered among individuals with head and neck cancer complicated by osteoradionecrosis. The data elucidate the extensive impact of such fractures on functional capacity, facial aesthetics, and psychological well-being, further aggravated by comorbidities and complications, including fistulae formation and impaired wound healing. Surgical intervention remains the principal therapeutic approach, individualized according to patient-specific factors. Technological advances, such as high-resolution imaging and virtual surgical planning, have notably contributed to improved outcomes. Nevertheless, the absence of standardized treatment protocols and a universally recognized classification system for mandibular pathological fractures constitutes a significant deficiency in the existing literature. There is a pressing need for future research to establish comprehensive management algorithms and undertake prospective, multicenter investigations aimed at optimizing therapeutic strategies and enhancing patient quality of life.

**Author Contributions:** Conceptualization, G.C. and K.P.; methodology, G.C., D.T., S.P. and K.P.; validation, A.S. and N.K.; investigation, A.S. and N.K.; data curation, A.S. and N.K.; writing—original draft preparation, G.C.; writing—review and editing, G.C., D.T. and S.P.; supervision, K.P. All authors have read and agreed to the published version of the manuscript.

**Funding:** This research received no external funding.

**Institutional Review Board Statement:** This study was conducted in accordance with the Declaration of Helsinki, and ethical review and approval from the local Scientific Committee of the Hospital were obtained (Protocol No. 332/5-5-2025, 5 May 2025).

**Informed Consent Statement:** Patient consent was waived due to personal data, information, or patient photographs not being used in the present article.

**Data Availability Statement:** Data are available upon request.

**Conflicts of Interest:** The authors declare no conflicts of interest.

## Abbreviations

The following abbreviations are used in this manuscript:

| | |
|---|---|
| MRONJ | Medication-Related Osteonecrosis of the Jaws |
| OPG | Orthopantomogram |
| 3D | Three-Dimensional |
| CT | Computed Tomography |
| NSAIDs | Nonsteroidal Anti-Inflammatory Drugs |
| MMF | Maxillo-Mandibular Fixation |
| CAD/CAM | Computer-Aided Design/Computer-Aided Manufacturing |
| COPD | Chronic Obstructive Pulmonary Disease |

## References

1. Ezsias, A.; Sugar, A.W. Pathological fractures of the mandible: A diagnostic and treatment dilemma. *Br. J. Oral Maxillofac. Surg.* **1994**, *32*, 303–306. [CrossRef] [PubMed]
2. Hiraoka, Y.; Akashi, M.; Wanifuchi, S.; Kusumoto, J.; Shigeoka, M.; Hasegawa, T.; Hashikawa, K.; Terashi, H.; Komori, T. Association between pain severity and clinicohistopathologic findings in the mandibular canal and inferior alveolar nerve of patients with advanced mandibular osteoradionecrosis. *Oral. Surg. Oral Med. Oral Pathol. Oral Radiol.* **2018**, *126*, 264–271. [CrossRef] [PubMed]
3. Khafif, A.; Posen, J.; Yagil, Y.; Beiser, M.; Gil, Z.; Ben-Yosef, R.; Landsberg, R.; Fliss, D.M. Quality of life in patients older than 75 years following major head and neck surgery. *Head Neck* **2007**, *29*, 932–939. [CrossRef] [PubMed]
4. Reuther, T.; Schuster, T.; Mende, U.; Kübler, A.C. Osteoradionecrosis of the jaws as a side effect of radiotherapy of head and neck tumour patients—A report of a thirty year retrospective review. *Int. J. Oral Maxillofac. Surg.* **2003**, *32*, 289–295. [CrossRef]
5. Niewald, M.; Fleckenstein, J.; Mang, K.; Holtmann, H.; Spitzer, W.J.; Rübe, C. Dental status, dental rehabilitation procedures, demographic and oncological data as potential risk factors for infected osteoradionecrosis of the lower jaw after radiotherapy for oral neoplasms: A retrospective evaluation. *Radiat. Oncol.* **2013**, *8*, 227. [CrossRef]
6. Nelke, K.H.; Pawlak, W.; Gerber, H.; Leszczyszyn, J. Head and neck cancer patients' quality of life. *Adv. Clin. Exp. Med.* **2014**, *23*, 1019–1027. [CrossRef]
7. Reyes, I.M.; Arenilla, M.J.; Alarcón, D.; Jaenes, J.C.; Trujillo, M. Psychological impact after treatment in patients with head and neck cancer. *Med. Oral Patol. Oral Cir. Bucal* **2023**, *28*, e467. [CrossRef]
8. Jimenez-Labaig, P.; Aymerich, C.; Braña, I.; Rullan, A.; Cacicedo, J.; González-Torres, M.Á.; Harrington, K.J.; Catalan, A. A comprehensive examination of mental health in patients with head and neck cancer: Systematic review and meta-analysis. *JNCI Cancer Spectr.* **2024**, *8*, pkae031. [CrossRef]

9. Lin, L.; Lin, H.; Zhou, R.; Liu, B.; Liu, K.; Jiang, R. Surviving and thriving: Assessing quality of life and psychosocial interventions in mental health of head and neck cancer patients. *Asian. J. Surg.* **2025**, *48*, 1634–1642. [CrossRef]
10. Rizzo, S.E.; Kenan, S. *Pathologic Fractures*; StatPearls Publishing: Treasure Island, FL, USA, 2025.
11. Biermann, J.S.; Holt, G.E.; Lewis, V.O.; Schwartz, H.S.; Yaszemski, M.J. Metastatic bone disease: Diagnosis, evaluation, and treatment. *J. Bone Jt. Surg. Am.* **2009**, *91*, 1518–1530.
12. Gerhards, F.; Kuffner, H.D.; Wagner, W. Pathological fractures of the mandible. A review of the etiology and treatment. *Int. J. Oral Maxillofac. Surg.* **1998**, *27*, 186–190. [CrossRef] [PubMed]
13. Ohori, H.; Iwata, E.; Takeda, D.; Kusumoto, J.; Hasegawa, T.; Akashi, M. Risk factors for pathological fracture in patients with mandibular osteoradionecrosis. *Sci. Rep.* **2023**, *13*, 5367. [CrossRef] [PubMed]
14. Grau-Mancls, V.; Gargallo-Albiol, J.; Almendros-Marqus, N.; Gay-Escoda, C. Mandibular fractures related to the surgical extraction of impacted lower third molars: A report of 11 cases. *J. Oral Maxillofac. Surg.* **2011**, *69*, 1286–1290. [CrossRef]
15. Bourhis, J.; Overgaard, J.; Audry, H.; Ang, K.K.; Saunders, M.; Bernier, J.; Horiot, J.C.; Le Maître, A.; Pajak, T.F.; Poulsen, M.G.; et al. Hyperfractionated or accelerated radiotherapy in head and neck cancer: A meta-analysis. *Lancet* **2006**, *368*, 843–854. [CrossRef] [PubMed]
16. Boffano, P.; Roccia, F.; Gallesio, C.; Berrone, S. Pathological mandibular fractures: A review of the literature of the last two decades. *Dent. Traumatol.* **2013**, *29*, 185–196. [CrossRef]
17. Coletti, D.; Ord, R.A. Treatment rationale for pathological fractures of the mandible: A series of 44 fractures. *Int. J. Oral Maxillofac. Surg.* **2008**, *37*, 215–222. [CrossRef]
18. Joshi, A.; Goel, M.; Thorat, A. Identifying the risk factors causing iatrogenic mandibular fractures associated with exodontia: A systemic meta-analysis of 200 cases from 1953 to 2015. *Oral Maxillofac. Surg.* **2016**, *20*, 391–396. [CrossRef]
19. Willaert, R.; Nevens, D.; Laenen, A.; Batstone, M.; Politis, C.; Nuyts, S. Does intensity-modulated radiation therapy lower the risk of osteoradionecrosis of the jaw? A long-term comparative analysis. *Int. J. Oral Maxillofac. Surg.* **2019**, *48*, 1387–1393. [CrossRef]
20. Kubota, H.; Miyawaki, D.; Mukumoto, N.; Ishihara, T.; Matsumura, M.; Hasegawa, T.; Akashi, M.; Kiyota, N.; Shinomiya, H.; Teshima, M.; et al. Risk factors for osteoradionecrosis of the jaw in patients with head and neck squamous cell carcinoma. *Radiat. Oncol.* **2021**, *16*, 1. [CrossRef]
21. Owosho, A.A.; Tsai, C.J.; Lee, R.S.; Freymiller, H.; Kadempour, A.; Varthis, S.; Sax, A.Z.; Rosen, E.B.; Yom, S.K.; Randazzo, J.; et al. The Prevalence and Risk Factors Associated with Osteoradionecrosis of the Jaw in Oral and Oropharyngeal Cancer Patients Treated with Intensity-Modulated Radiation Therapy (IMRT): The Memorial Sloan Kettering Cancer Center Experience. *Oral Oncol.* **2016**, *64*, 44. [CrossRef]
22. Dhanda, J.; Pasquier, D.; Newman, L.; Shaw, R. Current Concepts in Osteoradionecrosis After Head and Neck Radiotherapy. *Clin. Oncol.* **2016**, *28*, 459–466. [CrossRef] [PubMed]
23. Singh, A.; Huryn, J.M.; Kronstadt, K.L.; Yom, S.H.K.; Randazzo, J.R.; Estilo, C.L. Osteoradionecrosis of the jaw: A mini review. *Front. Oral Heal.* **2022**, *3*, 980786. [CrossRef] [PubMed]
24. Zhao, Y.; Li, R.F.; Sun, Y.F.; Liu, B.; Jia, J. Pathological Fractures of the Mandible: A Report of 27 Cases. *Clin. Surg.* **2017**, *2*, 1839.
25. Carlsen, A.; Marcussen, M. Spontaneous fractures of the mandible concept & treatment strategy. *Med. Oral Patol. Oral Cir. Bucal.* **2016**, *21*, e88–e94.
26. Sawhney, R.; Ducic, Y. Management of pathologic fractures of the mandible secondary to osteoradionecrosis. *Otolaryngol. Head. Neck Surg.* **2013**, *148*, 54–58. [CrossRef]
27. Alam, D.S.; Nuara, M.; Christian, J. Analysis of outcomes of vascularized flap reconstruction in patients with advanced mandibular osteoradionecrosis. *Otolaryngol. Head Neck Surg.* **2009**, *141*, 196–201. [CrossRef] [PubMed]
28. Zaghi, S.; Danesh, J.; Hendizadeh, L.; Nabili, V.; Blackwell, K.E. Changing indications for maxillomandibular reconstruction with osseous free flaps: A 17-year experience with 620 consecutive cases at UCLA and the impact of osteoradionecrosis. *Laryngoscope* **2014**, *124*, 1329–1335. [CrossRef] [PubMed]
29. Tso, T.V.; Blackwell, K.E.; Sung, E.C. Predictive factors of osteoradionecrosis necessitating segmental mandibulectomy: A descriptive study. *Oral Surg. Oral Med. Oral Pathol. Oral Radiol.* **2022**, *134*, e8–e13. [CrossRef]
30. Hirsch, D.L.; Bell, R.B.; Dierks, E.J.; Potter, J.K.; Potter, B.E. Analysis of Microvascular Free Flaps for Reconstruction of Advanced Mandibular Osteoradionecrosis: A Retrospective Cohort Study. *J. Oral Maxillofac. Surg.* **2008**, *66*, 2545–2556. [CrossRef]
31. Lee, M.; Chin, R.Y.; Eslick, G.D.; Sritharan, N.; Paramaesvaran, S. Outcomes of microvascular free flap reconstruction for mandibular osteoradionecrosis: A systematic review. *J. Cranio-Maxillofac. Surg.* **2015**, *43*, 2026–2033. [CrossRef]
32. Cannady, S.B.; Dean, N.; Kroeker, A.; Albert, T.A.; Rosenthal, E.L.; Wax, M.K. Free flap reconstruction for osteoradionecrosis of the jaws-Outcomes and predictive factors for success. *Head Neck* **2011**, *33*, 424–428. [CrossRef] [PubMed]

33. Ma, C.; Gao, W.; Liu, Z.; Zhu, D.; Zhu, F.; Li, X.; He, Y. Radiation-Induced Soft Tissue Injuries in Patients with Advanced Mandibular Osteoradionecrosis: A Preliminary Evaluation and Management of Various Soft Tissue Problems Around Radiation-Induced Osteonecrosis Lesions. *Front. Oncol.* **2021**, *11*, 641061. [CrossRef]
34. D'Souza, J.; Lowe, D.; Rogers, S.N. Changing trends and the role of medical management on the outcome of patients treated for osteoradionecrosis of the mandible: Experience from a regional head and neck unit. *Br. J. Oral Maxillofac. Surg.* **2014**, *52*, 356–362. [CrossRef]
35. Freiberger, J.J.; Yoo, D.S.; de Lisle Dear, G.; McGraw, T.A.; Blakey, G.H.; Padilla Burgos, R.; Kraft, K.; Nelson, J.W.; Moon, R.E.; Piantadosi, C.A. MultiModality Surgical and Hyperbaric Management of Mandibular Osteoradionecrosis. *Int. J. Radiat. Oncol. Biol. Phys.* **2009**, *75*, 717–724. [CrossRef]
36. Sweeny, L.; Lancaster, W.P.; Dean, N.R.; Magnuson, J.S.; Carroll, W.R.; Louis, P.J.; Rosenthal, E.L. Use of recombinant bone morphogenetic protein 2 in free flap reconstruction for osteonecrosis of the mandible. *J. Oral Maxillofac. Surg.* **2012**, *70*, 1991–1996. [CrossRef]
37. Nabil, S.; Samman, N. Incidence and prevention of osteoradionecrosis after dental extraction in irradiated patients: A systematic review. *Int. J. Oral Maxillofac. Surg.* **2011**, *40*, 229–243. [CrossRef] [PubMed]
38. Peterson, D.E.; Koyfman, S.A.; Yarom, N.; Lynggaard, C.D.; Ismaila, N.; Forner, L.E.; Fuller, C.D.; Mowery, Y.M.; Murphy, B.A.; Watson, E.; et al. Prevention and Management of Osteoradionecrosis in Patients with Head and Neck Cancer Treated with Radiation Therapy: ISOO-MASCC-ASCO Guideline. *J. Clin. Oncol.* **2024**, *42*, 1975–1996. [CrossRef] [PubMed]
39. Contrera, K.J.; Chinn, S.B.; Weber, R.S.; Roberts, D.; Myers, J.N.; Lai, S.Y.; Lewis, C.M.; Hessel, A.C.; Gillenwater, A.M.; Mulcahy, C.F.; et al. Outcomes after definitive surgery for mandibular osteoradionecrosis. *Head Neck* **2022**, *44*, 1313–1323. [CrossRef]
40. Gevorgyan, A.; Wong, K.; Poon, I.; Blanas, N.; Enepekides, D.J.; Higgins, K.M. Osteoradionecrosis of the mandible: A case series at a single institution. *J. Otolaryngol. Head Neck Surg.* **2013**, *42*, 46. [CrossRef]
41. Mayland, E.; Curry, J.M.; Wax, M.K.; Thomas, C.M.; Swendseid, B.P.; Kejner, A.E.; Kain, J.J.; Cannady, S.B.; Miles, B.A.; DiLeo, M.; et al. Impact of preoperative and intraoperative management on outcomes in osteoradionecrosis requiring free flap reconstruction. *Head Neck* **2022**, *44*, 698–709. [CrossRef]
42. Wu, R.T.; Lin, J.A.J.; Su, C.C.L.; Wei, F.C. Quality of Life for Osteoradionecrosis Reconstruction in the Head and Neck: A Longitudinal Framework and Risk Factors. *Plast. Reconstr. Surg.* **2025**, *1*, 55. [CrossRef] [PubMed]
43. Diarra, D.; Chen, J.; Lin, H.; Zeng, B.; Man, Q.; Deng, W.; Nyimi, B.F.; Wu, T.; Liu, B. Retrospective study of morphological and functional analysis of mandibular reconstructions using iliac and fibular flaps. *J. Stomatol. Oral Maxillofac. Surg.* **2025**, 102322. [CrossRef] [PubMed]
44. He, Y.; Liu, Z.; Tian, Z.; Dai, T.; Qiu, W.; Zhang, Z. Retrospective analysis of osteoradionecrosis of the mandible: Proposing a novel clinical classification and staging system. *Int. J. Oral Maxillofac. Surg.* **2015**, *44*, 1547–1557. [CrossRef] [PubMed]
45. Tatsis, D.; Kowa, X.Y.; Sinha, D.; Kalavrezos, N. Does Combined Access Mandibulotomy, Rim Mandibulectomy and Neck Dissection Compound the Late Effects of Radiotherapy? *Plast. Reconstr. Surg.–Glob. Open* **2023**, *11*, E5081. [CrossRef]
46. Frohwitter, G.; Rau, A.; Kesting, M.R.; Fichter, A. Microvascular reconstruction in the vessel depleted neck—A systematic review. *J. Cranio. Maxillofac. Surg.* **2018**, *46*, 1652–1658. [CrossRef]
47. Prince, A.D.P.; Broderick, M.T.; Heft Neal, M.E.; Spector, M.E. Head and Neck Reconstruction in the Vessel Depleted Neck. *Front. Oral Maxillofac. Med.* **2020**, *2*, 13. [CrossRef]
48. Toriumi, S.; Kobayashi, A.; Uesawa, Y. Comprehensive Study of the Risk Factors for Medication-Related Osteonecrosis of the Jaw Based on the Japanese Adverse Drug Event Report Database. *Pharmaceuticals* **2020**, *13*, 467. [CrossRef]
49. Vahtsevanos, K.; Kyrgidis, A.; Verrou, E.; Katodritou, E.; Triaridis, S.; Andreadis, C.G.; Boukovinas, I.; Koloutsos, G.E.; Teleioudis, Z.; Kitikidou, K.; et al. Longitudinal cohort study of risk factors in cancer patients of bisphosphonate-related osteonecrosis of the jaw. *J. Clin. Oncol.* **2009**, *27*, 5356–5362. [CrossRef]
50. Pichardo, S.E.C.; ten Broek, F.W.; van Merkesteyn, M.J.P. Treatment of pathologic fractures of the mandible in stage III medication-related osteonecrosis of the jaw-an observational study. *J. Craniomaxillofac. Surg.* **2018**, *46*, 1241–1246. [CrossRef]
51. Kim, H.J.; Park, T.J.; Ahn, K.M. Bisphosphonate-related osteonecrosis of the jaw in metastatic breast cancer patients: A review of 25 cases. *Maxillofac. Plast. Reconstr. Surg.* **2016**, *38*, 8. [CrossRef]
52. Nardi, C.; Vignoli, C.; Pietragalla, M.; Tonelli, P.; Calistri, L.; Franchi, L.; Preda, L.; Colagrande, S. Imaging of mandibular fractures: A pictorial review. *Insights Imaging* **2020**, *11*, 30. [CrossRef] [PubMed]
53. Dreizin, D.; Nam, A.J.; Tirada, N.; Levin, M.D.; Stein, D.M.; Bodanapally, U.K.; Mirvis, S.E.; Munera, F. Multidetector CT of Mandibular Fractures, Reductions, and Complications: A Clinically Relevant Primer for the Radiologist. *Radiography* **2016**, *36*, 1539–1564. [CrossRef] [PubMed]
54. May, M.M.; Howe, B.M.; O'Byrne, T.J.; Alexander, A.E.; Morris, J.M.; Moore, E.J.; Kasperbauer, J.L.; Janus, J.R.; Van Abel, K.M.; Dickens, H.J.; et al. Short and long-term outcomes of three-dimensional printed surgical guides and virtual surgical planning

versus conventional methods for fibula free flap reconstruction of the mandible: Decreased nonunion and complication rates. *Head Neck* **2021**, *43*, 2342–2352. [CrossRef] [PubMed]
55. Castro-Núñez, J.; Shelton, J.M.; Snyder, S.; Sickels, J.V. Virtual Surgical Planning for the Management of Severe Atrophic Mandible Fractures. *Craniomaxillofac. Trauma Reconstr.* **2017**, *11*, 150. [CrossRef]
56. Van Camp, N.; Verhelst, P.J.; Nicot, R.; Ferri, J.; Politis, C. Impaired Callus Formation in Pathological Mandibular Fractures in Medication-Related Osteonecrosis of the Jaw and Osteoradionecrosis. *J. Oral Maxillofac. Surg.* **2021**, *79*, 1892–1901. [CrossRef]
57. Jonasson, G.; Sundh, V.; Hakeberg, M.; Hassani-Nejad, A.; Lissner, L.; Ahlqwist, M. Mandibular bone changes in 24 years and skeletal fracture prediction. *Clin. Oral Investig.* **2013**, *17*, 565–572. [CrossRef]
58. Mohandas, R.; Mohapatra, S.; Narkhede, R.; Kheur, S. Effectiveness of Hyperbaric Oxygen Therapy in the Management of Osteoradionecrosis of the Jaw: A Systematic Review. *J. Health Allied Sci. NU* **2024**, *14*, 295–302. [CrossRef]
59. Forner, L.E.; Dieleman, F.J.; Shaw, R.J.; Kanatas, A.; Butterworth, C.J.; Kjeller, G.; Alsner, J.; Overgaard, J.; Hillerup, S.; Hyldegaard, O.; et al. Hyperbaric oxygen treatment of mandibular osteoradionecrosis: Combined data from the two randomized clinical trials DAHANCA-21 and NWHHT2009-1. *Radiother. Oncol.* **2022**, *166*, 137–144. [CrossRef]
60. Sultan, A.; Hanna, G.J.; Margalit, D.N.; Chau, N.; Goguen, L.A.; Marty, F.M.; Rabinowits, G.; Schoenfeld, J.D.; Sonis, S.T.; Thomas, T.; et al. The Use of Hyperbaric Oxygen for the Prevention and Management of Osteoradionecrosis of the Jaw: A Dana-Farber/Brigham and Women's Cancer Center Multidisciplinary Guideline. *Oncologist* **2017**, *22*, 343. [CrossRef]
61. Korambayil, P.M.; Ambookan, P.V.; Pillai, S.; Karangath, R.R.; George, D. Role of Hyperbaric Medicine for Osteoradionecrosis and Post Irradiation Wounds: An Institutional Experience. *Indian J. Surg. Oncol.* **2020**, *11*, 469. [CrossRef]
62. Banjar, A.; Patel, V.; Abed, H. Pentoxifylline and tocopherol (vitamin E) with/without clodronate for the management of osteoradionecrosis: A scoping review. *Oral Dis.* **2023**, *29*, 29–39. [CrossRef] [PubMed]
63. Arqueros-Lemus, M.; Mariño-Recabarren, D.; Niklander, S.; Martínez-Flores, R.; Moraga, V. Pentoxifylline and tocopherol for the treatment of osteoradionecrosis of the jaws. A. systematic. review. *Med. Oral Patol. Oral Cir. Bucal* **2023**, *28*, e293. [CrossRef] [PubMed]
64. Lyons, A.J.; Brennan, P.A. Pentoxifylline—A review of its use in osteoradionecrosis. *Br. J. Oral Maxillofac. Surg.* **2017**, *55*, 230–234. [CrossRef] [PubMed]

diagnostics

MDPI

*Case Report*

# Exploring Atypical Origins of Trismus: Surgical Solutions for Rare Pathologies—Insights from Rare Clinical Cases

**Ioanna Kalaitsidou [1,*], Mathieu Gass [1], Dimitris Tatsis [2], Sherin Khalil [1], Christian Schedeit [1], Simon David Marjanowski [1], Sarah Wiegner [1] and Benoît Schaller [1]**

[1] Department of Cranio-Maxillofacial Surgery, Inselspital, Bern University Hospital, University of Bern, CH-3010 Bern, Switzerland; mathieu.gass@insel.ch (M.G.)

[2] Department of Oral and Maxillofacial Surgery, Aristotle University of Thessaloniki, 54124 Thessaloniki, Greece; dtatsis@outlook.com

* Correspondence: ikalaitsidou@gmail.com or ioanna.kalaitsidou@insel.ch

**Abstract: Background**: Trismus, or restricted mouth opening, can present significant challenges in oral and maxillofacial surgery and trigger substantial functional and psychosocial disabilities. Intra-articular causes, such as temporomandibular joint ankylosis and arthritis, are thoroughly described; however, extra-articular pathologies like neoplastic, traumatic, infectious, and fibrotic conditions of adjacent soft and hard tissues are less frequently reported and present distinct diagnostic complexities and therapeutic hurdles. This retrospective study aims to investigate the difficulties encountered in diagnosis and surgical interventions associated with rare extra-articular causes of trismus. **Material and Methods**: This article describes five rare causes of extra-articular trismus. The cases range from benign pathologies like coronoid hyperplasia and osteomas to more complex diagnoses of myositis ossificans, external auditory canal abscess, and chronic osteomyelitis. A thorough diagnostic workup was performed for each patient, and specific surgical interventions were administered based on their pathology. **Results**: All five patients showed significant improvements in mouth opening after surgery. Diagnostic accuracy was ensured with advanced imaging modalities and innovative surgical techniques, and adequate postoperative care translated the favorable outcome. **Conclusions**: Although based on individual case descriptions, this study emphasizes the potential importance of early diagnosis, a multidisciplinary approach, and individualized treatment planning in managing rare extra-articular causes of trismus. These cases suggest a basis for a more organized system for the timely identification and treatment of such conditions. Additional research is needed to improve diagnostic accuracy, optimize surgical management, and develop evidence-based aftercare treatment to improve patient care and quality of life.

**Keywords:** trismus; osteoma; hyperplasia; myositis ossificans; osteomyelitis; abscess; ear canal

## 1. Introduction

Trismus, or restricted mouth opening, is a common problem encountered in oral and maxillofacial surgery [1]. The term originates from the Greek word "τρισμός" (trismos), meaning gnashing or grinding, and is described as a sustained, tetanic spasm of the mastication muscles that hinders normal jaw movement [2,3]. It is often considered both a symptom and a complication of temporomandibular disorders (TMDs), a collective term encompassing clinical conditions affecting the temporomandibular joint (TMJ), the masticatory muscles, and associated structures. TMDs are among the most prevalent musculoskeletal disorders in the craniofacial region, affecting approximately 31% to 34% of the population, with higher prevalence reported in women and individuals aged 20–40 years [4,5].

The normal range of mouth opening is variable, usually between 40 and 60 mm; an interincisal distance of less than 35 mm is often associated with severe functional disturbance [6]. Patients with trismus experience considerable difficulties in eating, speaking, and maintaining oral hygiene, which can severely impact their psychosocial well-being and quality of life [7].

The etiology of trismus has a wide range, including both intra-articular and extra-articular causes. Intra-articular pathologies, such as temporomandibular joint ankylosis or arthritis, are well-documented and often recognized early, whereas extra-articular causes are rare and often present a challenge for the clinician in the diagnosis process due to their low prevalence and heterogeneity. The uncommon causes involve neoplastic, traumatic, infectious, or fibrotic processes in the surrounding soft and hard tissues [2,8].

Knowledge of the underlying pathology, along with appropriate management and treatment, is essential, and prolonged treatable delay and inappropriate treatment lead to progressive functional decline, decreased quality of life, and worse prognosis [9,10]. The previously available literature on this topic is limited and primarily consists of isolated case reports, probably due to the uncommonness of extra-articular causes, despite the advancements in imaging and surgical techniques. This discrepancy highlights the importance of a holistic perspective on the diagnosis, categorization, and management of such infrequent diagnoses [10].

We describe several uncommon extra-articular causes of trismus and the challenges encountered while diagnosing and managing each entity. By presenting five rare clinical cases, we aim to contribute to understanding these unusual pathologies and enhance a systematic approach to their management. These conditions are individually infrequent, with the existing literature largely limited to isolated case reports or small case series. The scarcity of comprehensive epidemiological data reflects the inherent difficulty in studying such rare entities; nevertheless, their potential to cause significant functional impairment underscores the importance of early recognition and individualized treatment.

We hypothesize that such rare extra-articular causes of trismus are frequently under-recognized and that their structured presentation can contribute to earlier diagnosis and more effective treatment strategies.

## 2. Materials and Methods

A retrospective review was performed on patients diagnosed with rare extra-articular causes of trismus, treated at the Department of Oral and Maxillofacial Surgery from January 2018 to December 2024. The inclusion criteria discussed are those of cases with reduced mouth opening (defined as an interincisal distance of less than 35 mm) [3,7], secondary to extra-articular pathologies, which were confirmed by clinical assessment and imaging. This level of reduction was associated with significant functional impairment in daily activities, such as eating, speaking, and maintaining oral hygiene. Cases with intra-articular causes of trismus or incomplete medical records were excluded from the study.

Demographic details, clinical presentation, radiological findings, type of pathology, surgical approach performed, and postoperative outcome in mouth opening (interincisal distance) were available from the records. All patients underwent diagnostic imaging (CT or MRI) and received personalized surgical management depending on their specific diagnosis.

The study complied with the ethical principles of the Declaration of Helsinki (1964) (revised 2024).

Case 1

A 48-year-old male patient was referred to the Department of Oral and Maxillofacial Surgery with a complaint of progressive limitation of mouth opening for the past six months. The main complaint of the patient was recurrent difficulty in eating, which significantly affected his daily life. Past medical history was unremarkable, and the patient had experienced no previous trauma to the oral or maxillofacial region, nor did he report any related symptoms, including pain, swelling, or joint noises. Clinical examination revealed a maximum interincisal mouth opening of 19 mm, which is less than normal. No other abnormalities were found in the intraoral examination with respect to the mucosa (i.e., no lesions or masses) or signs of infection.

A panoramic radiograph was performed to investigate the limited mouth opening, which showed a well-defined radiopaque mass at the right coronoid process. A computed tomography (CT) scan was performed to further characterize the lesion and its relationship with surrounding structures. CT images showed an enlarged and elongated right coronoid process with its superior margin extending posteriorly and directly posterior to the zygomatic bone (Figure 1). This abnormal positioning indicated a mechanical obstruction in jaw movement, reducing mouth opening. Based on the imaging findings and the clinical history of slow symptom progression, a provisional diagnosis of a benign osseous neoplasm, likely an osteoma of the right mandibular coronoid process, was made.

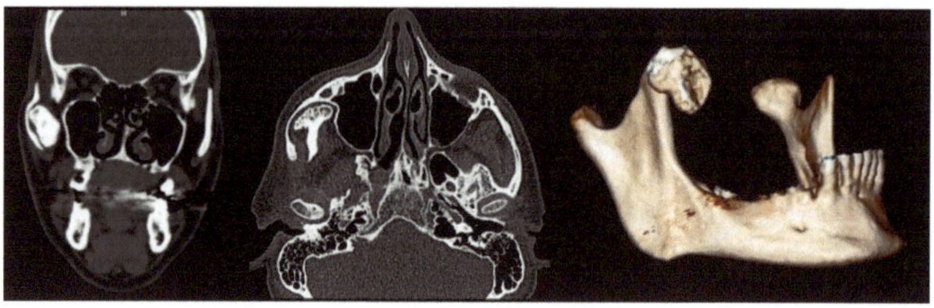

**Figure 1.** Coronal (**left**), axial (**center**), and 3D reconstructed (**right**) CT images demonstrating an enlarged and elongated right coronoid process.

Due to a marked restriction of mouth opening, a surgical reconstruction was planned after detailed preoperative planning. The procedure was conducted under general anesthesia with nasotracheal intubation for an unobstructed surgical field. An intraoral approach, combined with an extraoral approach, was deemed appropriate to access the lesion and obtain complete excision of the affected coronoid process.

The intraoral approach began with a similar incision to that performed for the sagittal split osteotomy. This technique offered direct access to the coronoid process. The periosteum and masseter muscle were meticulously elevated on the ascending ramus of the mandible to provide access to the coronoid process. For coronoid process detachment, the temporalis muscle insertion along the anterior border of the ramus was released, and the tendon was dissected and separated from the coronoid process. One channel retractor was introduced into the sigmoid notch to stabilize the field, and a ramus clamp was applied to push and secure the coronoid process. A low coronoidectomy was completed using a reciprocating saw from the sigmoid notch to the anterior oblique ridge. Despite these attempts, the coronoid process could not be resected due to the proximity to the zygomatic arch and lack of intraoral access.

Given the intraoperative difficulties, an additional extraoral approach was undertaken. Direct access to the zygomatic arch was achieved with a hemi-coronal incision with preauricular extension (Figure 2). Following the elevation of the periosteum, osteotomy of the zygomatic arch was performed at two different points to obtain broad access to the coronoid process. Prior to the osteotomy, a 1.5 mm titanium plate was placed to stabilize the anatomical positioning of the arch during the postoperative period. Once the coronoid process was fully exposed, it was successfully removed. The zygomatic arch was then repositioned anatomically and stabilized using the preplaced titanium plate.

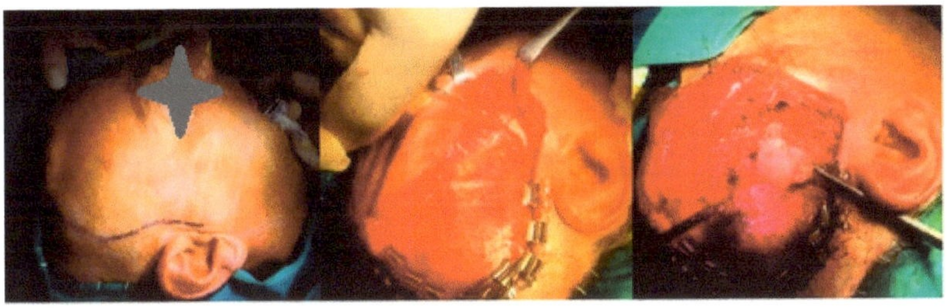

**Figure 2.** Intraoperative photographs demonstrating the additional extraoral approach. (**Left**) Marking of the hemi-coronal incision with preauricular extension. (**Middle**) Dissection to expose the zygomatic arch. (**Right**) Direct visualization and access to the coronoid process through the extended approach, allowing improved surgical access due to intraoperative limitations encountered during the initial phase.

The resected specimen was a bony mushroom-shaped mass (approximately 2.5 cm × 3 cm × 3 cm) (Figure 3). Histopathological examination of the lesion showed a highly cellular collagenized stroma in continuity with interspersed bony trabeculae. At higher magnification, cancellous lamellated bone was evident, with lacunae containing osteocytes and osteoblastic rimming. These findings were consistent with the diagnosis of an osteoma, a benign bone-forming tumor.

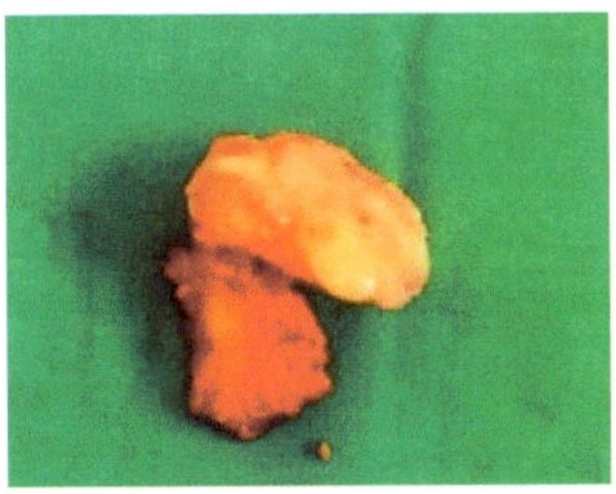

**Figure 3.** The resected specimen shows a bony, mushroom-shaped mass.

The postoperative recovery was uneventful, with no immediate complications like infection, nerve injury, or malocclusion. The patient showed a marked improvement in mouth opening, which increased to 36 mm. He was also counseled to initiate physiotherapy and mouth-opening exercises to improve the function of the mandible and to prevent fibrosis postoperatively. At the three-month follow-up, the patient's mouth opening improved to 39 mm (Figure 4). A 1-year follow-up examination revealed stability of surgical results without signs of recurrence or functional impairment.

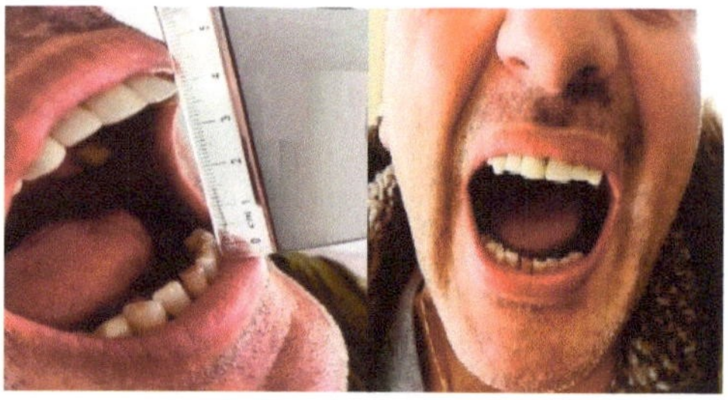

**Figure 4.** Postoperative clinical photographs showing improved mouth opening. (**Left**) Measurement of interincisal distance at three-month follow-up demonstrates an opening of 39 mm. (**Right**) One-year follow-up confirms stability of surgical results with maintained mouth opening and no signs of recurrence or functional limitation.

Case 2

A 10-year-old female patient was referred to the Department of Oral and Maxillofacial Surgery by her pediatrician due to a progressive limitation in mouth opening. The patient had difficulty with activities like eating and speaking without any associated pain. Intraoral examination showed a maximum interincisal opening (MIO) of 17 mm, which was remarkably limited for her age. Her medical history was unremarkable, and no injuries, infections, or systemic illnesses were documented. There was no family history of similar symptoms, and an examination of the temporomandibular joints showed no sounds, pain, or signs of dysfunction.

Initial panoramic radiography showed bilateral elongation of the coronoid processes (Figure 5), indicating structural abnormalities as the cause of her restricted mouth opening.

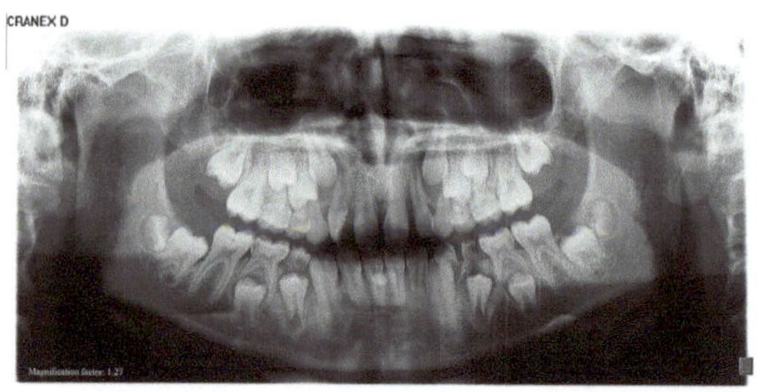


**Figure 5.** Initial panoramic radiograph showing bilateral elongation of the coronoid processes. The structural abnormality is evident on both sides and correlates clinically with the patient's restricted mouth opening.

Computed tomography (CT) imaging offered enhanced visualization, confirming the elongation of the bilateral coronoid processes and revealing the presence of heterotopic bone on the medial and inferior surfaces of the bilateral zygomatic arches (Figure 6). These findings indicated mechanical interference between the coronoid processes and the zygomatic arches during mandibular movement. Based on the clinical and imaging findings, as well as the history of slow symptom progression, a diagnosis of coronoid impingement syndrome (CIS) was established.

Surgical treatment was planned in order to restore functional mouth opening. Nasotracheal intubation was expected to be challenging because of the significant restriction of the mouth opening. General anesthesia was achieved, and nasotracheal intubation was conducted with a fiberoptic scope because the head-scope-guided approach was impossible. An intraoral approach was used for the bilateral coronoidectomies to reduce external scarring and postoperative morbidity. Bilateral buccal mucosa incisions at the level of the ascending ramus of the mandible were made to expose the coronoid processes. The periosteum and surrounding soft tissues were elevated, exposing the elongated coronoid processes. Performing the procedure with a reciprocating saw, the coronoid processes were resected (Figure 7) entirely on both sides to remove mechanical interference with the zygomatic arches. Adequate hemostasis was obtained during the procedure.

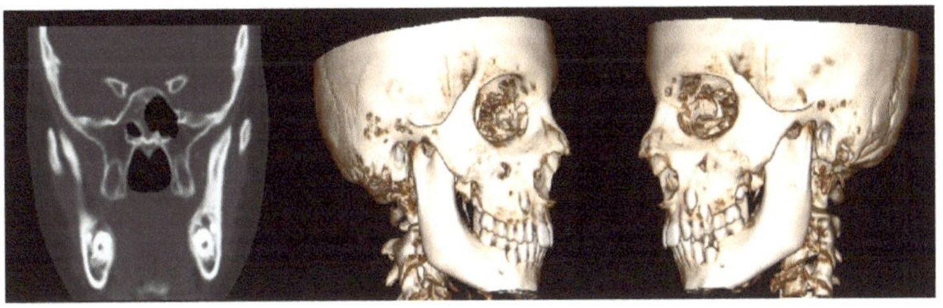

**Figure 6.** Coronal CT slice (**left**) and 3D reconstructed views (**center** and **right**) demonstrating bilateral elongation of the coronoid processes. Additionally, heterotopic bone formation is visible on the medial and inferior surfaces of the bilateral zygomatic arches, contributing to the patient's limited mouth opening.

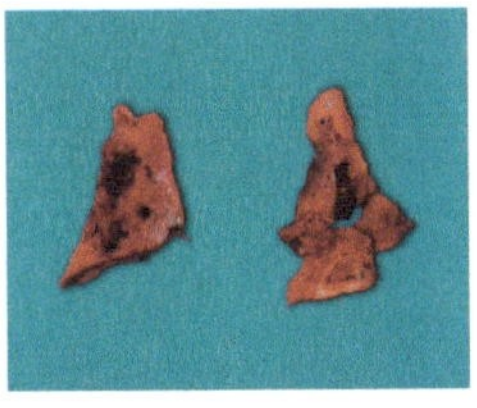

**Figure 7.** Resected bilateral coronoid processes.

Immediately following surgery, the operating room's maximal interincisal opening increased to 37 mm. This immediate improvement confirmed the restriction's mechanical nature and the intervention's success. Postoperative recovery was uneventful, without any complications. The patient was discharged with instructions to begin a structured physiotherapy program, including mouth-opening exercises, starting four weeks postoperatively to prevent fibrosis and maintain functional improvement.

At the ten-month follow-up, the maximal interincisal opening had improved to 45 mm, reflecting sustained functional gains. At the one-year follow-up, the patient exhibited stable and satisfactory mouth opening with no signs of recurrence or postoperative complications. The surgical outcome was highly successful, and the patient had fully recovered.

Case 3

A 34-year-old male patient was referred by his dentist to the Department of Oral and Maxillofacial Surgery, complaining of reduced mouth opening that had started about a month earlier. The clinical examination showed a maximal incisal opening (MIO) of 15 mm (Figure 8). The patient's medical history was notable for a facial injury on the right side sustained three months prior. There was no past medical history of systemic disease or other pertinent conditions.

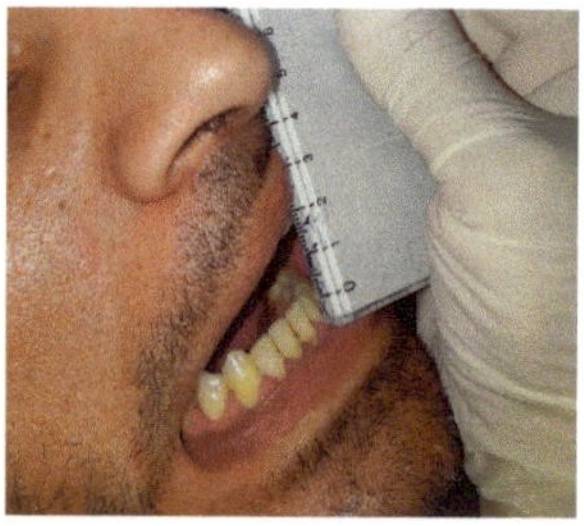

**Figure 8.** Preoperative clinical photograph showing a maximal incisal opening (MIO) of 15 mm, indicating a significant limitation in mouth opening.

Imaging studies were performed to assess the restricted mouth opening. Orthopantomography and computed tomography (CT) showed a well-defined calcified mass in the right masseter muscle (Figure 9). There was no evidence of fractures or abnormality of the cranial visceral bones. Laboratory tests showed normal serum calcium, phosphorus, and parathyroid hormone levels, excluding systemic metabolic causes of calcification. Given the clinical history and imaging findings, along with the background of previous trauma with gradual symptom development, a provisional diagnosis of myositis ossificans traumatica (MOT) was made.

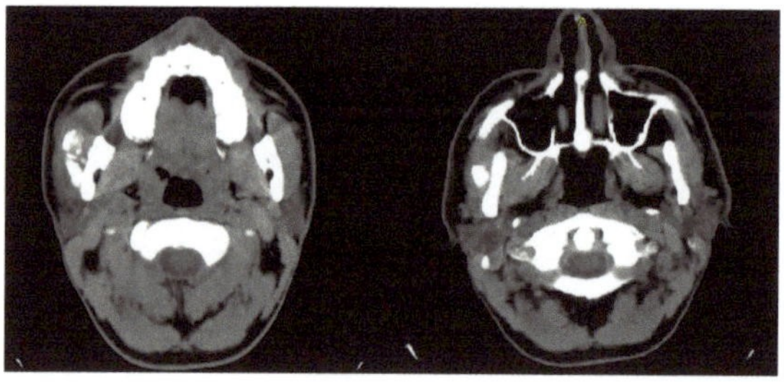

**Figure 9.** Axial CT images revealing a well-defined calcified mass within the right masseter muscle.

Surgical intervention was indicated, and the patient was transferred to the operating room. Under general anesthesia, fiberoptic-assisted nasotracheal intubation was performed owing to the limited opening of the mouth. The calcified mass in the right masseter muscle was excised through the intraoral approach to avoid excessive visible scarring. The lesion was circumscribed and measured 2.6 cm at its largest diameter, allowing for excision. Histopathological examination showed alternating lamellar bone with fat cells, fibrous tissue, and thin-walled vascular spaces, consistent with a diagnosis of MOT.

The patient had an uneventful immediate postoperative recovery without any complications. Upon discharge, the MIO had improved to approximately 34 mm. A regimen of forced physical therapy and mouth-opening exercises was recommended to prevent fibrosis and maintain an improved range of motion.

Two months after surgery, the patient returned to the department complaining of a new reduction in mouth opening. Clinical examination revealed an MIO of 20 mm. Imaging studies, including CT scans, identified a well-defined calcified lesion within the left masseter muscle, distinct from the previous surgical site (Figure 10). Given the recurrence of symptoms, a second surgical intervention was planned. Surgery was performed under general anesthesia with fiberoptic-assisted nasotracheal intubation, and the calcified mass in the left masseter muscle was excised by the intraoral approach.

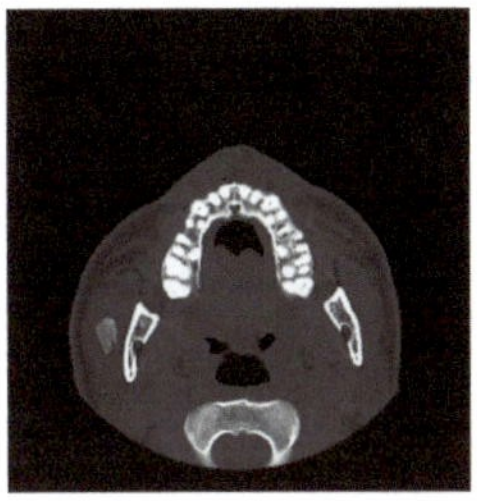

**Figure 10.** An axial CT scan showed a well-defined calcified lesion within the left masseter muscle, anatomically distinct from the previous surgical site. The radiologic appearance is consistent with recurrent or new-onset myositis ossificans.

Histological analysis of the excised lesion described a central zone of bone tissue with abundant osteoblasts surrounded by mature bone, findings consistent with myositis ossificans. The edges of the specimen were free of tumor or other pathological findings, ensuring complete excision.

The postoperative course was again uneventful, and the patient demonstrated a significant improvement in mouth opening, with an MIO of 36 mm achieved soon after surgery. He was once more advised to perform mouth-opening exercises and continue physiotherapy. At the six-month follow-up, the patient's MIO had increased to 52 mm (Figure 11), reflecting excellent functional recovery. At the one-year follow-up, the patient remained asymptomatic, with no signs of recurrence and stable mouth-opening capacity, indicating a successful surgical outcome and long-term resolution of the condition.

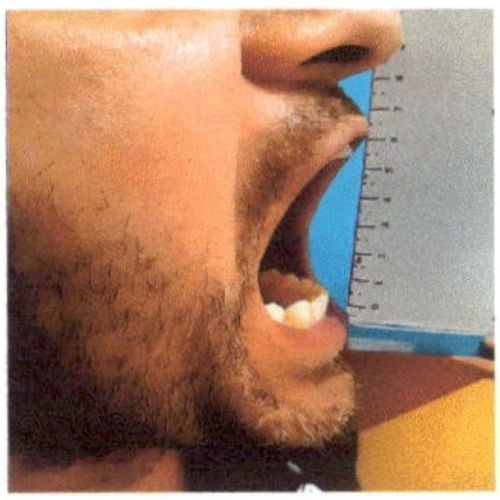

**Figure 11.** Clinical photograph at six-month follow-up showing a maximal incisal opening (MIO) of 52 mm, demonstrating excellent functional recovery and restoration of normal mandibular mobility.

Case 4

A 44-year-old healthy male patient was referred to the Craniomaxillofacial Surgery Department by his physiotherapist due to severe restriction of mouth opening. The patient reported a history of extraction of an impacted mandibular third molar (#38) three years prior. According to the patient, the extraction was straightforward and without immediate complications. As per his medical history, the onset of reduced mouth opening occurred suddenly and without apparent cause. Initial clinical and imaging evaluations by the patient's dentist prompted a referral to a specialized physiotherapy center within our hospital.

Despite undergoing nine physiotherapy sessions, there was no improvement in the patient's condition. During this period, the patient developed episodic intermittent hypoesthesia of the left inferior alveolar nerve. Given the inadequate response following therapy, he was referred to our clinic for further evaluation and management. On presentation, the patient exhibited no abnormal swelling, facial asymmetry, or hypertrophy of the masticatory muscles. The temporomandibular joint (TMJ) showed no frictional sounds, and no compression pain was elicited upon palpation of the joint areas bilaterally. The maximal incisal opening (MIO) was limited to 13 mm, and the posterior dental contacts were symmetrical.

A panoramic radiograph demonstrated normal TMJ articulation bilaterally, with no evidence of odontogenic infection or structural abnormalities (Figure 12). Magnetic resonance imaging (MRI) revealed mild bilateral anterior disc dislocation with arthropathy, more pronounced on the left side, and incomplete translation of the disc on mouth opening. No intracranial pathology or secondary cause of head and facial pain was identified. A computed tomography (CT) scan ruled out any pathological findings in the mandible.

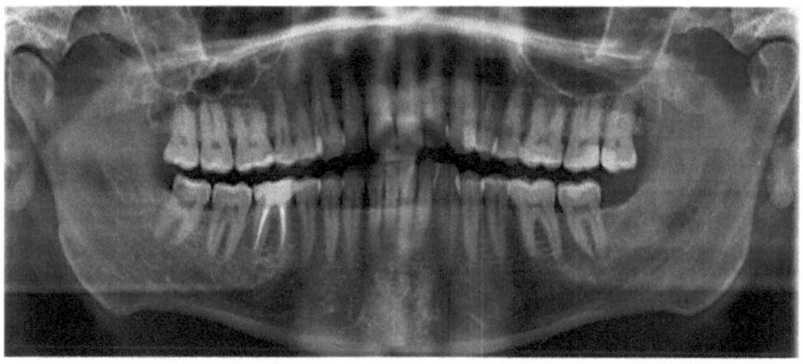

**Figure 12.** Postoperative panoramic radiograph showing normal bilateral temporomandibular joint (TMJ) articulation. No signs of odontogenic infection, recurrence, or structural abnormalities are present.

Based on the findings, a provisional diagnosis of tendomyopathy of the masseter muscles was established. The patient was started on tizanidine (4 mg) and re-referred for ongoing physiotherapy. After 1 week, the patient stopped taking the medication because of dizziness and muscle limpness. He also did not want to continue with physiotherapy. Tolperisone (150 mg) replaced tizanidine, which slightly improved trismus. Three months later, the patient presented with worsening symptoms. Mouth opening had further reduced to 2 mm, and he presented with swelling in the region of the left mandibular angle. The hypoesthesia of the inferior alveolar nerve, which had been intermittent, was now persistent. The patient was afebrile and reported no difficulty swallowing. An MRI revealed findings suggesting a developing abscess adjacent to focal cortical defects on the lateral side of the distal mandibular ramus, with possible incipient abscess formation medially (Figure 13). The masticatory musculature was associated with diffuse edematous or phlegmonous swelling, particularly the masseter and medial pterygoid muscles on the left side. The distal mandibular ramus also showed an increased bone marrow signal, corresponding to acute osteomyelitis.

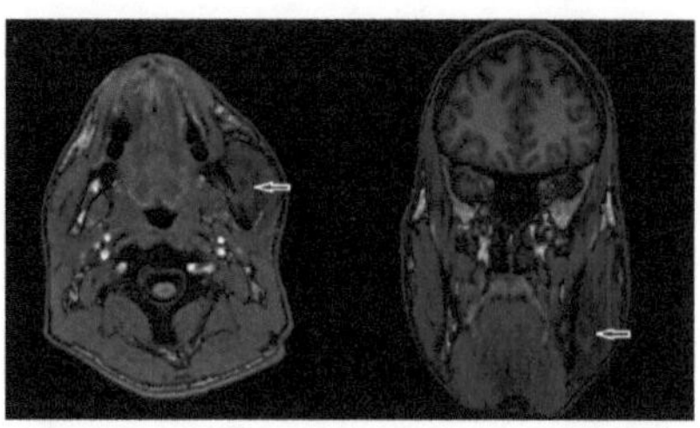

**Figure 13.** Axial (**left**) and coronal (**right**) T1-weighted MRI images showing a hyperintense lesion adjacent to the lateral aspect of the distal mandibular ramus (white arrows), suggestive of a developing abscess.

Surgical management by incision and drainage of the abscess and surgical curettage was performed under local anesthesia. Gram stain, culture, and sensitivity testing of swabs taken during the procedure showed a polymicrobial anaerobic population primarily composed of the *Streptococcus milleri* group. The histopathological study showed foci of chronic inflammatory infiltration and medullary fibrosis, leading to the diagnosis of late-diagnosed chronic osteomyelitis of the mandible. Pharmaceutical management consisted of a combination of amoxicillin (875 mg)/clavulanic acid (125 mg) and ibuprofen (600 mg) for anti-inflammatory. Fifteen days postoperatively, during a follow-up examination, the patient presented with a marked mouth opening measuring 39 mm, lower swelling in the mandibular angle region, and significant pain relief.

Further CT imaging disclosed a localized osteolysis area in the left mandibular corpus at the height of the mandibular canal (Figure 14), along with slight bony dehiscence of the medial and lateral compacta. No residual or adjacent soft tissue swelling was evident. The antibiotic was continued for another 15 days, and the patient showed marked improvement. At the end of treatment, the patient showed a mouth opening of 48 mm and remained pain-free.

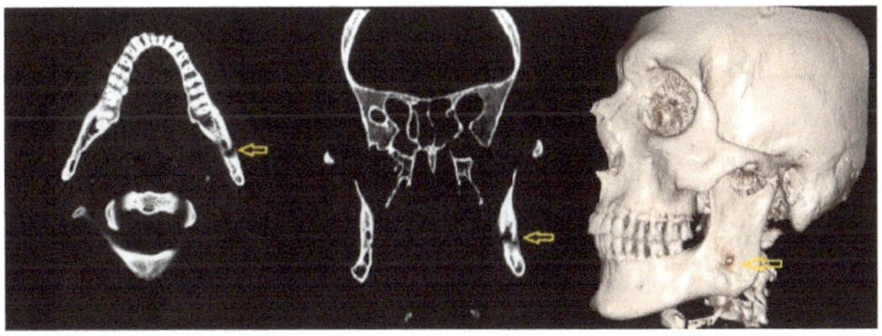

**Figure 14.** Axial (**left**), coronal (**middle**), and 3D reconstructed (**right**) CT images showing a localized area of osteolysis in the left mandibular body at the level of the mandibular canal (yellow arrows).

Case 5

A 45-year-old female patient was referred to the Craniomaxillofacial Surgery Department by the otorhinolaryngology (ENT) team with severe restriction of mouth opening and temporomandibular joint (TMJ) dysfunction. The patient presented with left otalgia and reduced mouth opening for three days and was initially diagnosed with otitis externa. Her symptoms persisted despite being treated with local antibiotic drops, leading to further evaluation. On examination, there was no evidence of swelling, erythema, or fluctuation near the TMJ. Severe tenderness was noted over the left TMJ. There was the restriction of maximal incisal opening (MIO) to 10 mm with right-sided mandibular deviation on occlusion. There were no visible mucosal abnormalities or evidence of odontogenic infection.

Panoramic radiographs indicated bilateral normal TMJ articulation without signs of odontogenic infection or structural changes (Figure 15).

A CT scan shows subluxation of the left TMJ (Figure 16), with soft tissue swelling up to the external auditory canal, but no evidence of abscess or joint arthrosis was found.

Magnetic resonance imaging (MRI) revealed TMJ effusion with phlegmonous changes posterior to the mandibular condyle and a small suspected abscess measuring $4 \times 5$ mm (Figure 17).

Surgical intervention was performed under local anesthesia, including incision and drainage of an abscess in the anterior external ear canal wall (Figure 18), followed by placement of a medicated Meche with gentamicin cream. Systemic antibiotics were initiated with Co-Amoxicillin. Swabs collected during the procedure revealed methicillin-resistant *Staphylococcus aureus* (MRSA), prompting a switch to Clindamycin (600 mg) thrice daily.

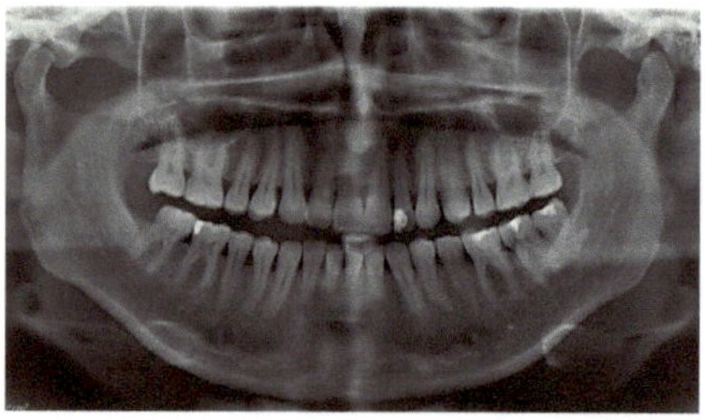

**Figure 15.** Panoramic radiograph demonstrating normal bilateral temporomandibular joint (TMJ) articulation. No evidence of odontogenic infection, pathological lesions, or structural abnormalities is observed.

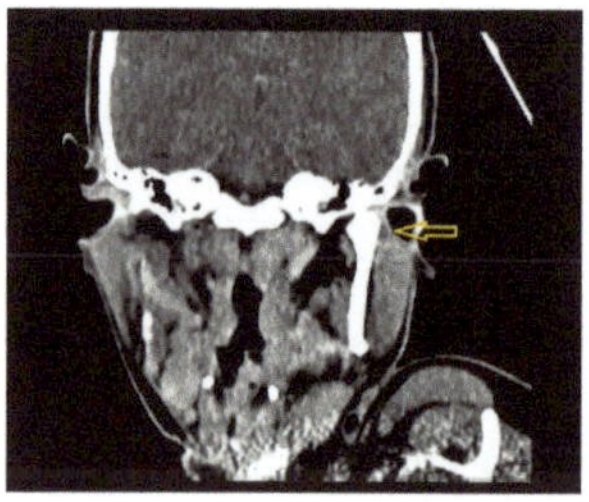

**Figure 16.** Coronal CT image showing subluxation of the left temporomandibular joint (TMJ), accompanied by surrounding soft tissue swelling extending toward the external auditory canal (yellow arrow).

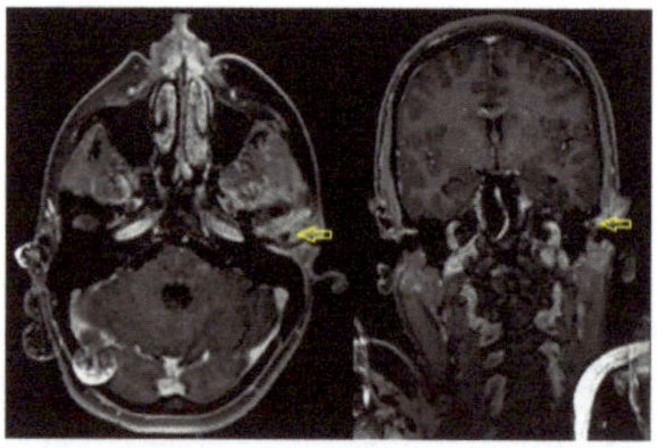

**Figure 17.** Axial (**left**) and coronal (**right**) contrast-enhanced MRI images showing effusion in the left temporomandibular joint (TMJ) and surrounding phlegmonous inflammatory changes (yellow arrows).

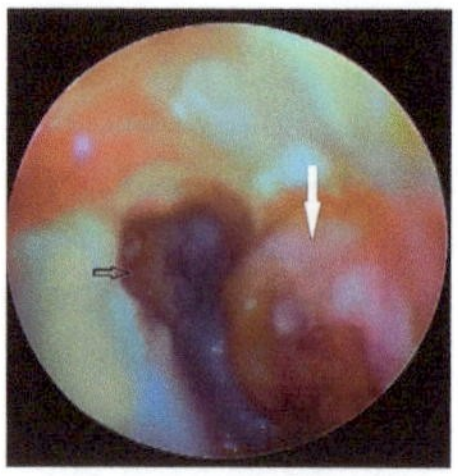

**Figure 18.** Otoscopic view showing the tympanic membrane (black arrow) and a bulging abscess (white arrow) in the anterior wall of the external auditory canal.

Gradually, over the subsequent weeks, the patient's pain intensity decreased, and mouth opening improved to 25 mm. At 15 days postoperatively, the patient had marked improvement in pain, and mouth opening had improved to 42 mm. She was advised to perform mouth-opening exercises and continue physiotherapy. Mouth opening was further improved at the end of treatment to 51 mm while the patient remained pain-free with no evidence of residual infection or complications.

## 3. Results

Five rare causes of extra-articular trismus were included. The pathologies were coronoid process hyperplasia and osteoma, myositis ossificans traumatica, chronic suppurative osteomyelitis of the ramus mandible, and deep-space abscess originating from the external auditory canal. Detailed diagnosis was made through various high-resolution imaging modalities, including computed tomography (CT) and magnetic resonance imaging (MRI), to localize and characterize the lesions appropriately. Surgical management was guided by each case's etiology and anatomical complexity and included coronoidectomy, local excision of ossified or infected tissue, and drainage of deep-seated abscesses. All five patients in this study showed significant improvement in mouth opening following surgery, with the interincisal distances increasing from less than 20 mm before the operation to more than 35 mm after it. Structured physiotherapy and regular follow-up further strengthened this functional recovery to achieve gradual and sustained recovery (Table 1).

**Table 1.** Patients with extra-articular causes of trismus.

| | Sex | Age | Etiology | Imaging | Preoperative Interincisal Distance | Operative Intervention | Postperative Interincisal Distance |
|---|---|---|---|---|---|---|---|
| 1 | Male | 48 | Osteoma of the coronoid process | OPG CT | 19 mm | Coronoidectomy | 39 mm |
| 2 | Female | 10 | Bilateral hyperplasia of the coronoid processes | OPG CT | 17 mm | Bilateral coronoidectomy | 45 mm |
| 3 | Male | 34 | Myositis ossificans traumatica | CT | 15 mm | Excision of calcified mass | 52 mm |
| 4 | Male | 44 | Chronic osteomyelitis of the mandible | OPG CT/MRI | 13 mm | Incision and drainage of the abscess and surgical curettage | 48 mm |
| 5 | Female | 45 | External auditory canal abscess | OPG CT/MRI | 10 mm | Incision and drainage of the abscess | 51 mm |

## 4. Discussion

Trismus, known as "locked jaw," is frequently encountered in oral and maxillofacial surgery and can have a devastating impact on the quality of life of a patient [9,11]. Although the normal range of interincisal distance varies among individuals and has been found to be between 40 and 60 mm [9,11], any significant decrease in this should be considered as a possible underlying disease and should be treated accordingly [12].

Trismus has a broad etiologic spectrum, which can be classified as intra-articular and extra-articular [1,9,10]. Intra-articular causes include pathologies of the temporomandibular joint (TMJ) itself, such as ankylosis, arthritis, synovitis, and meniscal derangements. These include several structural abnormalities or inflammatory processes directly affecting the joint [13]. The extra-articular causes, however, are numerous and may affect the adjacent structures, such as the masticatory muscles, coronoid processes, and soft tissues of the oral cavity [14,15]. These can be categorized further into congenital [16] and acquired conditions, with the acquired causes typically being trauma [17,18], infection [19,20], tumors [21,22], and fibrotic changes [23,24]. The table below (Table 2) summarizes the most common causes for trismus based on accepted classifications.

**Table 2.** Patients with extra-articular causes of trismus.

| Category | Etiology | Examples |
| --- | --- | --- |
| Intra-articular | Structural abnormalities or inflammation | TMJ ankylosis, arthritis, synovitis, Discus pathology |
| Extra-articular | Neoplastic | Osteoma, sarcoma, lymphoma |
| | Traumatic | Myositis ossificans, mandibular fractures |
| | Infectious | Peritonsillar abscess, mandibular osteomyelitis |
| | Fibrotic | Submucous fibrosis, radiation-induced fibrosis |
| | Neurological | Tetanus, dystonia |
| | Iatrogenic | Postoperative complications, TMJ surgeries |

Less commonly, trismus could be caused by tumors that involve the coronoid process of the mandible [25]. Notably, osteomas, benign bone tumors, can develop in this area and lead to restricted mouth opening by physically preventing mandibular movement against the zygomatic arch [26]. To date, only a few cases of coronoid osteoma have been reported in the literature since Lewars' first report in 1959 [27]. Petronis et al. (2024) recently addressed the difficulty in diagnosing coronoid osteomas because they are often asymptomatic in the early stages [28]. These tumors are generally diagnosed by clinical examination and imaging studies, including computed tomography (CT) and magnetic resonance imaging (MRI), supported by histopathological evaluation [29–31]. In our patient, the tumor was classified as a peripheral and cancellous variant of osteoma, originating from the periosteum of the coronoid process. Notably, no association with Gardner's syndrome [32]—identified by colorectal polyposis, skeletal abnormalities, and supernumerary teeth—was recognized in this patient.

Osteomas usually appear in adults older than 40 years and show a male predominance (a male-to-female ratio of approximately 2:1) [33]. The pathogenesis of etiology is still a matter of debate. Some investigators regard osteomas to be true neoplasms, while others believe they are developmental anomalies or reactive lesions in response to trauma or infection [31]. However, in the absence of trauma or infection, as in our case, the etiology is unknown. Differential diagnoses for osteomas are osteochondroma, fibrous dysplasia, Paget's disease, and ossifying fibroma [34,35]. They are generally benign and asymptomatic, but the surgery is often indicated if they cause functional disturbance, as in our patient who underwent intraoral coronoidectomy. This approach minimizes scarring and postoperative morbidity [35]. At the one-year follow-up, the patient had fully recovered without any recurrence.

Another rare etiology of trismus is bilateral coronoid process hyperplasia [36]. This condition, which is the exception, is seen in approximately 5% of mandibular hypomobility cases and is described by the abnormal elongation of the coronoid processes [37,38]. This elongation protrudes against the temporal surface of the zygomatic bone or the medial surface of the zygomatic arch while moving the mandible [39,40]. According to the study by Goh et al. (2020), most cases occur in men, and the average age of onset is 23 years [39]. However, it is rare in children under the age of 10 [40]. Our case of a 10-year-old female patient with bilateral coronoid process hyperplasia underscores the progressive and painless nature associated with the condition. Reduced mouth opening can be insidious, often undetected, until the function is seriously impaired and identified, in this case, during a routine pediatric check-up.

Coronoid hyperplasia has an obscure etiology. Possible explanations include genetics, trauma, overactivity of the temporalis muscle, and hormone ratios [41,42]. However, none of these factors were found in our patient. The most common treatment is to surgically remove the coronoid processes by performing a coronoidectomy through intraoral or extraoral approaches [43]. Intraoral coronoidectomy is often preferred due to its lower risk of complications, like facial nerve injury and external scarring [43]. These findings are consistent with those reported by Nogueira et al. (2015) in their retrospective analysis of similar cases [44]. The authors emphasized the importance of early intervention and physiotherapy. Postoperative physiotherapy is important to maintain an adequate range of motion and prevent recurrence [45,46]. In our case, the patient also reported considerable improvement and absence of recurrence at the one-year follow-up.

Myositis ossificans traumatica (MOT) is another rare etiology of trismus. MOT is described as the ectopic ossification of skeletal muscle and usually occurs after trauma [47]. Although it most often presents in the quadriceps or brachialis muscles, the masseter muscle in the head and neck region is not an unprecedented involvement [48]. Similar cases have been reported in the literature [49–52] discussing the diagnostic and therapeutic dilemmas of MOT. Trauma is a commonly accepted primary precipitating factor, although the exact pathogenesis of MOT is unclear. Proposed mechanisms include migrating osteoprogenitor cells to soft tissues and detaining periosteal fragments or differentiated cells exposed to bone morphogenic proteins [53]. Histopathological assessment of MOT lesions commonly indicates a three-zone arrangement, encompassing a peripheral layer of mature lamellar bone, an intermediate zone of immature osteoid and cartilage, and a central zone of granulation tissue and muscle necrosis [48].

In our case, a patient presented with trismus following trauma to the right side of the face. Imaging studies showed a calcified mass in the masseter muscle, and MOT was confirmed histopathologically. Subsequently, the lesion was surgically excised, and intensive physiotherapy was pursued. However, the patient experienced recurrence two months later, necessitating a second surgical intervention. This fact underscores the difficulty in managing MOT, including the best time for surgical intervention and how to maximize compliance with postoperative physiotherapy to prevent recurrence. Jović et al. (2021) also reported a high recurrence rate in cases of incomplete excision or insufficient rehabilitation [50]. Other treatments for MOT, including non-steroidal anti-inflammatory drugs, bisphosphonates, and low-dose radiation therapy, have also been investigated, but the evidence of their effectiveness is inconsistent [47–54].

Chronic osteomyelitis of the mandible is a challenging and often underdiagnosed condition that can significantly impact a patient's quality of life, particularly when diagnosed late [55]. Its insidious onset and nonspecific symptoms (pain, swelling, and restricted mouth opening) make an early diagnosis and treatment difficult [56]. In our case, a patient was presented initially with unexplained trismus and intermittent hypoesthesia of the inferior alveolar nerve, which are both red flags for more profound pathological processes. Over time, the disease progressed to include swelling, abscess formation, and cortical bone defects on imaging modalities. In the current case, magnetic resonance imaging (MRI) was instrumental in demonstrating inflammatory changes in the masticatory muscles and changes in the mandibular bone marrow signal that suggest acute-on-chronic osteomyelitis [57]. These results, together with findings from CT imaging, provide further evidence that comprehensive imaging plays an important role in the diagnosis and management of patients with mandibular osteomyelitis. The delay in diagnosis that is common in such cases illustrates the need for osteomyelitis to be part of the differential diagnosis in people who present with progressive trismus, once more common causes have been excluded [56].

Management of chronic osteomyelitis requires a multimodal approach. Surgery seeks to contain the infection and eliminate sources of persistent inflammation [58]. In this case, surgical management encompasses the exact methods for draining abscesses and curettage of the involved area, all of which match standard practices, such as sequestrectomy, saucerization, and decortication. Resection and subsequent reconstruction may be indicated in refractory cases [59]. The microbiological analysis in our case identified *Streptococcus milleri* as the predominant organism. This abscess-forming pathogen belongs to the Streptococcus anginosus group and is characterized by its tendency for deep infections, such as osteomyelitis [60]. Identification of *S. milleri* guided antibiotic therapy, which was critical in the eventual resolution of infection.

This case illustrates the importance of a high index of suspicion for chronic osteomyelitis in patients presenting with progressive trismus and nonspecific symptoms. Trismus is a clinical entity that needs a comprehensive diagnostic workup involving clinical assessment and advanced imaging. Panoramic radiography, CT, and MRI are important for detecting the underlying cause and for treatment planning. Physiotherapy following surgery is vital for the return of mandibular function and prevention of recurrence. Imaging studies, like open-mouth panoramic radiography, should be repeated periodically to follow recovery with time [61,62].

External auditory canal abscess or inflammation can be a rare but clinically significant cause of temporomandibular joint (TMJ) dysfunction and trismus [63]. Both structures are susceptible to secondary involvement due to their close anatomical relationship, with the external auditory canal neighboring the mandibular condyle. Infection in the external auditory canal can directly extend to the TMJ or compress adjacent tissues as a result of abscess expansion, resulting in pain, decreased movement, and dysfunction of the jaw [64]. Such cases often require advanced imaging to assess the extent of the pathology and ascertain the diagnosis to allow for appropriate management [64,65].

In the presented case, microbiological analysis revealed methicillin-resistant *Staphylococcus aureus* (MRSA) as the causative pathogen. MRSA's virulent behavior, resistance mechanisms, and association with healthcare settings are well described. The ability to create biofilms and infiltrate host tissues makes treatment challenging, often necessitating a dual method of surgical drainage and specific antibiotic therapy [66]. In our case, MRSA identification after the first 48 h of the Co-Amoxicillin led to changing the antibiotic to Clindamycin; this choice is a frequent option for its excellent effectiveness against MRSA and good penetration in bone and soft tissues. Therefore, this specific antimicrobial approach, together with immediate surgical treatment, is necessary to control the infections of the TMJ and adjacent parts [67].

Imaging was crucial to exposing the extent of the disease. Computed tomography (CT) demonstrated subluxation of the TMJ with surrounding soft tissue swelling. At the same time, magnetic resonance imaging (MRI) showed joint effusion, phlegmonous change, and a small abscess adjacent to the anterior wall of the external auditory canal, with no abnormality noted on panoramic radiographs. This emphasizes the role of CT and MRI in head and neck infections with complex inflammatory anatomical microenvironments [65].

Management consisted of incision and drainage of the abscess, followed by medicated dressing and systemic antibiotics. That approach effectively reduced infection and restored function. The resolution of the symptoms and the improvement in maximal incisal opening to 51 mm at the end of the treatment emphasize the effectiveness of early aggressive intervention.

Rehabilitation of trismus is the major phase after its treatment, and it requires a multidisciplinary approach to manage and achieve optimal recovery along with comprehensive prevention of future recurrences. These multidisciplinary teams usually consist of oral and maxillofacial surgeons, physiotherapists, and speech therapists, all of whom are integral in managing the functional and structural consequences of trismus [68].

The mainstay of rehabilitation is physiotherapy, which consists of active and passive stretching exercises to enhance the range of mandibular movement progressively [69]. These exercises are normally augmented through the use of dynamic devices, similar to continuous passive motion machines, and specialized implements, together with bite blocks, jaw stretchers, or mouth screws [70]. Individualized splints are specialized aids that help apply uniform lengthening to the masticatory muscles and prevent re-apposition. Regular physiotherapy and following a prescribed routine are essential for having a better recovery, and relapse can be prevented as it tends to fix the recovery in the jaw. For certain conditions, such as hyperplasia of the coronoid process or myositis ossificans, early initiation of physiotherapy—often immediately after surgical fixation—has been shown to improve outcomes. Early mobilization preserves the functional mobility of the temporomandibular joint and surrounding structures and prevents postoperative fibrosis or scarring, limiting recovery [68,70].

Speech therapy may then also be initiated, especially when trismus impairs swallowing, speech articulation, or oral functions. A holistic approach that covers functional and mechanical aspects while rehabbing a patient from trismus is vital to ensure the patient regains function and quality of life [71].

## 5. Conclusions

In conclusion, trismus may result from various aetiologies, including benign osteomas, coronoid process hyperplasia, myositis ossificans, and chronic osteomyelitis. The cases presented in this study emphasize the clinical complexity associated with such rare extra-articular causes and highlight the importance of early diagnosis, multidisciplinary evaluation, and customized surgical planning. Early intervention and structured postoperative care are essential in achieving functional outcomes. Although the results are derived from selected clinical scenarios, these findings report pivotal management areas and advocate the requirement for continued research to improve diagnostic care, develop surgical interventions, and standardize rehabilitation protocols to improve patient management.

**Author Contributions:** Conceptualization: I.K. and M.G.; methodology, I.K.; validation, I.K.; investigation, I.K. and M.G.; resources, I.K.; data curation, I.K., M.G., S.K., C.S., S.D.M., S.W. and D.T.; writing—original draft preparation, I.K., M.G. and D.T.; writing—review and editing, I.K. and D.T.; supervision, I.K. and B.S. All authors have read and agreed to the published version of the manuscript.

**Funding:** This research received no external funding.

**Institutional Review Board Statement:** This manuscript presents a retrospective description of five clinical cases combined with a literature review. According to our institution's guidelines and applicable regulations, such retrospective case series that do not constitute systematic investigations aimed at contributing to generalizable knowledge are not considered research and therefore do not require approval by an Institutional Review Board (IRB) or Ethics Committee. Nevertheless, written informed consent for participation and publication was obtained from all patients involved.

**Informed Consent Statement:** Written informed consent has been obtained from the patients to publish this paper.

**Data Availability Statement:** The data presented in this study are available on request from the corresponding author.

**Conflicts of Interest:** The authors declare no conflicts of interest.

## Abbreviations

The following abbreviations are used in this manuscript:

| | |
|---|---|
| CT | Computed tomography |
| MRI | Magnetic Resonance Imaging |
| OPG | Orthopantomogramm |
| TMJ | Temporomandibular joint |
| MIO | Maximum interincisal opening |
| CIS | Coronoid impingement syndrome |
| MOT | Myositis ossificans traumatica |
| MRSA | Methicillin-resistant *Staphylococcus aureus* |
| SAG | *Streptococcus anginosus* group |
| ENT | Otorhinolaryngology (ear, nose, throat) |

## References

1. Poornima, G.; Poornima, C. Trismus. *J. Health Sci. Res.* **2014**, *5*, 15–20. [CrossRef]
2. Dhanrajani, P.J.; Jonaidel, O. Trismus: Aetiology, Differential Diagnosis and Treatment. Diagnosis and Treatment. *Dent. Update* **2002**, *29*, 88–94. [CrossRef] [PubMed]
3. Rapidis, A.D.; Dijkstra, P.U.; Roodenburg, J.L.N.; Rodrigo, J.P.; Rinaldo, A.; Strojan, P.; Ferlito, A. Trismus in patients with head and neck cancer: Etiopathogenesis, diagnosis and management. *Clin. Otolaryngol.* **2015**, *40*, 516–526. [CrossRef]
4. Valesan, L.F.; Da-Cas, C.D.; Réus, J.C.; Denardin, A.C.S.; Garanhani, R.R.; Bonotto, D.; Januzzi, E.; de Souza, B.D.M. Prevalence of temporomandibular joint disorders: A systematic review and meta-analysis. *Clin. Oral Investig.* **2021**, *25*, 441–453. [CrossRef]
5. Zieliński, G.; Pająk-Zielińska, B.; Ginszt, M. A Meta-Analysis of the Global Prevalence of Temporomandibular Disorders. *J. Clin. Med.* **2024**, *13*, 1365. [CrossRef]
6. Mezitis, M.; Rallis, G.; Zacharides, N. The normal range of mouth opening. *J. Oral Maxillofac. Surg.* **1984**, *47*, 1028–1029. [CrossRef] [PubMed]
7. Johnson, J.; Johansson, M.; Rydén, A.; Houltz, E.; Finizia, C. Impact of trismus on health-related quality of life and mental health. *Head Neck* **2015**, *37*, 1672–1679. [CrossRef]
8. Luyk, N.H.; Steinberg, B. Aetiology and diagnosis of clinically evident jaw trismus. *Aust. Dent. J.* **1990**, *35*, 523–529. [CrossRef]
9. Amin, B.; Chandra, S.B. Recognizing trismus symptoms, prevention, and treatment. *Med. Sci.* **2019**, *8*, 766–769. [CrossRef]
10. Tveterås, K.; Kristense, S. The aetiology and pathogenesis of trismus. *Clin. Otolaryngol. Allied Sci.* **1986**, *11*, 383–387. [CrossRef]
11. Siddiqui, L.; Khan, H.F.; Kanwal, S.S.; Mustafa, K.M. Evaluating the Impact of temporo-mandibular joint disorders on oral health related quality of life; A literature review. *Int. Ann. Health Sci.* **2024**, *3*, 4–11. [CrossRef]
12. Małgorzata, P.; Małgorzata, K.M.; Karolina, C.; Gala, A. Diagnostic of Temporomandibular Disorders and Other Facial Pain Conditions-Narrative Review and Personal Experience. *Medicina* **2020**, *56*, 472. [CrossRef] [PubMed]
13. Tanaka, E.; Detamore, M.S.; Mercuri, L.G. Degenerative disorders of the temporomandibular joint: Etiology, diagnosis, and treatment. *J. Dent. Res.* **2008**, *87*, 296–307. [CrossRef] [PubMed]
14. Hilaire, H.; Weber, W.; Ramer, M.; Lumerman, H. Clinicopathologic conference: Trismus following dental treatment. *Oral Surg. Oral Med. Oral Pathol. Oral Radiol. Endod.* **2004**, *98*, 261–266. [CrossRef]
15. Skinner, A.M.; Rees, M.J. Congenital trismus secondary to masseteric fibrous bands: A 7-year follow-up report as an approach to management. *J. Craniofac. Surg.* **2004**, *15*, 709–713. [CrossRef]
16. Hong, C.J.; Caulley, L.; Kohlert, S.; Graham, G.E.; McMillan, H.J.; Michaud, J.; Vaccani, J.P. Congenital Trismus From Brainstem Dysgenesis: Case Report and Review of Literature. *Pediatrics* **2016**, *138*, e20154605. [CrossRef]
17. Campanella, G.; Artuso, G.; Murgia, M.S.; Orrù, G.; Casu, C. Severe Post-Traumatic Trismus Unresponsive to Drug Therapy in a 12-Year-Old Patient Treated with a Capacitive-Resistive Electrical Transfer Therapy: A Case Report. *Oral* **2022**, *2*, 173–181. [CrossRef]
18. Managutti, A.; Patel, N.; Menat, S.; Kamala, R.; Patel, H. Post-traumatic-Zygomaticocoronoid Ankylosis: A Rare Clinical Case Report. *IJSS Case Rep. Rev.* **2015**, *1*, 4–6.
19. Obradovic, B. Intraoral management of odontogenic infection associated with severe trismus under local anesthesia. *Ann. Ital. Chir.* **2021**, *92*, 116–118.
20. Kim, H.-Y.; Chung, J.-W. Infectious Myositis of the Jaw Presenting as Trismus of Unknown Origin. *J. Oral Med. Pain* **2020**, *45*, 115–119. [CrossRef]

21. Satheeshkumar, P.S.; Mohan, M.P.; Jacob, J. Restricted mouth opening and trismus in oral oncology. *Oral Surg. Oral Med. Oral Pathol. Oral Radiol.* **2014**, *117*, 709–715. [CrossRef] [PubMed]
22. Anand, A.; Mathew, A.; Balasubramanian, D. Trismus in Head and Neck Cancer: Causes and Management. In *Dysphagia Management in Head and Neck Cancers*; Thankappan, K., Iyer, S., Menon, J., Eds.; Springer: Singapore, 2018; pp. 161–172. [CrossRef]
23. Bouman, M.A.; Dijkstra, P.U.; Reintsema, H.; Roodenburg, J.L.; Werker, P.M. Surgery for extra-articular trismus: A systematic review. *Br. J. Oral Maxillofac. Surg.* **2016**, *54*, 253–259. [CrossRef]
24. Shen, Y.W.; Shih, Y.H.; Fuh, L.J.; Shieh, T.M. Oral Submucous Fibrosis: A Review on Biomarkers, Pathogenic Mechanisms, and Treatments. *Int. J. Mol. Sci.* **2020**, *21*, 7231. [CrossRef]
25. Chen, Y.-K.; Lin, L.-M.; Lin, C.-C. Osteoma of the mandibular coronoid process. *Int. J. Oral Maxillofac. Surg.* **1998**, *27*, 222–223. [CrossRef] [PubMed]
26. Saikrishna, D.; Das, A.; Jha, C. Management of a case of osteoma of coronoid: A rare case report. *Natl. J. Maxillofac. Surg.* **2021**, *12*, 276–279. [CrossRef] [PubMed]
27. Lewars, L.J. Osteomas of the coronoid process. *Oral Surg. Oral Med. Oral Pathol.* **1959**, *12*, 490–496.
28. Petronis, Z.; Janovskiene, A.; Leketas, M. Cancellous osteoma of the coronoid process: A literature review and rare case report. *J. Oral Facial Pain Headache* **2024**, *38*, 126–130. [CrossRef]
29. Vashishth, S.; Garg, K.; Patil, P.; Sreenivasan, V. An unusual cause for trismus caused by mandibular coronoid osteoma: A case report. *Imaging Sci. Dent.* **2013**, *43*, 45–48. [CrossRef]
30. Nah, K.S. Osteomas of the craniofacial region. *Imaging Sci. Dent.* **2011**, *41*, 107–113. [CrossRef]
31. Jundt, G.; Bertoni, F.; Unni, K.K.; Saito, K.; Dehne, L.P. Benign tumours of bone and cartilage. In *WHO Classification of Tumors: Pathology and Genetics of Head and Neck Tumours*; Barnes, L., Eveson, J.W., Reichart, P., Sidransky, D., Eds.; IARC: Lyon, France, 2005; pp. 54–55.
32. Wesley, R.K.; Cullen, C.L.; Bloom, W.S. Gardner's syndrome with bilateral osteomas of coronoid process resulting in limited opening. *Pediatr. Dentl.* **1987**, *9*, 53–57.
33. Woldenberg, Y.; Nash, M.; Bodner, L. Peripheral osteoma of the maxillofacial region. Diagnosis and management: A study of 14 cases. *Med. Oral Patol. Oral Cir. Bucal.* **2005**, *10* (Suppl. S2), E139–E142. [PubMed]
34. Dandriyal, R.; Giri, K.Y.; Pant, S.; Alam, S.; Joshi, A. Giant osteochondroma of the coronoid process. *J. Maxillofac. Oral Surg.* **2015**, *14* (Suppl. S1), 412–416. [CrossRef] [PubMed]
35. Lan, T.; Liu, X.; Liang, P.S.; Tao, Q. Osteochondroma of the coronoid process: A case report and review of the literature. *Oncol. Lett.* **2019**, *18*, 2270–2277. [CrossRef]
36. Ghazizadeh, M.; Sheikhi, M.; Salehi, M.; Khaleghi, A. Bilateral coronoid hyperplasia causing painless limitation of mandibular movement. *Radiol Case Rep.* **2017**, *13*, 112–117. [CrossRef] [PubMed]
37. Cha, J.; Chung, J.W. Coronoid Process Hyperplasia: A Rare Case of Restricted Mouth Opening Masquerading as Temporomandibular Disorder. *J. Oral Med. Pain* **2023**, *48*, 112–117. [CrossRef]
38. Tavassol, F.; Spalthoff, S.; Essig, H.; Bredt, M.; Gellrich, N.C.; Kokemüller, H. Elongated coronoid process: CT-based quantitative analysis of the coronoid process and review of literature. *Int. J. Oral Maxillofac. Surg.* **2012**, *41*, 331–338. [CrossRef]
39. Goh, Y.C.; Tan, C.C.; Lim, D. Coronoid hyperplasia: A review. *J. Stomatol. Oral Maxillofac. Surg.* **2020**, *121*, 397–403. [CrossRef] [PubMed]
40. Farronato, M.; Lucchina, A.G.; Mortellaro, C.; Fama, A.; Galbiati, G.; Farronato, G.; Maspero, C. Bilateral Hyperplasia of the Coronoid Process in Pediatric Patients: What is the Gold Standard for Treatment? *J. Craniofac. Surg.* **2019**, *30*, 1058–1063. [CrossRef]
41. Puche, M.; Guijarro-Martínez, R.; Pérez-Herrezuelo, G.; Miragall, L.; Iglesias, M.E.; Martínez-Costa, C. The hypothetical role of congenital hypotonia in the development of early coronoid hyperplasia. *J. Craniomaxillofac. Surg.* **2012**, *40*, e155–e158. [CrossRef]
42. Khandavilli, S.D.; Pattni, N.; Naredla, P.R.; Williams, R. First case of bilateral coronoid hyperplasia in monozygotic twin sisters-a new aetiological perspective? *Oral Maxillofac. Surg.* **2016**, *20*, 441–443. [CrossRef]
43. Parmentier, G.I.; Nys, M.; Verstraete, L.; Politis, C. A systematic review of treatment and outcomes in patients with mandibular coronoid process hyperplasia. *J. Korean Assoc. Oral Maxillofac. Surg.* **2022**, *48*, 133–148. [CrossRef] [PubMed]
44. Nogueira, E.F.C.; Maranhão, C.M.C.T.; Almeida, R.A.C.; Torres, B.C.A. Treatment of hyperplasia of the coronoid process of the mandible in adults: Analysis of 42 literature reports and illustrative case. *RGO Rev. Gaúch Odontol.* **2021**, *69*, e20210033. [CrossRef]
45. Ozkaya, O.; Colak, O.; Sutcu, M.; Akan, M. The outcome of coronoidectomy in bilateral coronoid process hyperplasia. *Cranio* **2018**, *36*, 53–60. [CrossRef] [PubMed]
46. Fernández Ferro, M.; Fernández Sanromán, J.; Sandoval Gutierrez, J.; Costas López, A.; López de Sánchez, A.; Etayo Pérez, A. Treatment of bilateral hyperplasia of the coronoid process of the mandible. Presentation of a case and review of the literature. *Med. Oral Patol. Oral Cir. Bucal.* **2008**, *13*, E595–E598.

47. Hanisch, M.; Hanisch, L.; Fröhlich, L.F.; Werkmeister, R.; Bohner, L.; Kleinheinz, J. Myositis ossificans traumatica of the masticatory muscles: Etiology, diagnosis and treatment. *Head Face Med.* **2018**, *14*, 23. [CrossRef] [PubMed]
48. Palla, B.; Han, M.D.; Callahan, N. Myositis Ossificans Traumatica of the Head and Neck in a Child. *J. Dent. Child.* **2020**, *87*, 120–123.
49. Anshika, R.; Hoogar, M.B.; Shilpi, S. Myositis ossificans of masseter muscle: A rare case. *Int. J. Health Sci. Res.* **2021**, *11*, 105–108. Available online: https://www.ijhsr.org/IJHSR_Vol.11_Issue.2_Feb2021/IJHSR015.pdf (accessed on 2 February 2021).
50. Jović, S.; Brajković, D.; Borilović, M.; Marjanović, U.; Brkić, M.; Kozomara, R.; Stošić, S. Recurring myositis ossificans traumatica of temporal muscle: A case report. *Vojnosanit. Pregl.* **2021**, *78*, 255–260. [CrossRef]
51. Spinzia, A.; Moscato, G.; Broccardo, E.; Castelletti, L.; Maglitto, F.; Orabona, G.D.; Piombino, P. A rare isolated unilateral myositis ossificans traumatica of the lateral pterygoid muscle: A case report. *J. Med. Case Rep.* **2014**, *8*, 230. [CrossRef]
52. Torres, A.M.; Nardis, A.C.; da Silva, R.A.; Savioli, C. Myositis ossificans traumatica of the medial pterygoid muscle following a third molar extraction. *Int. J. Oral Maxillofac. Surg.* **2015**, *44*, 488–490. [CrossRef]
53. Abbasi, A.J.; Taheri, M.M.; Asadi, A.; Bahrami, R.; Nikparto, N. Myositis ossificans traumatica of masticatory muscles: A case report and review of the literature. *Oral Maxillofac. Surg. Cases* **2024**, *10*, 100361. [CrossRef]
54. Fité-Trepat, L.; Martos-Fernández, M.; Alberola-Ferranti, M.; Romanini-Montecino, C.; Saez-Barba, M.; Bescós-Atín, C. Myositis ossificans of the masseter muscle: A rare location. Report of a case and review of literature. *J. Clin. Exp. Dent.* **2016**, *8*, e210–e213. [CrossRef]
55. Baur, D.A.; Altay, M.A.; Flores-Hidalgo, A.; Ort, Y.; Quereshy, F.A. Chronic osteomyelitis of the mandible: Diagnosis and management--an institution's experience over 7 years. *J. Oral Maxillofac. Surg.* **2015**, *73*, 655–665. [CrossRef]
56. Chun, J.Y.; Shim, Y.J. Osteomyelitis of the Mandibular Coronoid Process Mimicking a Temporomandibular Joint Disorder: A Case Report. *J. Oral Med. Pain* **2024**, *49*, 35–39. [CrossRef]
57. Muraoka, H.; Ito, K.; Hirahara, N.; Ichiki, S.; Kondo, T.; Kaneda, T. Magnetic resonance imaging texture analysis in the quantitative evaluation of acute osteomyelitis of the mandibular bone. *Dentomaxillofac. Radiol.* **2022**, *51*, 20210321. [CrossRef] [PubMed]
58. Gudmundsson, T.; Torkov, P.; Thygesen, T.H. Diagnosis and Treatment of Osteomyelitis of the Jaw—A Systematic Review (2002–2015) of the Literature. *J. Dent. Oral Disord.* **2017**, *3*, 1066. [CrossRef]
59. Vargas-Rojas, D.C.; Rodriguez-Flores, A.; Moreno-Villalobos, D.; Chumpitaz-Cerrate, V.; Chávez-Rimache, L. Radical Surgical Approach to Chronic Suppurative Osteomyelitis: Case Report. *Odovtos-Int. J. Dent. Sci.* **2023**, *26*, 14–20. [CrossRef]
60. Griffin, A.T.; Timbrook, T.; Harting, J.; Christensen, D. Streptococcus anginosus group and osteomyelitis: A single centre clinical experience. *Postgrad. Med. J.* **2013**, *89*, 262–265. [CrossRef]
61. Tiwari, P.; Bera, R.N.; Kanojia, S.; Chauhan, N.; Hirani, M.S. Assessing the optimal imaging modality in the diagnosis of jaw osteomyelitis. A meta-analysis. *Br. J. Oral Maxillofac. Surg.* **2021**, *59*, 982–992. [CrossRef]
62. Park, M.S.; Eo, M.Y.; Myoung, H.; Kim, S.M.; Lee, J.H. Early diagnosis of jaw osteomyelitis by easy digitalized panoramic analysis. *Maxillofac. Plast. Reconstr. Surg.* **2019**, *41*, 6. [CrossRef]
63. Salimi, F.; Motter, D.; Salimi, Z. Temporomandibular joint (TMJ) disorders as first clinical manifestations in external auditory canal cholesteatoma. A case report. *Ann. Med. Surg.* **2022**, *74*, 103287. [CrossRef] [PubMed]
64. Mardinger, O.; Rosen, D.; Minkow, B.; Tulzinsky, Z.; Ophir, D.; Hirshberg, A. Temporomandibular joint involvement in malignant external otitis. *Oral Surg. Oral Med. Oral Pathol. Oral Radiol. Endod.* **2003**, *96*, 398–403. [CrossRef] [PubMed]
65. Tsuno, N.S.G.; Tsuno, M.Y.; Coelho Neto, C.A.F.; Noujaim, S.E.; Decnop, M.; Pacheco, F.T.; Souza, S.A.; Fonseca, A.P.A.; Garcia, M.R.T. Imaging the External Ear: Practical Approach to Normal and Pathologic Conditions. *Radiographics* **2022**, *42*, 522–540. [CrossRef]
66. Abebe, A.A.; Birhanu, A.G. Methicillin Resistant Staphylococcus aureus: Molecular Mechanisms Underlying Drug Resistance Development and Novel Strategies to Combat. *Infect Drug Resist.* **2023**, *16*, 7641–7662. [CrossRef] [PubMed]
67. Tuon, F.F.; Suss, P.H.; Telles, J.P.; Dantas, L.R.; Borges, N.H.; Ribeiro, V.S.T. Antimicrobial Treatment of Staphylococcus aureus Biofilms. *Antibiotics* **2023**, *12*, 87. [CrossRef]
68. Weden, A.; Haig, H. Current thinking in physiotherapy for the management of idiopathic and postsurgical temporomandibular disorders: A narrative review. *Br. J. Oral Maxillofac. Surg.* **2024**, *62*, 588–593. [CrossRef]
69. Sidebottom, A.J. How do I manage restricted mouth opening secondary to problems with the temporomandibular joint? *Br. J. Oral Maxillofac. Surg.* **2013**, *51*, 469–472. [CrossRef]
70. Shulman, D.H.; Shipman, B.; Willis, F.B. Treating trismus with dynamic splinting: A cohort, case series. *Adv. Ther.* **2008**, *25*, 9–16. [CrossRef]
71. Harris, B.N.; Kuhn, M.; Evangelista, L.; Davis, S. Speech and Swallow Therapy. In *Complex Head and Neck Microvascular Surgery*; Quimby, A., Parmar, S., Fernandes, R., Eds.; Springer: Cham, Switzerland, 2023; pp. 231–248. [CrossRef]

diagnostics

MDPI

Article

# Mucoscopic Features of Oral Lichen Planus: A Retrospective Comparative Study with Inflammatory Mimickers

**Mihaela Paula Toader [1], Oana Mihaela Condurache Hritcu [1], Cristina Colac Botoc [2,*], Antonia Elena Hutanu [2], Catalina Anca Munteanu [2], Roxana Paraschiva Ciobanu [2], Stefan Vasile Toader [3], Alin Gabriel Colac [4], Victor Vlad Costan [4], Elena Porumb Andrese [5] and Daciana Elena Branisteanu [5]**

1 Discipline of Oral Medicine, Oral Dermatology, Grigore T. Popa University of Medicine and Pharmacy, 16 Universitatii Street, 700115 Iasi, Romania; mihaela.toader@umfiasi.ro (M.P.T.); oana.condurache-hritcu@umfiasi.ro (O.M.C.H.)

2 Dermatology Clinic, University Clinical Railways Hospital, 1 Garabet Ibraileanu Street, 700115 Iasi, Romania; antoniaclivet@yahoo.com (A.E.H.); anca.munteanu2@yahoo.com (C.A.M.); r.p.ciobanu@gmail.com (R.P.C.)

3 Discipline of Physiopathology, Grigore T. Popa University of Medicine and Pharmacy, 16 Universitatii Street, 700115 Iasi, Romania; stefan.toader@umfiasi.ro

4 Department of Oral and Maxillofacial Surgery, 'Grigore T. Popa' University of Medicine and Pharmacy, 700115 Iasi, Romania; colac.alin@yahoo.com (A.G.C.); victorcostan@gmail.com (V.V.C.)

5 Discipline of Dermatology, Grigore T. Popa University of Medicine and Pharmacy, 16 Universitatii Street, 700115 Iasi, Romania; andrese.elena@yahoo.com (E.P.A.); debranisteanu@yahoo.com (D.E.B.)

* Correspondence: cristina.botoc28@gmail.com; Tel.: +40-04743777206

**Abstract: Background/Objectives**: Oral lichen planus (OLP) is a chronic inflammatory mucocutaneous disorder with a recognized potential for malignant transformation. While histopathological examination remains the diagnostic gold standard, mucoscopy has emerged as a valuable non-invasive tool for assessing striae patterns, vascular features, and pigmentary alterations. This study aimed to evaluate the mucoscopic characteristics of OLP across different oral mucosal sites and to compare them with other inflammatory oral conditions, assessing their diagnostic relevance. **Methods**: A retrospective comparative study was conducted on 106 patients, including 33 with histopathologically confirmed OLP and 73 with other inflammatory oral conditions (pemphigus vulgaris, chronic cheilitis, hyperplastic oral candidiasis, leukoplakia, squamous cell carcinoma, pachyonychia congenita, morsicatio buccarum). Mucoscopic evaluation focused on the buccal mucosa, vermilion, and lingual mucosa. Features assessed included background color, white striae patterns, vascular morphology, the presence of erosions, and other features like blunting of the lingual papillae and scales on the vermilion. Statistical analysis was carried out using SPSS 29.0. **Results**: Reticular striae were highly specific to OLP, particularly on the buccal mucosa (90.9%, $p < 0.001$). Leukoplakia-like lesions were most prevalent on the lingual mucosa and significantly associated with dotted ($p = 0.027$) and looped vessels ($p = 0.002$). Erosions correlated significantly with both dotted ($p < 0.001$) and linear vessels ($p = 0.011$), especially in lingual and vermilion lesions. In comparison, control group lesions displayed significantly more globular structures ($p < 0.001$), veil-like patterns ($p < 0.001$), and diffuse vascular distributions ($p = 0.018$), particularly in cheilitis and candidiasis cases. **Conclusions**: Mucoscopy reveals distinct site-specific patterns in OLP, supporting its role as a non-invasive diagnostic aid. Comparative analysis highlights its utility in differentiating OLP from other inflammatory oral conditions and in identifying lesions with features suggestive of malignant potential. These findings support the integration of mucoscopy into routine clinical practice and warrant further validation through larger, prospective studies.

**Keywords:** oral lichen planus; dermoscopy; mucoscopy; white striae; erosions; vascularity

## 1. Introduction

Oral lichen planus (OLP) is a rare, chronic inflammatory disorder, with a prevalence ranging between 0.5% and 2.2%, with notable female predilection. It primarily occurs in middle-aged and older adults and is characterized by white, lace-like reticular lesions, most commonly on the buccal mucosa [1–4].

OLP is classified as an oral potentially malignant disorder, with the highest risk of progression to oral squamous cell carcinoma related to clinically red lesions (erosive or atrophic), location on the borders of the tongue and fewer mucosal sites involved [5]. Recent studies have reported an overall malignant transformation rate of 1.39% for OLP over an average follow-up of 5.8 years, while the erosive subtype showed a significantly higher rate of 5.98% [5,6].

Oral manifestations of lichen planus (LP) may present alongside cutaneous lesions or may be the sole clinical manifestation of the disease. These lesions are thought to result from a T-cell-mediated autoimmune response triggered by various antigens, including dental restorative materials, certain medications (particularly antihypertensive drugs), mechanical trauma, or viral infections such as hepatitis C virus. This immune response induces apoptosis of basal keratinocytes and promotes chronic mucosal inflammation, ultimately contributing to the clinical presentation of the disease [7–12].

Clinically, OLP lesions can be divided into six distinct subtypes: reticular, bullous, atrophic, plaque-like, papular, and erosive [13].

The reticular form is the most frequently observed, characterized by interlacing white striae known as Wickham's striae (WS), which may also be present in cutaneous LP [13]. These asymptomatic lesions can appear anywhere in the oral cavity, but predominantly on the posterior buccal mucosa [14]. In contrast, the erosive form (EOLP), presenting as one or multiple erosions on an erythematous base, often causes pain and difficulty in mastication. EOLP follows a chronic, recurrent course, requiring periodic follow-up. Although malignant transformation in OLP is rare, it remains a clinically significant concern, particularly in the erosive subtype. Transformation is thought to result from chronic mucosal inflammation and sustained immune-mediated epithelial damage, promoting dysplastic changes and, ultimately, progression to oral squamous cell carcinoma (SCC). Clinically, features suggestive of malignant transformation include the emergence of persistent, non-healing ulcers, induration, nodular or exophytic growths, and increased symptom severity. Histopathologically, early malignant changes are marked by epithelial dysplasia, characterized by nuclear pleomorphism, loss of basal cell polarity, abnormal mitotic figures, and architectural disarray, while advanced transformation may exhibit stromal invasion consistent with oral squamous cell carcinoma. These findings highlight the necessity for vigilant follow-up and prompt biopsy of suspicious lesions to ensure early detection and management [15–17].

The World Health Organization (WHO) established diagnostic criteria in 1978 to distinguish OLP from clinically similar conditions, which were subsequently revised in 2003 to address the inconsistencies between clinical and histopathological diagnoses [14,18].

Clinical criteria:

1. Bilateral, more or less symmetrical lesions;
2. Presence of a lace-like network of slightly elevated gray-white striae (reticular pattern);
3. Erosive, atrophic, bullous, and plaque-type lesions are considered subtypes only if the reticular lesions are concurrently present elsewhere in the oral mucosa;
4. In cases where the lesions resemble OLP but do not fully meet these criteria, the term "clinically compatible with OLP" should be used.

Histopathological criteria:

1. A well-demarcated, band-like infiltrate of lymphocytes confined to the superficial connective tissue;
2. Evidence of basal cell-layer liquefaction degeneration;
3. Absence of epithelial dysplasia;
4. When histopathologic findings are suggestive but not definite, the term "histopathologically compatible with OLP" should be applied.

A definitive diagnosis of OLP requires the fulfillment of both clinical and histopathological criteria. The term "oral lichenoid lesions" should be used in the following scenarios:

1. Clinically characteristic of OLP but histopathologically only compatible with OLP;
2. Histopathologically characteristic of OLP but clinically only compatible with OLP;
3. Clinically and histopathologically compatible with OLP.

Certain variants of OLP can present diagnostic challenges. The plaque-like form predominantly affects the posterior tongue and buccal mucosa and it may mimic oral leukoplakia. The atrophic form is characterized by diffuse erythematous lesions mixed with reticular features. The bullous form is the least common, presenting as fluid-filled vesicles that can rupture, leading to ulceration and a symptomatology similar to EOLP [19,20]. In ambiguous cases, direct immunofluorescence can be employed to differentiate OLP from autoimmune mucosal disorders, aiding in diagnostic accuracy [21]. Recent advancements in artificial intelligence (AI) technologies have positioned AI as a promising adjunctive tool in the diagnosis of OLP, with targeted training significantly enhancing diagnostic accuracy and efficiency. Nonetheless, variability in performance across platforms and anatomical sites underscores the need for continued optimization and cautious integration into clinical workflows [22,23].

Dermoscopy is a non-invasive, in vivo imaging technique that allows the visualization of intraepithelial and subepithelial structures, otherwise not visible during the clinical examination. It has proven especially valuable in dermatology for the evaluation of pigmented lesions, inflammatory disorders, and early malignancies. This is achieved by using a magnification lens and light to visualize intraepidermal and superficial dermal structures. It employs polarized light or a contact fluid to reduce reflection, achieving magnifications of 10× or higher [24]. Mucoscopy, the application of dermoscopy on mucosal sites, may offer diagnostic clues that support clinical differential diagnosis. As a digital tool, when the dermatoscope is attached to a smartphone for image acquisition and further magnification, mucoscopy contributes to improved diagnostic accuracy, guides biopsy site selection, and facilitates documentation and monitoring over time. Its portability, accessibility, and ability to provide real-time insights make it an increasingly relevant adjunct in the examination and diagnosis of oral mucosal lesions, including oral lichen planus and its mimickers [25]. Mucoscopic features of OLP are not yet standardized and based on case reports and case series. They include a lace-like network of gray-white lines (WS), typically seen around papules or ring-shaped structures. The erosive form presents with an atrophic appearance, characterized by areas of erosion, an erythematous background, and keratotic white striae arranged in a network pattern. Atrophic lesions represent a combination of the reticular and erosive forms, showing striae surrounded by erythematous mucosa. The plaque-like subtype is described mucoscopically as resembling leukoplakia [26,27]. However, because clinical and mucoscopic features may overlap with those of other inflammatory oral conditions such as pemphigus vulgaris, chronic cheilitis, candidiasis, and oral leukoplakia, a comparative analysis is essential. Identifying mucoscopy-specific features of OLP could improve the clinical diagnostic orientation, forgoing the need for ancillary tests to exclude autoimmune conditions that may present with similar clinical features.

While mucoscopy may offer significant diagnostic advantages, histopathological analysis remains the gold standard for confirming the diagnosis of OLP [18].

This study aims to describe the mucoscopic features of OLP and to perform a comparative analysis between OLP and other inflammatory oral conditions on mucoscopy. By evaluating specific patterns such as white lesion morphology, vascular structures and distribution, and other changes across various oral mucosal sites, it seeks to identify distinguishing mucoscopic characteristics of OLP. To our knowledge, this is the first study to include a site-specific comparison between OLP and a control group comprising other inflammatory oral disorders, each diagnosed according to established clinical, histopathological, or specific diagnostic criteria (e.g., mycological examination for candidiasis). This approach enhances the diagnostic utility of mucoscopy in differentiating OLP from its mimickers and contributes to the development of a standardized, non-invasive mucoscopic assessment algorithm to support clinical decision-making and biopsy guidance.

## 2. Materials and Methods

A retrospective, observational, comparative study was conducted on 106 patients. Cases included were collected from admissions to the Department of Dermatology of Clinical Railways Hospital of Iasi, as well as from presentations to the Dermatology Outpatient Department, between January 2021 and December 2024. A total of 106 patients were included. The study group comprised 33 patients with histopathologically confirmed OLP. The control group included 73 patients confirmed with other inflammatory oral conditions—chronic cheilitis [actinic ($n$ = 20), exfoliative ($n$ = 5), eczematous ($n$ = 3)], oral pemphigus vulgaris (PV) ($n$ = 15), lip squamous cell carcinoma ($n$ = 2), oral leukoplakia ($n$ = 2), pachyonychia congenital ($n$ = 1), hyperplastic oral candidiasis ($n$ = 25), and morsicatio buccarum ($n$ = 2). To facilitate the comparative analysis with OLP, mucoscopic features of the following conditions were assessed by anatomical site: cheilitis and squamous cell carcinoma of the lip on the vermilion; PV, morsicatio buccarum, and hyperplastic candidiasis on the buccal mucosa; and hyperplastic candidiasis, oral leukoplakia, pachyonychia congenita, and PV on the lingual mucosa. Several patients with either oral PV or hyperplastic oral candidiasis were considered as controls on multiple mucosal sites. The case number distribution of control group patients according to mucosal site can be found in Table 1.

**Table 1.** Distribution of cases in the control group by diagnosis and mucosal site.

| Mucosal Site | Diagnosis | No. |
|---|---|---|
| Vermilion ($n$ = 30) | Chronic cheilitis | |
| | • Actinic | 20 |
| | • Exfoliative | 5 |
| | • Eczematous | 3 |
| | Lip squamous cell carcinoma | 2 |
| Buccal mucosa ($n$ = 20) | Oral PV | 15 |
| | Hyperplastic oral candidiasis | 3 |
| | Morsicatio buccarum | 2 |
| Lingual mucosa ($n$ = 30) | Hyperplastic oral candidiasis | 25 |
| | Oral leukoplakia | 2 |
| | Oral PV | 2 |
| | Pachyonychia congenita | 1 |

Inclusion criteria:

- Patients diagnosed clinically and histopathologically with OLP according to the WHO criteria;
- Patients diagnosed with other inflammatory oral conditions according to the individual protocol:
  - Pemphigus vulgaris: diagnosis based on clinical, histopathological, and immunological criteria;
  - Oral leukoplakia: diagnosis based on clinical and histopathological findings;
  - Chronic cheilitis: diagnosis based on clinical and histopathological evaluation;
  - Lip squamous cell carcinoma: diagnosis based on clinical and immunological testing;
  - Hyperplastic candidiasis: diagnosis based on clinical and direct mycological examination and mycological culture;
  - Pachynonychia congenita: diagnosis based on clinical and genetic testing.

Exclusion criteria:

- Patients who did not meet the OLP criteria according to the WHO criteria;
- Patients diagnosed with oral lichenoid reactions;
- Patients with only clinical suspicion of other inflammatory oral conditions, lacking immunological or histopathological confirmation.

Each patient underwent a comprehensive intraoral examination, focusing on three primary anatomical sites: buccal mucosa, vermilion border of the lips, and lingual mucosa.

Mucoscopic evaluations were performed using a handheld polarized dermatoscope (Dermlite DL4 and Dermlite DL5, 3Gen, San Juan Capistrano, CA, USA) with 10× magnification, attached to a smartphone via a magnetic adapter, with additional 5× magnification for image acquisition and storage. A non-contact technique using polarized light was employed for all examinations in order to avoid blunting of the lingual papillae or altering the appearance of vascular structures. The following features were recorded for each lesion:

1. Background color—pink, erythematous, violaceous;

2. White lesions—radial striae, linear striae, reticular striae, annular striae, leaf-venation, globular, dotted, veil, rosette, leukoplakia-like (the term is used to describe the mucoscopic appearance of the lesion);

3. Vascular patterns—linear, dotted, looped, sea anemone-like;

4. Distribution of vascular structures—radial at the periphery or diffuse regular;

5. Presence/absence of erosions;

6. Other features—scaling, blunting of lingual papillae.

Mucoscopic images were taken for each mucosal site and analyzed by two dermoscopists. The results are presented comparatively, emphasizing the differences and similarities in mucoscopic findings between OLP and the other evaluated inflammatory oral conditions.

*Statistical Analysis*

The statistical analysis was carried out in SPSS 29.0. Data were recorded and analyzed using descriptive and inferential statistical methods. Categorical variables were expressed as frequencies and percentages. To assess potential associations between white lesions and vascular patterns, Pearson's Chi-square test was performed. A $p$-value $< 0.05$ was considered statistically significant and a $p$-value $< 0.01$ was considered statistically highly significant.

## 3. Results

### 3.1. Demographic Characteristics of the Study Group

The study group included a total of 33 patients diagnosed with OLP, with a female predominance (72.2%, $n = 24/33$) compared to males (27.3%, $n = 9/33$). The mean age of the study population was 53.03 years (SD = 15.52), with a median age of 53 years. Female patients had a higher mean age (54.71 ± 14.81 years) compared to males (48.56 ± 17.37 years) (Table 2).

**Table 2.** Demographic data of the study population.

| | | n/33 | % |
|---|---|---|---|
| **Gender** | M | 9 | 27.3 |
| | F | 24 | 72.7 |
| **Age** | <30 ys | 3 | 9.1 |
| | 31–50 ys | 11 | 33.3 |
| | 51–70 ys | 14 | 42.4 |
| | >70 ys | 5 | 15.2 |
| **Total** | | 33 | 100.0 |

The clinical presentation of OLP in the study cohort predominantly included the reticular form (54.5%, $n = 18/33$), with the erosive form observed in 45.5% ($n = 15/33$). Concomitant cutaneous involvement was noted in 42.4% ($n = 14/33$) of cases, whereas 57.5% ($n = 19$) showed lesions limited to the oral mucosa (Table 3).

**Table 3.** Clinical features of the OLP study population.

| | | n/33 | % |
|---|---|---|---|
| **Clinical aspect** | Erosive | 15/33 | 45.5 |
| | Reticular | 18/33 | 54.5 |
| **Associated cutaneous lesions** | No | 19/33 | 57.6 |
| | Yes | 14/33 | 42.4 |
| **Total** | | 33/33 | 100.0 |

### 3.2. Descriptive Analysis of Mucoscopic Features of OLP

To better illustrate the mucoscopic profile within the OLP cohort, we analyzed the overall frequency of each feature across the 33 patients, acknowledging that multiple features could be present in the same individual. The most common background color observed was pink (96.9%, $n = 32/33$), followed by erythematous (51.5%, $n = 17/33$) and violaceous (33.3%, $n = 11/33$) tones. Among white lesions, reticular striae were most prevalent (93.9%, $n = 31/33$), followed by linear striae (84.8%, $n = 28/33$), leukoplakia-like lesions (60.6%, $n = 20/33$), and veil-like patterns (57.5%, $n = 19/33$). Less frequently observed patterns included leaf venation (21.2%, $n = 7/33$), annular striae (15.1%, $n = 5/33$), globular structures (18.1%, $n = 6/33$), dotted white areas (15.1%, $n = 5/33$), and rosettes (3.0%, $n = 1/33$).

In terms of vascular features, dotted vessels were the most frequent (69.6%, $n = 23/33$), followed by linear (57.5%, $n = 19/33$) and looped vessels (24.2%, $n = 8/33$), with sea anemone-like patterns observed in one case (3.0%, $n = 1/33$). The distribution of vessels was most often radial at the periphery (63.6%, $n = 21/33$), while a diffuse regular pattern was observed in 27.3% ($n = 9/33$) of cases. Additional findings included erosions in 48.4%

of patients ($n$ = 16/33), scales in 42.4% ($n$ = 14/33), and blunting of lingual papillae in 60.6% of cases ($n$ = 20/33). A schematic distribution of mucoscopic features of the OLP study cohort is summarized in Tables 4 and 5.

**Table 4.** Overall distribution of the mucoscopic features in the OLP study cohort ($n$ = 33).

| Parameter Investigated | | Number of Patients ($n$/33) | Percentages (%) |
|---|---|---|---|
| **Background color** | Erythematous | 17/33 | 51.5 |
| | Violaceous | 11/33 | 33.3 |
| **White lesions** | Radial striae | 15/33 | 45.4 |
| | Linear striae | 28/33 | 84.8 |
| | Reticular striae | 31/33 | 93.9 |
| | Leaf venation | 7/33 | 21.2 |
| | Annular striae | 5/33 | 15.1 |
| | Globular | 6/33 | 18.1 |
| | Dotted | 5/33 | 15.1 |
| | Veil | 19/33 | 57.5 |
| | Rosette | 1/33 | 3.0 |
| | Leukoplakia-like | 20/33 | 60.6 |
| **Blood vessels** | Linear | 19/33 | 57.5 |
| | Dotted | 23/33 | 69.6 |
| | Looped | 8/33 | 24.2 |
| | Sea anemone-like | 1/33 | 3.0 |
| **Distribution of blood vessels** | Radial at the perifery | 21/33 | 63.6 |
| | Diffuse regular | 9/33 | 27.2 |
| **Erosions** | | 16/33 | 48.4 |
| **Scales** | | 14/33 | 42.4 |
| **Blunting of lingual papillae** | | 20/33 | 60.6 |

The predominant background color observed in mucoscopic examination varied across anatomical regions. A pink background was the most common, observed in 69.7% of lesions on the vermilion ($n$ = 23/33), 63.6% of lingual lesions ($n$ = 21/33), and 90.9% ($n$ = 30/33) of buccal mucosa lesions. An erythematous background was present in 30.3% ($n$ = 10/33) of vermilion lesions, 33.3% ($n$ = 11/33) of lingual lesions, and 24.2% ($n$ = 8/33) of buccal lesions. A violaceous background was detected in 27.3% ($n$ = 9/33) of vermilion lesions but was rarely observed in lingual mucosa (9.1%) ($n$ = 3/33) and absent in buccal mucosa (Table 5).

White structures were present in various patterns. Reticular striae were most frequently found on the buccal mucosa (90.9%, $n$ = 30/33), while they were less prevalent on the vermilion (39.4%, $n$ = 13/33) and the lingual mucosa (18.2%, $n$ = 6/33). Linear striae were predominant on the vermilion (81.8%, $n$ = 27/33) but were less common on the lingual (12.1%, $n$ = 4/33) and buccal mucosa (21.2%, $n$ = 7/33). Radial striae were most frequently observed on the buccal mucosa (21.2%, $n$ = 7/33), followed by the vermilion (15.2%, $n$ = 5/33) and lingual mucosa (9.1%, $n$ = 3/33). Annular striae were rare, occurring in 9.1% ($n$ = 3/33) of vermilion lesions, 6.1% ($n$ = 2/33) of lingual lesions, and 3.0% ($n$ = 1/33) of buccal lesions. Globular patterns were identified in 6.1% ($n$ = 2/33) of vermilion lesions, 12.1% ($n$ = 4/33) of lingual lesions, and 3.0% ($n$ = 1/33) of buccal lesions. Leukoplakia-like patterns were more frequently detected on the lingual mucosa (48.5%, $n = 16/33$) compared to the vermilion (18.2%, $n = 6/33$) and buccal mucosa (15.2%, $n = 5/33$) (Table 5).

**Table 5.** Mucoscopic features of OLP and distribution in different oral sites.

| | | Vermilion | | Lingual | | Buccal | |
|---|---|---|---|---|---|---|---|
| | | $n/33$ | % | $n/33$ | % | $n/33$ | % |
| **Background color** | Pink | 23/33 | 69.7 | 21/33 | 63.6 | 30/33 | 90.9 |
| | Erythematous | 10/33 | 30.3 | 11/33 | 33.3 | 8/33 | 24.2 |
| | Violaceous | 9/33 | 27.3 | 3/33 | 9.1 | - | - |
| **White lesions** | Radial striae | 5/33 | 15.2 | 3/33 | 9.1 | 7/33 | 21.2 |
| | Linear striae | 27/33 | 81.8 | 4/33 | 12.1 | 7/33 | 21.2 |
| | Reticular striae | 13/33 | 39.4 | 6/33 | 18.2 | 30/33 | 90.9 |
| | Leaf venation | 1/33 | 3.0 | - | - | 6/33 | 18.2 |
| | Annular striae | 3/33 | 9.1 | 2/33 | 6.1 | 1/33 | 3.0 |
| | Globular | 2/33 | 6.1 | 4/33 | 12.1 | 1/33 | 3.0 |
| | Dotted | 1/33 | 3.0 | 1/33 | 3.0 | 3/33 | 9.1 |
| | Veil | 5/33 | 15.2 | 14/33 | 42.4 | 7/33 | 21.2 |
| | Rosette | 1/33 | 3.0 | - | - | - | - |
| | Leukoplakia-like | 6/33 | 18.2 | 16/33 | 48.5 | 5/33 | 15.2 |
| **Blood vessels** | Linear | 13/33 | 39.4 | 12/33 | 36.4 | 5/33 | 15.2 |
| | Dotted | 19/33 | 57.6 | 12/33 | 36.4 | 5/33 | 15.2 |
| | Looped | 5/33 | 15.2 | 4/33 | 12.1 | 2/33 | 6.1 |
| | Sea anemone-like | - | - | 1/33 | 3.0 | 1/33 | 3.0 |
| **Distribution of blood vessels** | Radial at the perifery | 16/33 | 48.5 | 16/33 | 48.5 | 7/33 | 21.2 |
| | Diffuse regular | 10/33 | 30.3 | 2/33 | 6.1 | 2/33 | 6.1 |
| **Erosions** | | 13/33 | 39.4 | 14/33 | 42.4 | 12/33 | 36.4 |
| **Scales** | | 16/33 | 48.5 | - | - | - | - |
| **Blunting of lingual papillae** | | 0 | 0 | 20/33 | 60.6 | - | - |

Dotted blood vessels were the most frequently encountered vascular feature, observed in 57.6% ($n = 19/33$) of vermilion lesions, 36.4% ($n = 12/33$) of lingual lesions, and 15.2% ($n = 5/33$) of buccal lesions. Linear vessels were more frequently seen on the vermilion (39.4%, $n = 13/33$) than on the buccal mucosa (15.2%, $n = 5/33$). Looped vessels were identified in 15.2% ($n = 5/33$) of vermilion lesions, 12.1% ($n = 4/33$) of lingual lesions, and 6.1% ($n = 2/33$) of buccal lesions. Radial peripheral vascular distribution was noted in 48.5% ($n = 16/33$) of lingual and vermilion mucosa lesions, whereas it was less frequent on the buccal mucosa (21.2%, $n = 7/33$). A diffuse regular vascular pattern was present in 30.3% ($n = 10/33$) of vermilion lesions, 6.1% ($n = 2/33$) of lingual lesions, and 6.1% ($n = 2/33$) of buccal mucosa lesions. The rare sea anemone-like vascular pattern was noted in 3.0% ($n = 1/33$) of lingual and buccal mucosa lesions (Tables 4 and 5).

Erosions were observed in 39.4% ($n = 13/33$) of vermilion lesions, 42.4% ($n = 14/33$) of lingual lesions, and 36.4% ($n = 12/33$) of buccal mucosa lesions. Scaling was noted exclusively on the vermilion (48.5%, $n = 16/33$). Blunting of lingual papillae was observed in 60.6% ($n = 20/33$) of lingual lesions (Tables 4 and 5).

Statistical analysis revealed significant associations between certain white or erosive lesions and vascular features (Appendix A):

1. Leukoplakia-like lesions were significantly associated with dotted blood vessels ($p = 0.027$), suggesting increased vascularization in hyperkeratotic lesions.

2. A significant association was found between the presence of erosions and dotted blood vessels ($p < 0.001$), as well as between erosions and linear vessels ($p = 0.011$), indicating a stronger angiogenic component in erosive OLP.

3. A trend toward significance was noted between annular striae and dotted blood vessels ($p = 0.053$) and between radial striae and linear vessels ($p = 0.057$).

4. Leukoplakia-like lesions were also significantly associated with looped vessels on the lingual mucosa ($p = 0.002$) and dotted vessels in the buccal mucosa ($p = 0.044$), reinforcing their potential role in advanced disease stages.

### 3.3. Comparative Analysis of Mucoscopic Features According to Mucosal Sites

#### 3.3.1. Vermilion

On the vermilion, an erythematous background was significantly more common in the control group (80.0%, $n = 24/30$) compared to the OLP group (30.3%, $n = 10/33$) ($p < 0.001$), whereas the violaceous background showed no significant difference (27.3%, $n = 9/33$ vs. 30.0%, $n = 9/30$, $p = 0.811$).

Regarding white lesions, radial striae were observed in 15.2% ($n = 5/33$) of OLP cases and 13.3% ($n = 4/30$) of controls ($p = 1.000$), while linear striae (Figure 1a,b) were present in 81.8% ($n = 27/33$) of OLP patients and 66.7% ($n = 20/30$) of controls ($p = 0.168$). Reticular striae (Figure 1a) were detected exclusively in OLP cases (39.4%, $n = 13/33$, $p < 0.001$). Leaf venation and annular striae were rare and found only in OLP (3.0%, $n = 1/33$ and 9.1%, $n = 3/33$, respectively), but without statistical significance. Globular structures were significantly more frequent in the controls (30.0%, $n = 9/30$) than in OLP (6.1%, $n = 2/33$, $p = 0.012$), and dotted structures were more common in controls (20.0%, $n = 6/30$) than OLP (3.0%, $n = 1/33$), although not statistically significant ($p = 0.052$). The veil pattern was markedly more frequent in the controls (66.7%, $n = 20/30$) compared to OLP (15.2%, $n = 5/33$, $p < 0.001$), and leukoplakia-like lesions were also more prevalent among the controls (50.0%, $n = 15/30$) than OLP patients (18.2%, $n = 6/33$, $p = 0.007$). Rosettes were rare and identified only in one OLP case (3.0%, $n = 1/33$).

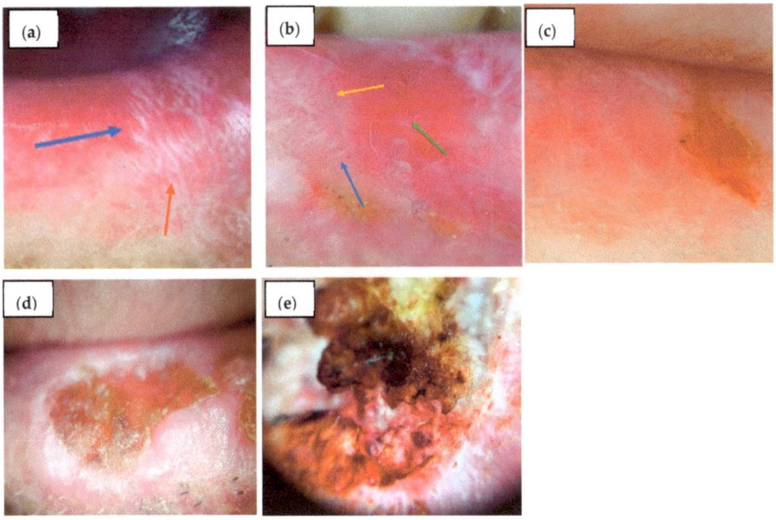


**Figure 1.** Mucoscopic features on the vermilion: (**a**) OLP: Blue arrow—white linear striae; Red arrow—reticular white striae; (**b**) OLP: Blue arrow—linear striae; Orange arrow—dotted vessels; Green arrow—erosion; (**c**) Eczematous cheilitis—dotted vessels, white veil, scales, and an erosion on a pink background; (**d**) Actinic chronic cheilitis—leukoplakia-like lesion and erosions; (**e**) SCC—erosion surrounded by polymorphous vessels; leukoplakia-like lesion, crusts.

Linear and dotted blood vessels (Figure 1b) were comparably distributed in both groups (39.4%, $n = 13/33$ vs. 40.0%, $n = 12/30$, $p = 0.961$ and 57.6%, $n = 19/33$ vs. 76.7%, $n = 23/30$, $p = 0.108$, respectively). Looped vessels showed no significant difference (15.2%, $n = 5/33$ vs. 13.3% $n = 4/30$, $p = 1.000$), and sea anemone–like vessels were observed in only one control subject (3.3%, $n = 1/30$). Radial distribution of vessels at the periphery was seen in 48.5% ($n = 16/33$) of OLP and 30.0% ($n = 9/30$) of controls ($p = 0.134$), while diffuse regular vascular distribution was significantly more frequent in the controls (60.0%, $n = 18/30$) than in OLP (30.3%, $n = 10/33$, $p = 0.018$). Erosions were observed in 39.4% ($n = 13/33$) of OLP (Figure 1b) and 53.3% ($n = 16/30$) of controls ($p = 0.268$) (Figure 1c–e). Scales were significantly more common in controls (100%, $n = 3/300$) than in OLP (48.5%, $n = 16/33$, $p < 0.001$). Comparative mucoscopic features between OLP and controls on the vermilion are presented in Table 6.

**Table 6.** Mucoscopic features of OLP compared to the control group on the vermilion border of the lips.

| | Group | | | | Total | | Pearson Chi-Squared Test |
|---|---|---|---|---|---|---|---|
| | OLP | | Control | | | | |
| | N | % | N | % | N | % | p-Value |
| **Background color** | | | | | | | |
| Erythematous | 10 | 30.3% | 24 | 80.0% | 34 | 54.0% | <0.001 ** |
| Violaceous | 9 | 27.3% | 9 | 30.0% | 18 | 28.6% | 0.811 |
| **White lesions** | | | | | | | |
| Radial striae | 5 | 15.2% | 4 | 13.3% | 9 | 14.3% | 1.000 |
| Linear striae | 27 | 81.8% | 20 | 66.7% | 47 | 74.6% | 0.168 |
| Reticular striae | 13 | 39.4% | - | - | 13 | 20.6% | <0.001 ** |
| Leaf venation | 1 | 3.0% | - | - | 1 | 1.6% | 1.000 |
| Annular striae | 3 | 9.1% | - | - | 3 | 4.8% | 0.240 |
| Globular | 2 | 6.1% | 9 | 30.0% | 11 | 17.5% | 0.012 * |
| Dotted | 1 | 3.0% | 6 | 20.0% | 7 | 11.1% | 0.052 |
| Veil | 5 | 15.2% | 20 | 66.7% | 25 | 39.7% | <0.001 ** |
| Rosette | 1 | 3.0% | - | - | 1 | 1.6% | 1.000 |
| Leukoplakia-like | 6 | 18.2% | 15 | 50.0% | 21 | 33.3% | 0.007 ** |
| **Blood vessels** | | | | | | | |
| Linear | 13 | 39.4% | 12 | 40.0% | 25 | 39.7% | 0.961 |
| Dotted | 19 | 57.6% | 23 | 76.7% | 42 | 66.7% | 0.108 |
| Looped | 5 | 15.2% | 4 | 13.3% | 9 | 14.3% | 1.000 |
| Sea anemone-like | - | - | 1 | 3.3% | 1 | 1.6% | 0.476 |
| **Distribution of blood vessels** | | | | | | | |
| Radial at the perifery | 16 | 48.5% | 9 | 30.0% | 25 | 39.7% | 0.134 |
| Diffuse regular | 10 | 30.3% | 18 | 60.0% | 28 | 44.4% | 0.018 * |
| **Erosions** | 13 | 39.4% | 16 | 53.3% | 29 | 46.0% | 0.268 |
| **Scales** | 16 | 48.5% | 30 | 100.0% | 46 | 73.0% | <0.001 ** |

* Statistically significant, ** statistically highly significant.

### 3.3.2. Lingual Mucosa

Regarding the lingual lesions, an erythematous background was more frequent in the controls (70.0%, $n = 21/30$) than OLP patients (33.3%, $n = 11/33$, $p = 0.004$), while a violaceous background was present in 9.1% ($n = 3/33$) of OLP cases and absent in controls ($p = 0.240$). Radial striae (9.1%, $n = 3/33$ vs. 3.3%, $n = 1/30$, $p = 0.614$), linear striae (12.1%, $n = 4/33$, vs. 6.7%, $n = 2/30$, $p = 0.674$) (Figure 2a), and reticular striae (18.2%, $n = 6/33$, vs. 3.3%, $n = 1/30$, $p = 0.107$) were slightly more common in OLP but without statistical significance. Annular striae were found in 6.1% ($n = 2/33$) of OLP cases and none of the controls ($p = 0.493$), while leaf venation was absent in both groups. Globular structures were significantly more prevalent in controls (93.3%, $n = 28/30$) compared to OLP (12.1%, $n = 4/33$, $p < 0.001$), while dotted structures were rare in both groups (3.0%, $n = 1/33$ vs. 3.3%, $n = 1/30$, $p = 1.000$). Veil pattern was more common in OLP (42.4%, $n = 14/33$) than controls (20.0%, $n = 6/30$, $p = 0.056$). Leukoplakia-like lesions were found in 48.5% ($n = 16/33$) of OLP (Figure 2a) and 30.0% ($n = 9/30$) of controls ($p = 0.134$) (Figure 2b–d). Rosettes were not observed.

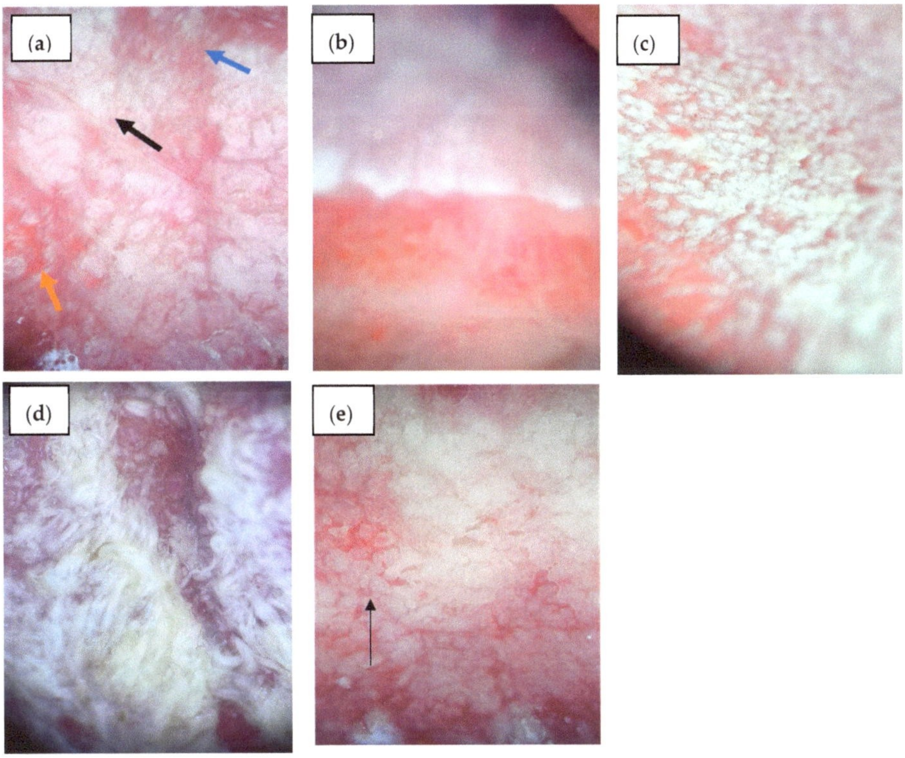


**Figure 2.** Mucoscopic aspects on the lingual mucosa: (**a**) OLP: Blue arrow—linear striae; OLP: Black arrow—blunted lingual papillae; Orange arrow—dotted vessels; (**b**) Leukoplakia—white structureless homogenous area; (**c**) Oral hyperplastic candidiasis—white hypertrophic filiform papillae; (**d**) Pachyonychia congenita—elongated white-yellow filiform papillae; (**e**) OLP: Black arrow- blunted lingual papillae.

Linear and dotted vessels were significantly more common in OLP (36.4% each, $n = 12/33$) (Figure 3) compared to controls, where they were absent or rare (0% and 3.3%, $n = 0/30$ and $n = 1/30$, respectively; $p < 0.001$ and $p = 0.001$). Looped vessels (12.1%, $n = 4/33$, 0% controls, $p = 0.115$) and sea anemone-like vessels (3.0%, $n = 1/33$, 0% controls, $p = 1.000$) were infrequent. Radial vascular distribution was present exclusively in OLP patients (48.5%, $n = 16/33$, $p < 0.001$), while diffuse regular distribution was seen in 6.1% ($n = 2/33$) of OLP and 3.3% ($n = 1/30$) of controls ($p = 1.000$). Erosions were significantly more common in OLP (42.4%, $n = 14/33$) than controls (16.7%, $n = 5/30$, $p = 0.026$). Scales were present in only 6.7% ($n = 2/30$) of controls and absent in OLP ($p = 0.223$). Blunting of lingual papillae was notably more frequent in OLP (60.6%, $n = 20/33$) (Figure 2e) versus controls (10.0%, $n = 3/30$, $p < 0.001$). Comparative mucoscopic features between OLP and controls on the lingual mucosa are presented in Table 7.

**Table 7.** Mucoscopic features of OLP compared to the control group on the lingual mucosa.

| | Group | | | | Total | | Pearson Chi-Squared Test p-Value |
|---|---|---|---|---|---|---|---|
| | OLP | | Control | | | | |
| | N | % | N | % | N | % | |
| **Background color** | | | | | | | |
| Erythematous | 11 | 33.3% | 21 | 70.0% | 32 | 50.8% | 0.004 ** |
| Violaceous | 3 | 9.1% | - | - | 3 | 4.8% | 0.240 |
| **White lesions** | | | | | | | |
| Radial striae | 3 | 9.1% | 1 | 3.3% | 4 | 6.3% | 0.614 |
| Linear striae | 4 | 12.1% | 2 | 6.7% | 6 | 9.5% | 0.674 |
| Reticular striae | 6 | 18.2% | 1 | 3.3% | 7 | 11.1% | 0.107 |
| Leaf venation | - | - | - | - | - | - | |
| Annular striae | 2 | 6.1% | - | - | 2 | 3.2% | 0.493 |
| Globular | 4 | 12.1% | 28 | 93.3% | 32 | 50.8% | <0.001 ** |
| Dotted | 1 | 3.0% | 1 | 3.3% | 2 | 3.2% | 1.000 |
| Veil | 14 | 42.4% | 6 | 20.0% | 20 | 31.7% | 0.056 |
| Rosette | - | - | - | - | - | - | |
| Leukoplakia-like | 16 | 48.5% | 9 | 30.0% | 25 | 39.7% | 0.134 |
| **Blood vessels** | | | | | | | |
| Linear | 12 | 36.4% | - | - | 12 | 19.0% | <0.001 ** |
| Dotted | 12 | 36.4% | 1 | 3.3% | 13 | 20.6% | 0.001 ** |
| Looped | 4 | 12.1% | - | - | 4 | 6.3% | 0.115 |
| Sea anemone-like | 1 | 3.0% | - | - | 1 | 1.6% | 1.000 |
| **Distribution of blood vessels** | | | | | | | |
| Radial at the perifery | 16 | 48.5% | - | - | 16 | 25.4% | <0.001 ** |
| Diffuse regular | 2 | 6.1% | 1 | 3.3% | 3 | 4.8% | 1.000 |
| **Erosions** | 14 | 42.4% | 5 | 16.7% | 19 | 30.2% | 0.026 * |
| **Blunting of lingual papillae** | 20 | 60.6% | 3 | 10.0% | 23 | 36.5% | <0.001 ** |

* Statistically significant, ** statistically highly significant.

### 3.3.3. Buccal Mucosa

As for the buccal mucosa lesions, an erythematous background was significantly more common in controls (85.0%, $n = 17/30$) compared to OLP patients (24.2%, $n = 8/30$, $p < 0.001$), while a violaceous background was not observed in either group. Radial striae were present in 21.2% ($n = 7/33$) of OLP and 25.0% ($n = 5/30$) of controls ($p = 0.748$), and linear striae were significantly more frequent in the controls (90.0%, $n = 18/30$) than OLP (21.2%, $n = 7/33$, $p < 0.001$) (Figure 3). Reticular striae were highly specific for OLP, being present in 90.9% ($n = 30/33$) of cases versus only 5.0% ($n = 1/30$) of controls ($p < 0.001$). Leaf venation was found in 18.2% ($n = 6/33$) of OLP and absent in controls ($p = 0.072$). Annular striae were observed in 3.0% ($n = 1/33$) of OLP and none in controls ($p = 1.000$). Globular structures were significantly more common in controls (75.0%, $n = 15/30$) than OLP (3.0%, $n = 1/33$, $p < 0.001$). Dotted structures were also more frequent in the controls (45.0%, $n = 9/30$) than OLP (9.1%, $n = 3/30$, $p = 0.005$), as was the veil pattern (55.0%, $n = 11/30$ vs. 21.2%, $n = 7/33$, $p = 0.012$) (Figure 3a,b). Leukoplakia-like lesions were observed in 30.0% ($n = 6/30$) of controls and 15.2% ($n = 5/33$) of OLP ($p = 0.296$) (Figure 3c). Rosettes were absent in both groups.

Among blood vessel morphologies, linear vessels were observed in 15.2% ($n = 5/33$) of OLP and 5.0% ($n = 1/30$) of controls ($p = 0.390$), and dotted vessels were significantly more frequent in the controls (65.0%, $n = 13/30$) than OLP (15.2%, $n = 5/33$, $p < 0.001$) (Figure 3a). Looped vessels were found in 6.1% ($n = 2/33$) of OLP and 5.0% ($n = 1/30$) of controls ($p = 1.000$). Sea anemone-like vessels were seen in one OLP patient (3.0%, $n = 1/33$). Radial peripheral vascular distribution was observed only in OLP (21.2%, $n = 7/33$, $p = 0.037$), while diffuse regular distribution was significantly more common in controls (65.0%, $n = 13/30$) than OLP (6.1%, $n = 2/33$, $p < 0.001$). Erosions were significantly more frequent in the controls (75.0%, $n = 15/30$) than OLP (36.4%, $n = 12/33$, $p = 0.006$), mainly because our control group consisted, for the most part, of pemphigus vulgaris with active lesions. Comparative mucoscopic features between OLP and controls on the buccal mucosa are presented in Table 8.

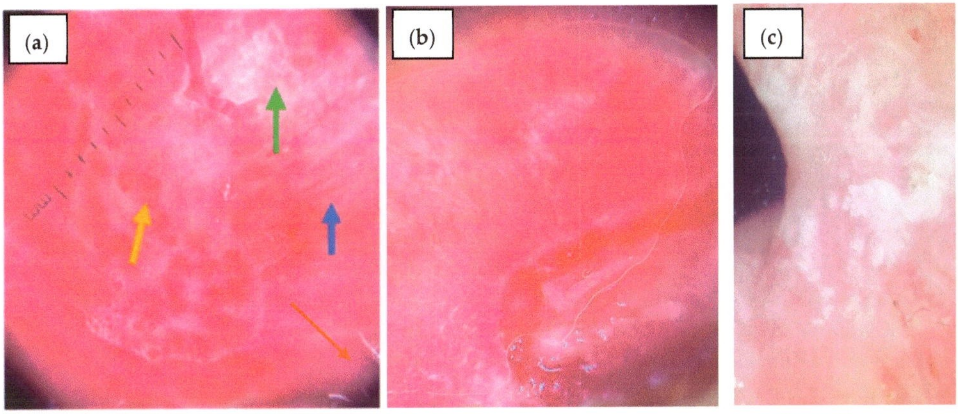


**Figure 3.** Mucoscopic features on the buccal mucosa: (**a**) OLP: Blue arrow—linear striae; Green arrow—reticular striae; Red arrow—white veil; Yellow arrow—dotted vessels; (**b**) PV—well demarcated erosion, scales, white parallel striae at the periphery of the erosion; (**c**) Morsicatio buccarum—white elevated structureless area, white corrugated bands.

**Table 8.** Mucoscopic features of OLP compared to the control group on the buccal mucosa.

| | Group | | | | Total | | Pearson Chi-Squared Test $p$-Value |
|---|---|---|---|---|---|---|---|
| | OLP | | Control | | | | |
| | N | % | N | % | N | % | |
| **Background color** | | | | | | | |
| Erythematous | 8 | 24.2% | 17 | 85.0% | 25 | 47.2% | <0.001 ** |
| Violaceous | - | - | - | - | - | - | |
| **White lesions** | | | | | | | |
| Radial striae | 7 | 21.2% | 5 | 25.0% | 12 | 22.6% | 0.748 |
| Linear striae | 7 | 21.2% | 18 | 90.0% | 25 | 47.2% | <0.001 ** |
| Reticular striae | 30 | 90.9% | 1 | 5.0% | 31 | 58.5% | <0.001 ** |
| Leaf venation | 6 | 18.2% | - | - | 6 | 11.3% | 0.072 |
| Annular striae | 1 | 3.0% | - | - | 1 | 1.9% | 1.000 |
| Globular | 1 | 3.0% | 15 | 75.0% | 16 | 30.2% | <0.001 ** |
| Dotted | 3 | 9.1% | 9 | 45.0% | 12 | 22.6% | 0.005 ** |
| Veil | 7 | 21.2% | 11 | 55.0% | 18 | 34.0% | 0.012 ** |
| Rosette | - | - | - | - | - | - | |
| Leukoplakia-like | 5 | 15.2% | 6 | 30.0% | 11 | 20.8% | 0.296 |
| **Blood vessels** | | | | | | | |
| Linear | 5 | 15.2% | 1 | 5.0% | 6 | 11.3% | 0.390 |
| Dotted | 5 | 15.2% | 13 | 65.0% | 18 | 34.0% | <0.001 ** |
| Looped | 2 | 6.1% | 1 | 5.0% | 3 | 5.7% | 1.000 |
| Sea anemone-like | 1 | 3.0% | - | - | 1 | 1.9% | 1.000 |
| **Distribution of blood vessels** | | | | | | | |
| Radial at the perifery | 7 | 21.2% | - | - | 7 | 13.2% | 0.037 * |
| Diffuse regular | 2 | 6.1% | 13 | 65.0% | 15 | 28.3% | <0.001 ** |
| **Erosions** | 12 | 36.4% | 15 | 75.0% | 27 | 50.9% | 0.006 ** |

* Statistically significant, ** statistically highly significant.

## 4. Discussion

Lip localization of LP lesions is quite rare, and the available literature does not provide sufficient mucoscopic patterns to draw a definitive conclusion in order to achieve a final diagnosis solely based on mucoscopy. Clinically, OLP on the lip can present as an erosive or papular form. The background color is reported to appear violaceous or erythematous, with WS in three different patterns: circular, radial, and linear, although isolated cases with different configurations have been mentioned (e.g., leaf venation-like). Additionally, diffuse scaling, pigmentation (in a streak or globule pattern), and various vascular arrangements (most frequently described as linear, hairpin, or dotted) have been identified in the few cases documented in the literature. There are also reports of rosettes identified at the lip margin, alongside erosions and bleeding spots. However, it is considered that the hallmarks of lip LP are represented by a mixture of WS, pigmentation, telangiectasia, and scales [28–30]. Our study aligns with previous findings, emphasizing linear striae as the most prevalent white lesion pattern on the vermilion and dotted vessels as the most frequently observed vascular feature. A radial peripheral vascular distribution was observed in 48.5% ($n = 16/33$) of OLP cases on the vermilion, which may serve as a useful differentiating pattern from other inflammatory lip conditions. When compared to the control group, several key differences emerged. In the control cases, globular structures, veil-like appearances, and a diffuse regular vascular distribution were significantly more prevalent. Moreover, scales were universally present in the control group, compared to 48.5% ($n = 16/33$) in OLP. These differences suggest that the combination of linear striae, dotted vessels, and radial vessel distribution may provide diagnostic specificity for OLP, especially in distinguishing it from chronic cheilitis. Erosions were observed in 39.4% ($n = 13/33$) of the vermilion lesions in OLP, and the background was most commonly pink, followed by erythematous and violaceous, which may reflect inflammation and vascular involvement.

The buccal mucosa is a common site for lesions of OLP and has drawn significant attention for mucoscopic analysis. Prior studies have predominantly described the background color as pinkish-brown, violaceous, or dull pink to dull red [25]. In our cohort, the most frequently observed background was erythematous, followed by a violaceous hue. Linear vascular structures were the most frequently observed pattern, with occasional sea anemone-like arrangements. Other vascular configurations, such as radial, hairpin, and dotted vessels, were described but less frequently reported [31]. In the control group, buccal mucosal lesions were significantly different, with a predominance of globular and dotted patterns, while reticular striae (present in 90.9%, $n = 30/33$ of OLP cases) were almost absent. Linear striae were paradoxically more frequent in the controls than in OLP, highlighting the need to interpret striae morphology alongside other features. Moreover, diffuse regular vascular distribution and dotted vessels were significantly more common in controls, while radial vascular patterns were specific to OLP. Veil-like structures and leukoplakia-like lesions were also more frequently identified in controls, suggesting their lower specificity for OLP.

On the lingual mucosa, OLP typically manifests as white patches, erosions, or ulcers, particularly on the dorsal or lateral surfaces. The literature describes WS in circular, structureless, veil-like patterns, often appearing gray-white to bluish-white, commonly on the dorsum of the tongue. These lesions can include leukoplakia-like areas and a smoothing or blunting of lingual papillae. Erosions on the tongue are well-defined, bright red, and often surrounded by a hyperkeratotic white rim. Pigmentation may appear as brown or blue-gray clods and globules [32–34]. In our cohort, the most common background color was pink, followed by erythematous. The most prevalent white lesion was leukoplakia-like, suggesting a higher degree of hyperkeratosis in lingual OLP. Reticular striae were also present but at a lower frequency than in the buccal mucosa. A radial peripheral vascular pattern and dotted vessels were prominent, reinforcing the vascular remodeling characteristic of lingual OLP. Erosions were frequently observed, along with blunting of the lingual papillae—a finding absent in the control group. Compared with the control group for the lingual mucosa, distinct differences were evident. Globular patterns were overwhelmingly more common in hypertrophic candidiasis than OLP ($p < 0.001$), while linear and dotted vessels, radial vascular arrangements, and blunting of papillae were unique to OLP. This contrast supports the diagnostic potential of mucoscopy in distinguishing lingual OLP from candidiasis, which typically lacks structured white striae and presents with diffuse erythema or pseudomembranous plaques.

Mucoscopy has emerged as an essential non-invasive tool in the early detection and differentiation of squamous cell carcinoma (SCC) of the lip and oral mucosa. Given the challenges of distinguishing potentially malignant disorders and malignant lesions from benign inflammatory conditions, mucoscopy provides enhanced visualization of vascular and structural alterations that may indicate malignant transformation. One of the most significant mucoscopic findings in oral SCC is the presence of irregular, polymorphous, or atypical vascular patterns, reflecting tumor-induced neovascularization. Linear-irregular vessels, dotted vessels, and glomerular vessels are commonly observed in early SCC, whereas polymorphous vascular arrangements suggest progression toward malignancy. Additionally, white structureless areas and keratinization indicate hyperproliferative activity, which, when combined with ulcerations and a milky red or erythematous background, strongly raises suspicion for invasive SCC. In cases of OLP with suspected malignant transformation, the loss of Wickham's striae, the appearance of disorganized pigmentation, and an increase in vascular density should prompt further histopathological evaluation. By integrating mucoscopy into routine oral examinations, clinicians can facilitate earlier biopsy decisions, improving early SCC detection and patient outcomes. Future studies should aim to standardize mucoscopic criteria for oral SCC and further investigate its role in monitoring high-risk lesions such as EOLP [35–41].

Our findings support the diagnostic utility of mucoscopy in the evaluation of OLP, especially in distinguishing it from clinically similar inflammatory oral conditions. This aligns with the conclusions of the American Academy of Oral and Maxillofacial Pathology, which emphasize the ongoing challenges in achieving a reliable diagnosis of OLP due to its overlapping clinical and histopathologic features with other lichenoid disorders and immune-mediated mucosal diseases. The current expert consensus emphasizes the necessity of thorough clinicopathologic correlation and ongoing follow-up, acknowledging the risk of disease progression or evolution into other lichenoid disorders. Within this framework, mucoscopy emerges as a valuable non-invasive diagnostic adjunct, capable of highlighting striae, vascular patterns, and erosions that may remain undetected during routine clinical examination. By identifying features such as leukoplakia-like plaques and associated vascular patterns, mucoscopy may contribute to earlier recognition of lesions with malignant potential and guide biopsy decisions. These observations support the call for more refined diagnostic approaches, as outlined by Cheng et al., and point to mucoscopy as a complementary tool to enhance both clinical accuracy and research reproducibility in OLP [42].

It is crucial to emphasize that, while mucoscopy exhibits high sensitivity and specificity in diagnosing OLP, it cannot currently serve as the sole method for a definitive diagnosis. This limitation stems from insufficient large-scale patient cohorts to validate mucoscopic criteria for conclusive diagnosis, as well as a lack of comparative studies between mucoscopic findings of OLP and similar conditions. Therefore, histopathological examination remains the gold standard for definitive diagnosis. Mucoscopy continues to serve as a primary non-invasive tool that supports clinical diagnosis and aids in monitoring the effectiveness of OLP treatments. It offers supplementary insights that assist clinicians in determining the necessity and the best site for biopsy or further evaluation. While reticular striae were highly specific to OLP in our study, particularly on the buccal mucosa (90.9%, $p < 0.001$), other mucoscopic features were rather important in association rather than individually. Thus, leukoplakia-like lesions were most prevalent on the lingual mucosa and significantly associated with dotted ($p = 0.027$) and looped vessels ($p = 0.002$). Erosions correlated significantly with both dotted ($p < 0.001$) and linear vessels ($p = 0.011$), especially in lingual and vermilion lesions.

This study has several limitations that should be acknowledged. The small sample size and single-center design may limit the generalizability of the findings, necessitating larger, multi-center studies for validation. Additionally, the study lacks longitudinal follow-up, preventing an assessment of mucoscopic changes over time and their potential role in predicting disease progression or malignant transformation. Another limitation is the potential for observer bias, as mucoscopic evaluations were performed by a limited number of examiners without interobserver agreement analysis. Future studies should focus on larger, prospective cohorts, direct histopathologic comparisons, and multi-observer evaluations to further refine the role of mucoscopy in OLP diagnosis and monitoring.

## 5. Conclusions

This study highlights the diagnostic value of mucoscopy in OLP, revealing site-specific patterns that contribute to distinguishing it from other oral inflammatory conditions. Buccal lesions predominantly showed classical reticular striae with minimal vascular changes, whereas vermilion and lingual sites exhibited more prominent vascular structures, scaling, and leukoplakia-like areas, suggesting increased inflammatory activity, chronicity, and epithelial alteration. Dotted and linear vessels were more frequently observed in erosive and hyperkeratotic lesions, supporting a potential role for angiogenesis in active disease. Compared to the control group, OLP lesions presented more structured and disease-specific features, while mimicking conditions showed diffuse, nonspecific patterns.

This study reinforces the diagnostic and prognostic role of mucoscopy in OLP, demonstrating site-specific mucoscopic variations that may aid in differentiating disease subtypes and identifying high-risk lesions. Future research should focus on longitudinal studies, standardized mucoscopic criteria, and AI-assisted image analysis to enhance the diagnostic accuracy and predictive value of mucoscopy in OLP and its malignant transformation.

**Author Contributions:** Conceptualization: M.P.T., C.C.B. and D.E.B., methodology: E.P.A., O.M.C.H., S.V.T. and A.G.C., software: A.E.H., R.P.C. and C.A.M.; validation: M.P.T. and D.E.B.; formal analysis: C.C.B. and O.M.C.H.; investigation: A.E.H., R.P.C., C.A.M., C.C.B. and V.V.C.; resources: A.E.H., R.P.C., C.A.M. and C.C.B.; data curation: M.P.T. and D.E.B.; writing—M.P.T. and C.C.B.; writing—review and editing: M.P.T., E.P.A. and D.E.B.; visualization, S.V.T. and A.G.C.; supervision: M.P.T. and D.E.B.; project administration: M.P.T. and D.E.B. All authors have read and agreed to the published version of the manuscript.

**Funding:** This research received no external funding.

**Institutional Review Board Statement:** This study was conducted according to the guidelines of the Declaration of Helsinki and approved by the Ethics Committee of University Clinical Railways Hospital, Iasi, Romania (Approval code DCF0005, Date of approval 12 December 2024).

**Informed Consent Statement:** Written informed consent was obtained from all patients prior to their inclusion in the study and was documented in each patient's observation chart, in accordance with institutional and ethical guidelines.

**Data Availability Statement:** The original contributions presented in this study are included in the article. Further inquiries can be directed to the corresponding authors.

**Conflicts of Interest:** The authors declare no conflicts of interest.

## Abbreviations

The following abbreviations are used in this manuscript:

| | |
|---|---|
| OLP | Oral Lichen Planus |
| LP | Lichen Planus |
| HCV | Hepatitis C Virus |
| EOLP | Erosive Oral Lichen Planus |
| WHO | World Health Organization |
| DIF | Direct Immunofluorescence |
| SD | Standard Deviation |
| PV | Pemphigus Vulgaris |
| AI | Artificial Intelligence |
| SCC | Squamous Cell Carcinoma |

## Appendix A

**Table A1.** The association between white lesions and blood vessel patterns of the vermilion.

| **VERMILION** | | **BLOOD VESSELS** | | | | | | | | | | | | | | | |
|---|---|---|---|---|---|---|---|---|---|---|---|---|---|---|---|---|---|
| | | **Linear** | | | | **Dotted** | | | | **Looped** | | | | **Sea Anemone-Like** | | | |
| **WHITE LESIONS** | | 0 | | 1 | | 0 | | 1 | | 0 | | 1 | | 0 | | 1 | |
| | | N | % | N | % | N | % | N | % | N | % | N | % | N | % | N | % |
| Radial striae | 0 | 17 | 85.0% | 11 | 84.6% | 14 | 100.0% | 14 | 73.7% | 24 | 85.7% | 4 | 80.0% | 28 | 84.8% | - | - |
| | 1 | 3 | 15.0% | 2 | 15.4% | | | 5 | 26.3% | 4 | 14.3% | 1 | 20.0% | 5 | 15.2% | - | - |
| | | $p = 1.000$ | | | | $p = 0.057$ * | | | | $p = 1.000$ | | | | - | | | |
| Linear striae | 0 | 5 | 25.0% | 1 | 7.7% | 5 | 35.7% | 1 | 5.3% | 6 | 21.4% | | | 6 | 18.2% | - | - |
| | 1 | 15 | 75.0% | 12 | 92.3% | 9 | 64.3% | 18 | 94.7% | 22 | 78.6% | 5 | 100.0% | 27 | 81.8% | - | - |
| | | $p = 0.364$ | | | | $p = 0.062$ | | | | $p = 0.556$ | | | | - | | | |
| Reticular striae | 0 | 13 | 65.0% | 7 | 53.8% | 6 | 42.9% | 14 | 73.7% | 16 | 57.1% | 4 | 80.0% | 20 | 60.6% | - | - |
| | 1 | 7 | 35.0% | 6 | 46.2% | 8 | 57.1% | 5 | 26.3% | 12 | 42.9% | 1 | 20.0% | 13 | 39.4% | - | - |
| | | $p = 0.522$ | | | | $p = 0.073$ | | | | $p = 0.625$ | | | | - | | | |
| Leaf venation | 0 | 20 | 100.0% | 12 | 92.3% | 14 | 100.0% | 18 | 94.7% | 28 | 100.0% | 4 | 80.0% | 32 | 97.0% | - | - |
| | 1 | | | 1 | 7.7% | | | 1 | 5.3% | | | 1 | 20.0% | 1 | 3.0% | - | - |
| | | $p = 0.394$ | | | | $p = 1.000$ | | | | $p = 0.152$ | | | | - | | | |
| Annular striae | 0 | 18 | 90.0% | 12 | 92.3% | 14 | 100.0% | 16 | 84.2% | 27 | 96.4% | 3 | 60.0% | 30 | 90.9% | - | - |
| | 1 | 2 | 10.0% | 1 | 7.7% | | | 3 | 15.8% | 1 | 3.6% | 2 | 40.0% | 3 | 9.1% | - | - |
| | | $p = 1.000$ | | | | $p = 0.244$ | | | | $p = 0.053$ * | | | | - | | | |
| Globular | 0 | 19 | 95.0% | 12 | 92.3% | 14 | 100.0% | 17 | 89.5% | 27 | 96.4% | 4 | 80.0% | 31 | 93.9% | - | - |
| | 1 | 1 | 5.0% | 1 | 7.7% | | | 2 | 10.5% | 1 | 3.6% | 1 | 20.0% | 2 | 6.1% | - | - |
| | | $p = 1.000$ | | | | $p = 0.496$ | | | | $p = 0.284$ | | | | - | | | |
| Dotted | 0 | 20 | 100.0% | 12 | 92.3% | 14 | 100.0% | 18 | 94.7% | 27 | 96.4% | 5 | 100.0% | 32 | 97.0% | - | - |
| | 1 | | | 1 | 7.7% | | | 1 | 5.3% | 1 | 3.6% | | | 1 | 3.0% | - | - |
| | | $p = 0.394$ | | | | $p = 1.000$ | | | | $p = 1.000$ | | | | - | | | |
| Veil | 0 | 16 | 80.0% | 12 | 92.3% | 11 | 78.6% | 17 | 89.5% | 24 | 85.7% | 4 | 80.0% | 28 | 84.8% | - | - |
| | 1 | 4 | 20.0% | 1 | 7.7% | 3 | 21.4% | 2 | 10.5% | 4 | 14.3% | 1 | 20.0% | 5 | 15.2% | - | - |
| | | $p = 0.625$ | | | | $p = 0.628$ | | | | $p = 1.000$ | | | | - | | | |
| Rosette | 0 | 19 | 95.0% | 13 | 100.0% | 14 | 100.0% | 18 | 94.7% | 27 | 96.4% | 5 | 100.0% | 32 | 97.0% | - | - |
| | 1 | 1 | 5.0% | | | | | 1 | 5.3% | 1 | 3.6% | | | 1 | 3.0% | - | - |
| | | $p = 1.000$ | | | | $p = 1.000$ | | | | $p = 1.000$ | | | | - | | | |
| Leukoplakia-like | 0 | 16 | 80.0% | 11 | 84.6% | 14 | 100.0% | 13 | 68.4% | 25 | 89.3% | 2 | 40.0% | 27 | 81.8% | - | - |
| | 1 | 4 | 20.0% | 2 | 15.4% | | | 6 | 31.6% | 3 | 10.7% | 3 | 60.0% | 6 | 18.2% | - | - |
| | | $p = 1.000$ | | | | $p = 0.027$ * | | | | $p = 0.031$ * | | | | - | | | |
| **Total** | | **20** | **100.0%** | **13** | **100.0%** | **14** | **100.0%** | **19** | **100.0%** | **28** | **100.0%** | **5** | **100.0%** | **33** | **100.0%** | **-** | **-** |

Pearson Chi-squared test. * Statistically significant.

**Table A2.** Association between vermilion erosions and blood vessels.

| VERMILION EROSION | | BLOOD VESSELS | | | | | | | | | | | | | | | |
|---|---|---|---|---|---|---|---|---|---|---|---|---|---|---|---|---|---|
| | | Linear | | | | Dotted | | | | Looped | | | | Sea Anemone-Like | | | |
| | | 0 | | 1 | | 0 | | 1 | | 0 | | 1 | | 0 | | 1 | |
| | | N | % | N | % | N | % | N | % | N | % | N | % | N | % | N | % |
| | 0 | 17 | 85.0% | 3 | 23.1% | 12 | 85.7% | 8 | 42.1% | 19 | 67.9% | 1 | 20.0% | 20 | 60.6% | - | - |
| | 1 | 3 | 15.0% | 10 | 76.9% | 2 | 14.3% | 11 | 57.9% | 9 | 32.1% | 4 | 80.0% | 13 | 39.4% | - | - |
| | | $p$ <0.001 ** | | | | $p$ = 0.011 ** | | | | $p$ = 0.066 * | | | | - | | | |
| **Total** | | **20** | **100.0%** | **13** | **100.0%** | **14** | **100.0%** | **19** | **100.0%** | **28** | **100.0%** | **5** | **100.0%** | **33** | **100.0%** | **-** | **-** |

Pearson Chi-squared test. * Statistically significant, ** statistically highly significant.

**Table A3.** Association between white lesions and blood vessel patterns of the lingual mucosa.

| LINGUAL WHITE LESIONS | | BLOOD VESSELS | | | | | | | | | | | | | | | |
|---|---|---|---|---|---|---|---|---|---|---|---|---|---|---|---|---|---|
| | | Linear | | | | Dotted | | | | Looped | | | | Sea Anemone-Like | | | |
| | | 0 | | 1 | | 0 | | 1 | | 0 | | 1 | | 0 | | 1 | |
| | | N | % | N | % | N | % | N | % | N | % | N | % | N | % | N | % |
| Radial striae | 0 | 20 | 95.2% | 10 | 83.3% | 20 | 95.2% | 10 | 83.3% | 27 | 93.1% | 3 | 75.0% | 29 | 90.6% | 1 | 100.0% |
| | 1 | 1 | 4.8% | 2 | 16.7% | 1 | 4.8% | 2 | 16.7% | 2 | 6.9% | 1 | 25.0% | 3 | 9.4% | | |
| | | $p$ = 0.538 | | | | $p$ = 0.538 | | | | $p$ = 0.330 | | | | $p$ = 1.000 | | | |
| Linear striae | 0 | 20 | 95.2% | 9 | 75.0% | 19 | 90.5% | 10 | 83.3% | 26 | 89.7% | 3 | 75.0% | 28 | 87.5% | 1 | 100.0% |
| | 1 | 1 | 4.8% | 3 | 25.0% | 2 | 9.5% | 2 | 16.7% | 3 | 10.3% | 1 | 25.0% | 4 | 12.5% | | |
| | | $p$ = 0.125 | | | | $p$ = 0.610 | | | | $p$ = 0.420 | | | | $p$ = 1.000 | | | |
| Reticular striae | 0 | 19 | 90.5% | 8 | 66.7% | 19 | 90.5% | 8 | 66.7% | 24 | 82.8% | 3 | 75.0% | 26 | 81.3% | 1 | 100.0% |
| | 1 | 2 | 9.5% | 4 | 33.3% | 2 | 9.5% | 4 | 33.3% | 5 | 17.2% | 1 | 25.0% | 6 | 18.8% | | |
| | | $p$ = 0.159 | | | | $p$ = 0.159 | | | | $p$ = 1.000 | | | | $p$ = 1.000 | | | |
| Leaf venation | 0 | 21 | 100.0% | 12 | 100.0% | 21 | 100.0% | 12 | 100.0% | 29 | 100.0% | 4 | 100.0% | 32 | 100.0% | 1 | 100.0% |
| | 1 | - | - | - | - | - | - | - | - | - | - | - | - | - | - | - | - |
| | | - | | | | - | | | | - | | | | - | | | |
| Annular striae | 0 | 21 | 100.0% | 10 | 83.3% | 20 | 95.2% | 11 | 91.7% | 28 | 96.6% | 3 | 75.0% | 30 | 93.8% | 1 | 100.0% |
| | 1 | | | 2 | 16.7% | 1 | 4.8% | 1 | 8.3% | 1 | 3.4% | 1 | 25.0% | 2 | 6.3% | | |
| | | $p$ = 0.125 | | | | $p$ = 1.000 | | | | $p$ = 0.231 | | | | $p$ = 1.000 | | | |
| Globular | 0 | 19 | 90.5% | 10 | 83.3% | 18 | 85.7% | 11 | 91.7% | 25 | 86.2% | 4 | 100.0% | 28 | 87.5% | 1 | 100.0% |
| | 1 | 2 | 9.5% | 2 | 16.7% | 3 | 14.3% | 1 | 8.3% | 4 | 13.8% | | | 4 | 12.5% | | |
| | | $p$ = 0.610 | | | | $p$ = 1.000 | | | | $p$ = 1.000 | | | | $p$ = 1.000 | | | |
| Dotted | 0 | 20 | 95.2% | 12 | 100.0% | 21 | 100.0% | 11 | 91.7% | 29 | 100.0% | 3 | 75.0% | 31 | 96.9% | 1 | 100.0% |
| | 1 | 1 | 4.8% | | | | | 1 | 8.3% | | | 1 | 25.0% | 1 | 3.1% | | |
| | | $p$ = 1.000 | | | | $p$ = 0.364 | | | | $p$ = 0.121 | | | | $p$ = 1.000 | | | |
| Veil | 0 | 14 | 66.7% | 5 | 41.7% | 14 | 66.7% | 5 | 41.7% | 19 | 65.5% | | | 19 | 59.4% | | |
| | 1 | 7 | 33.3% | 7 | 58.3% | 7 | 33.3% | 7 | 58.3% | 10 | 34.5% | 4 | 100.0% | 13 | 40.6% | 1 | 100.0% |
| | | $p$ = 0.162 | | | | $p$ = 0.162 | | | | $p$ = 0.024 * | | | | $p$ = 0.424 | | | |
| Rosette | 0 | 21 | 100.0% | 12 | 100.0% | 21 | 100.0% | 12 | 100.0% | 29 | 100.0% | 4 | 100.0% | 32 | 100.0% | 1 | 100.0% |
| | 1 | - | - | - | - | - | - | - | - | - | - | - | - | - | - | - | - |
| | | - | | | | - | | | | - | | | | - | | | |
| Leukoplakia-like | 0 | 14 | 66.7% | 3 | 25.0% | 15 | 71.4% | 2 | 16.7% | 17 | 58.6% | | | 17 | 53.1% | | |
| | 1 | 7 | 33.3% | 9 | 75.0% | 6 | 28.6% | 10 | 83.3% | 12 | 41.4% | 4 | 100.0% | 15 | 46.9% | 1 | 100.0% |
| | | $p$ = 0.021 * | | | | $p$ = 0.002 ** | | | | $p$ = 0.044 * | | | | $p$ = 0.485 | | | |
| **Total** | | **21** | **100.0%** | **12** | **100.0%** | **21** | **100.0%** | **12** | **100.0%** | **29** | **100.0%** | **4** | **100.0%** | **32** | **100.0%** | **1** | **100.0%** |

Pearson Chi-squared test. * Statistically significant, ** statistically highly significant.

**Table A4.** Association between lingual erosions and blood vessels.

| LINGUAL EROSION | | BLOOD VESSELS | | | | | | | | | | | | | | | |
|---|---|---|---|---|---|---|---|---|---|---|---|---|---|---|---|---|---|
| | | Linear | | | | Dotted | | | | Looped | | | | Sea Anemone-Like | | | |
| | | 0 | | 1 | | 0 | | 1 | | 0 | | 1 | | 0 | | 1 | |
| | | N | % | N | % | N | % | N | % | N | % | N | % | N | % | N | % |
| | 0 | 17 | 81.0% | 2 | 16.7% | 17 | 81.0% | 2 | 16.7% | 18 | 62.1% | 1 | 25.0% | 19 | 59.4% | | |
| | 1 | 4 | 19.0% | 10 | 83.3% | 4 | 19.0% | 10 | 83.3% | 11 | 37.9% | 3 | 75.0% | 13 | 40.6% | 1 | 100.0% |
| | | $p$ < 0.001 ** | | | | $p$ < 0.001 ** | | | | $p$ = 0.288 | | | | $p$ = 0.424 | | | |
| **Total** | | **21** | **100.0%** | **12** | **100.0%** | **21** | **100.0%** | **12** | **100.0%** | **29** | **100.0%** | **4** | **100.0%** | **32** | **100.0%** | **1** | **100.0%** |

Pearson Chi-squared test. ** statistically highly significant.

**Table A5.** Association between white lesions and blood vessel patterns of the buccal mucosa.

| BUCCAL | | BLOOD VESSELS | | | | | | | | | | | | | | | |
|---|---|---|---|---|---|---|---|---|---|---|---|---|---|---|---|---|---|
| | | Linear | | | | Dotted | | | | Looped | | | | Sea Anemone-Like | | | |
| WHITE LESIONS | | 0 | | 1 | | 0 | | 1 | | 0 | | 1 | | 0 | | 1 | |
| | | N | % | N | % | N | % | N | % | N | % | N | % | N | % | N | % |
| Radial striae | 0 | 23 | 82.1% | 3 | 60.0% | 22 | 78.6% | 4 | 80.0% | 24 | 77.4% | 2 | 100.0% | 26 | 81.3% | | |
| | 1 | 5 | 17.9% | 2 | 40.0% | 6 | 21.4% | 1 | 20.0% | 7 | 22.6% | | | 6 | 18.8% | 1 | 100.0% |
| | | $p = 0.282$ | | | | $p = 1.000$ | | | | $p = 1.000$ | | | | $p = 0.212$ | | | |
| Linear striae | 0 | 23 | 82.1% | 3 | 60.0% | 23 | 82.1% | 3 | 60.0% | 26 | 83.9% | | | 26 | 81.3% | | |
| | 1 | 5 | 17.9% | 2 | 40.0% | 5 | 17.9% | 2 | 40.0% | 5 | 16.1% | 2 | 100.0% | 6 | 18.8% | 1 | 100.0% |
| | | $p = 0.282$ | | | | $p = 0.282$ | | | | $p = 0.040$ * | | | | $p = 0.212$ | | | |
| Reticular striae | 0 | 1 | 3.6% | 2 | 40.0% | 3 | 10.7% | | | 2 | 6.5% | 1 | 50.0% | 3 | 9.4% | | |
| | 1 | 27 | 96.4% | 3 | 60.0% | 25 | 89.3% | 5 | 100.0% | 29 | 93.5% | 1 | 50.0% | 29 | 90.6% | 1 | 100.0% |
| | | $p = 0.053$ * | | | | $p = 1.000$ | | | | $p = 0.176$ | | | | $p = 1.000$ | | | |
| Leaf venation | 0 | 22 | 78.6% | 5 | 100.0% | 22 | 78.6% | 5 | 100.0% | 25 | 80.6% | 2 | 100.0% | 26 | 81.3% | 1 | 100.0% |
| | 1 | 6 | 21.4% | | | 6 | 21.4% | | | 6 | 19.4% | | | 6 | 18.8% | | |
| | | $p = 0.556$ | | | | $p = 0.556$ | | | | $p = 1.000$ | | | | $p = 1.000$ | | | |
| Annular striae | 0 | 28 | 100.0% | 4 | 80.0% | 27 | 96.4% | 5 | 100.0% | 31 | 100.0% | 1 | 50.0% | 31 | 96.9% | 1 | 100.0% |
| | 1 | | | 1 | 20.0% | 1 | 3.6% | | | | | 1 | 50.0% | 1 | 3.1% | | |
| | | $p = 0.152$ | | | | $p = 1.000$ | | | | $p = 0.061$ * | | | | $p = 1.000$ | | | |
| Globular | 0 | 28 | 100.0% | 4 | 80.0% | 27 | 96.4% | 5 | 100.0% | 31 | 100.0% | 1 | 50.0% | 31 | 96.9% | 1 | 100.0% |
| | 1 | | | 1 | 20.0% | 1 | 3.6% | | | | | 1 | 50.0% | 1 | 3.1% | | |
| | | $p = 0.152$ | | | | $p = 1.000$ | | | | $p = 0.061$ * | | | | $p = 1.000$ | | | |
| Dotted | 0 | 26 | 92.9% | 4 | 80.0% | 25 | 89.3% | 5 | 100.0% | 29 | 93.5% | 1 | 50.0% | 29 | 90.6% | 1 | 100.0% |
| | 1 | 2 | 7.1% | 1 | 20.0% | 3 | 10.7% | | | 2 | 6.5% | 1 | 50.0% | 3 | 9.4% | | |
| | | $p = 0.400$ | | | | $p = 1.000$ | | | | $p = 0.176$ | | | | $p = 1.000$ | | | |
| Veil | 0 | 22 | 78.6% | 4 | 80.0% | 24 | 85.7% | 2 | 40.0% | 25 | 80.6% | 1 | 50.0% | 26 | 81.3% | | |
| | 1 | 6 | 21.4% | 1 | 20.0% | 4 | 14.3% | 3 | 60.0% | 6 | 19.4% | 1 | 50.0% | 6 | 18.8% | 1 | 100.0% |
| | | $p = 1.000$ | | | | $p = 0.052$ * | | | | $p = 0.384$ | | | | $p = 0.212$ | | | |
| Rosette | 0 | 28 | 100.0% | 5 | 100.0% | 28 | 100.0% | 5 | 100.0% | 31 | 100.0% | 2 | 100.0% | 32 | 100.0% | 1 | 100.0% |
| | 1 | - | - | - | - | - | - | - | - | - | - | - | - | - | - | - | - |
| | | - | | | | - | | | | - | | | | - | | | |
| Leukoplakia-like | 0 | 25 | 89.3% | 3 | 60.0% | 25 | 89.3% | 3 | 60.0% | 27 | 87.1% | 1 | 50.0% | 27 | 84.4% | 1 | 100.0% |
| | 1 | 3 | 10.7% | 2 | 40.0% | 3 | 10.7% | 2 | 40.0% | 4 | 12.9% | 1 | 50.0% | 5 | 15.6% | | |
| | | $p = 0.155$ | | | | $p = 0.155$ | | | | $p = 0.284$ | | | | $p = 1.000$ | | | |
| **Total** | | **28** | **100.0%** | **5** | **100.0%** | **28** | **100.0%** | **5** | **100.0%** | **31** | **100.0%** | **2** | **100.0%** | **32** | **100.0%** | **1** | **100.0%** |

Pearson Chi-squared test. * Statistically significant.

**Table A6.** Association between buccal erosions and blood vessels.

| BUCCAL | BLOOD VESSELS | | | | | | | | | | | | | | | |
|---|---|---|---|---|---|---|---|---|---|---|---|---|---|---|---|---|
| | Linear | | | | Dotted | | | | Looped | | | | Sea Anemone-Like | | | |
| EROSION | 0 | | 1 | | 0 | | 1 | | 0 | | 1 | | 0 | | 1 | |
| | N | % | N | % | N | % | N | % | N | % | N | % | N | % | N | % |
| 0 | 21 | 75.0% | | | 19 | 67.9% | 2 | 40.0% | 20 | 64.5% | 1 | 50.0% | 21 | 65.6% | | |
| 1 | 7 | 25.0% | 5 | 100.0% | 9 | 32.1% | 3 | 60.0% | 11 | 35.5% | 1 | 50.0% | 11 | 34.4% | 1 | 100.0% |
| | $p = 0.003$ ** | | | | $p = 0.328$ | | | | $p = 1.000$ | | | | $p = 0.364$ | | | |
| **Total** | **28** | **100.0%** | **5** | **100.0%** | **28** | **100.0%** | **5** | **100.0%** | **31** | **100.0%** | **2** | **100.0%** | **32** | **100.0%** | **1** | **100.0%** |

Pearson Chi-squared test. ** statistically highly significant.

## References


1. Warnakulasuriya, S. Clinical Features and Presentation of Oral Potentially Malignant Disorders. *Oral Surg. Oral Med. Oral Pathol. Oral Radiol.* **2018**, *125*, 582–590. [CrossRef] [PubMed]
2. Lavanya, N.; Jayanthi, P.; Rao, U.K.; Ranganathan, K. Oral lichen planus: An update on pathogenesis and treatment. *J. Oral Maxillofac. Pathol.* **2011**, *15*, 127–132. [CrossRef] [PubMed]
3. Li, C.; Tang, X.; Zheng, X.; Ge, S.; Wen, H.; Lin, X.; Chen, Z.; Lu, L. Global Prevalence and Incidence Estimates of Oral Lichen Planus: A Systematic Review and Meta-analysis. *JAMA Dermatol.* **2020**, *156*, 172–181. [CrossRef] [PubMed]
4. Mohan, R.P.S.; Gupta, A.; Kamarthi, N.; Malik, S.; Goel, S.; Gupta, S. Incidence of Oral Lichen Planus in Perimenopausal Women: A Cross-sectional Study in Western Uttar Pradesh Population. *J. Midlife Health* **2017**, *8*, 70–74. [CrossRef]

5. Arduino, P.G.; Magliano, A.; Gambino, A.; Macciotta, A.; Carbone, M.; Conrotto, D.; Karimi, D.; Carrozzo, M.; Broccoletti, R. Risk of Malignant Transformation in 3173 Subjects with Histopathologically Confirmed Oral Lichen Planus: A 33-Year Cohort Study in Northern Italy. *Cancers* **2021**, *13*, 5740. [CrossRef]
6. González-Moles, M.Á.; Ramos-García, P. An Evidence-Based Update on the Potential for Malignancy of Oral Lichen Planus and Related Conditions: A Systematic Review and Meta-Analysis. *Cancers* **2024**, *16*, 608. [CrossRef]
7. Manchanda, Y.; Rathi, S.K.; Joshi, A.; Das, S. Oral Lichen Planus: An Updated Review of Etiopathogenesis, Clinical Presentation, and Management. *Indian Dermatol. Online J.* **2023**, *15*, 8–23. [CrossRef] [PubMed]
8. Adnane, S.; Mahad, C.; Haitami, S.; Yahya, I.B. Hepatitis C virus infection and oral lichen planus: A controversial association. *Adv. Oral Maxillofac. Surg.* **2022**, *6*, 100271. [CrossRef]
9. Rahat, S.; Kashetsky, N.; Bagit, A.; Sachdeva, M.; Lytvyn, Y.; Mufti, A.; Maibach, H.I.; Yeung, J. Can We Separate Oral Lichen Planus from Allergic Contact Dermatitis and Should We Patch Test? A Systematic Review of Chronic Oral Lichenoid Lesions. *Dermatitis* **2021**, *32*, 144–150. [CrossRef]
10. Teoh, L.; Moses, G.; McCullough, M.J. A review and guide to drug-associated oral adverse effects—Oral mucosal and lichenoid reactions. Part 2. *J. Oral Pathol. Med.* **2019**, *48*, 637–646. [CrossRef]
11. Gholizadeh, N.; Sadeghi, A.; Mirzaii-Dizgah, I.; Sheykhbahaei, N. Serum level of estrogen in Iranian patients with oral lichen planus. *Asian Biomed. (Res. Rev. News)* **2021**, *15*, 145–150. [CrossRef] [PubMed]
12. Ślebioda, Z.; Drożdżyńska, J.; Karpińska, A.; Krzyżaniak, A.; Kasperczak, M.; Tomoń, N.; Wiśniewska, P.; Wyganowska, M.L. Oral Lichen Planus: Clinical Presentation, Demographic Characteristics, and Risk Factors in a Retrospective Study of 186 Polish Patients. *J. Clin. Med.* **2024**, *13*, 7363. [CrossRef] [PubMed]
13. Arnold, D.L.; Krishnamurthy, K. Lichen Planus. [Updated 29 October 2024]. In *StatPearls*; StatPearls Publishing: Treasure Island, FL, USA, 2025. Available online: https://www.ncbi.nlm.nih.gov/books/NBK526126/ (accessed on 12 February 2025).
14. GunaShekhar, M.; Sudhakar, R.; Shahul, M.; Tenny, J.; Ravikanth, M.; Manikyakumar, N. Oral lichen planus in childhood: A rare case report. *Dermatol. Online J.* **2010**, *16*, 9. [CrossRef]
15. Gall, R.; Navarro-Fernandez, I.N. Lichen Planus Erosive Form. [Updated 24 July 2023]. In *StatPearls*; StatPearls Publishing: Treasure Island, FL, USA, 2025. Available online: https://www.ncbi.nlm.nih.gov/books/NBK560700/ (accessed on 8 February 2025).
16. Tampa, M.; Mitran, M.; Mitran, C.; Sarbu, I.; Rusu, L.-C.; Matei, C.; Constantin, C.; Neagu, M.; Georgescu, S.-R. Markers of Oral Lichen Planus Malignant Transformation. *Dis. Markers* **2018**, *2018*, 1959506. [CrossRef]
17. Idrees, M.; Kujan, O.; Shearston, K.; Farah, C.S. Oral lichen planus has a very low malignant transformation rate: A systematic review and meta-analysis using strict diagnostic and inclusion criteria. *J. Oral Pathol. Med.* **2021**, *50*, 287–298. [CrossRef]
18. Van Der, M.E.H.; Van Der, W.I. Lack of clinicopathologic correlation in the diagnosis of oral lichen planus based on the presently available diagnostic criteria and suggestions for modifications. *J. Oral Pathol. Med.* **2003**, *32*, 507–512. [CrossRef]
19. Batra, M.R.; Mohod, S.; Sawarbandhe, P. Oral Lichen Planus and Its Therapeutic Approaches: A Case Report. *Cureus* **2024**, *16*, e63192. [CrossRef]
20. Litaiem, N.; Mansour, Y.; Jones, M.; Zeglaoui, F. Dermoscopic signs of lichen planus. *BMJ Case Rep.* **2016**, *2016*, bcr2015213923. [CrossRef]
21. Buajeeb, W.; Okuma, N.; Thanakun, S.; Laothumthut, T. Direct Immunofluorescence in Oral Lichen Planus. *J. Clin. Diagn. Res.* **2015**, *9*, ZC34–ZC37. [CrossRef]
22. Yu, S.; Sun, W.; Mi, D.; Jin, S.; Wu, X.; Xin, B.; Zhang, H.; Wang, Y.; Sun, X.; He, X. Artificial Intelligence Diagnosing of Oral Lichen Planus: A Comparative Study. *Bioengineering* **2024**, *11*, 1159. [CrossRef]
23. Achararit, P.; Manaspon, C.; Jongwannasiri, C.; Phattarataratip, E.; Osathanon, T.; Sappayatosok, K. Artificial Intelligence-Based Diagnosis of Oral Lichen Planus Using Deep Convolutional Neural Networks. *Eur. J. Dent.* **2023**, *17*, 1275–1282. [CrossRef] [PubMed]
24. Chen, X.; Lu, Q.; Chen, C.; Jiang, G. Recent developments in dermoscopy for dermatology. *J. Cosmet. Dermatol.* **2021**, *20*, 1611–1617. [CrossRef] [PubMed]
25. Ashok, S. Dermatoscopy: A New Diagnostic Approach for Lesions on Mucous Membrane. In *Clinical Diagnosis and Management of Squamous Cell Carcinoma*; IntechOpen: London, UK, 2023. [CrossRef]
26. Rouai, M.; Litaiem, N.; Hammami, H.; Bacha, T.; Jones, M.; Ksontini, M.; Rammeh, S.; Mokni, M.; Zeglaoui, F. Dermoscopic features of mucosal lichen planus. *Int. J. Dermatol.* **2021**, *60*, 1368–1372. [CrossRef]
27. Singh, S.K.; Kharabanda, A.; Kundalia, A. Dermoscopic features in different types of lichen planus: A case series. *Int. J. Res. Dermatol.* **2025**, *11*, 151–156. [CrossRef]
28. Humberto, J.S.M.; Saia, R.S.; Costa, L.H.A.; Rocha, M.J.A.; Motta, A.C.F. Salivary cytokine profile in patients with oral lichen planus. *Odovtos Int. J. Dent. Sci.* **2024**, *26*, 128–140. [CrossRef]

29. Popa, C.; Sciuca, A.M.; Onofrei, B.-A.; Toader, S.; Hritcu, O.M.C.; Colac, C.B.; Andrese, E.P.; Brănișteanu, D.E.; Toader, M.P. Integrative Approaches for the Diagnosis and Management of Erosive Oral Lichen Planus. *Diagnostics* **2024**, *14*, 692. [CrossRef]
30. Mittal, S.; Vinitha, N.M.; Chaitra, V. Dermoscopy of Isolated Lip Lichen Planus. *Indian Dermatol. Online J.* **2022**, *13*, 165–166. [CrossRef]
31. Marcu, C.A.; Parlatescu, I.; Tovaru, S.; Nicolae, C.L.; Costache, M.; Tovaru, M. Lichen Planus of the Lip—Case Series and Review of the Literature. *Medicina* **2024**, *60*, 987. [CrossRef]
32. Rather, S.; Shah, A.A.; Shah, F.Y.; S, K.; Bhat, M.A.; Reyaz, S.; Hassan, I. Dermoscopy of Oral Mucosal Lesions: Experience from a Tertiary Care Center in North India and Review of Literature. *Indian Dermatol. Online J.* **2022**, *13*, 346–360. [CrossRef]
33. Sachdeva, S.; Sachdeva, S.; Kapoor, P. Wickham striae: Etiopathogenensis and clinical significance. *Indian J. Dermatol.* **2011**, *56*, 442–443. [CrossRef]
34. Makhecha, M.; Singh, T.; Malladi, N.; Rambhia, K. Dermoscopic features of various stages of lichen planus. *Indian J. Dermatol. Venereol. Leprol.* **2020**, *86*, 191–194. [CrossRef]
35. Sonthalia, S.; Varma, S.; Jha, A.K.; Jakhar, D.; Kaliyadan, F. Case Report: Dermoscopic features of oral lichen planus—The evolution of mucoscopy. *F1000Research* **2018**, *7*, 284. [CrossRef] [PubMed]
36. Jha, A.K.; Vinay, K.; Sławińska, M.; Sonthalia, S.; Sobjanek, M.; Kamińska-Winciorek, G.; Errichetti, E.; Kamat, D.; Chatterjee, D.; Apalla, Z.; et al. Application of mucous membrane dermoscopy (mucoscopy) in diagnostics of benign oral lesions—Literature review and preliminary observations from International Dermoscopy Society study. *Dermatol. Ther.* **2021**, *34*, e14478. [CrossRef]
37. Sousa, F.; Blumer Rosa, L. Oral lichen planus: Clinical and histopathological considerations. *Braz. J. Otorhinolaryngol.* **2008**, *74*, 284–292. [CrossRef] [PubMed]
38. Jose, S.C.; Kurien, G.V. Diagnostic dermoscopic features and the correlation between dermoscopic and histopathologic features in lichen planus. *Int. J. Res. Dermatol.* **2020**, *6*, 637–640. [CrossRef]
39. Peralta, R.; Salerni, G.; Sabban, E.C.; Marin, M.B.; Cabo, H. Dermoscopy of a Squamous Cell Carcinoma of the Lower Lip Showing Multiple Rosettes. *Dermatol. Pract. Concept.* **2019**, *10*, e2020022. [CrossRef]
40. Lallas, A.; Martínez, G.; Arceu, M.; Kyrgidis, A.; Liopyris, K.; Brancaccio, G.; Longo, C.; Errichetti, E.; Sgouros, D.; Papageorgiou, C.; et al. Clinical and dermatoscopic predictors of squamous cell carcinoma of the lips: A case-control, multicentric study. *J. Eur. Acad. Dermatol. Venereol.* **2022**, *36*, 222–227. [CrossRef]
41. Tsushima, F.; Sakurai, J.; Uesugi, A.; Oikawa, Y.; Ohsako, T.; Mochizuki, Y.; Hirai, H.; Kayamori, K.; Harada, H. Malignant transformation of oral lichen planus: A retrospective study of 565 Japanese patients. *BMC Oral Health* **2021**, *21*, 298. [CrossRef]
42. Cheng, Y.S.; Gould, A.; Kurago, Z.; Fantasia, J.; Muller, S. Diagnosis of oral lichen planus: A position paper of the American Academy of Oral and Maxillofacial Pathology. *Oral Surg. Oral Med. Oral Pathol. Oral Radiol.* **2016**, *122*, 332–354. [CrossRef]

*diagnostics*

MDPI

*Article*

# Discrepancy in the Histological Diagnoses of Oral Lichen Planus Based on WHO Criteria Versus the Newly Proposed Diagnostic Set of the American Academy of Oral and Maxillofacial Pathology

**Maria Zaharieva Mutafchieva [1,*] and Desislava Atanasova Tashkova [2,3]**

1 Department of Periodontology and Oral Mucosa Diseases, Faculty of Dental Medicine, Medical University of Plovdiv, 4000 Plovdiv, Bulgaria
2 Department of General and Clinical Pathology, Faculty of Medicine, Medical University of Plovdiv, 4000 Plovdiv, Bulgaria; desislava.tashkova@mu-plovdiv.bg
3 Department of Clinical Pathology, Oncology Centre—Plovdiv, Medical University of Plovdiv, 4000 Plovdiv, Bulgaria
* Correspondence: mariya.mutafchieva@mu-plovdiv.bg; Tel.: +359-883339644

**Abstract: Background/Objectives**: The diagnosis of oral lichen planus (OLP) is challenging because many other oral diseases demonstrate similar clinical and microscopic features. Clinicopathological discrepancy and inter- and intraobserver variability in the histological assessment of OLP have been shown in the literature, as there are no unified diagnostic criteria for the disease. In 2016, the American Academy of Oral and Maxillofacial Pathology (AAOMP) proposed a new diagnostic set for OLP. The aim of the study was to assess the reliability of the AAOMP histological criteria in diagnosing OLP. **Methods**: In this retrospective study, 34 histological sections, once diagnosed as OLP, were revised by a second pathologist using the WHO criteria. Then, all specimens were analyzed for the presence (P) or absence (A) of the criteria listed in the AAOMP diagnostic set. The reproducibility of the histological diagnosis of OLP when applying the different sets of diagnostic criteria was assessed. **Results**: From the AAOMP diagnostic criteria, hydropic degeneration was found in 35.2%, lymphocytic exocytosis in 32.3%, mild epithelial dysplasia in 2.9%, verrucous epithelial architectural change in 0% and band-like lymphocytic infiltrate, confined to the epithelium-lamina propria interface in 55.8% of the samples. Reproducibility of the histological diagnosis of OLP was achieved in only 19.3% of the cases when applying the 1978 WHO criteria versus the newly proposed AAOMP criteria. **Conclusions**: A large number of OLP cases failed to meet the AAOMP histological criteria in the present study. Further studies are needed to assess the validity of the proposed diagnostic set.

**Keywords:** oral lichen planus; OLP; American Academy of Oral and Maxillofacial Pathology (AAOMP) diagnostic set; histological assessment

## 1. Introduction

A number of dermatological diseases can affect the oral mucosa. Lichen planus (LP) is a common mucocutaneous disease. Classic LP on the skin presents as polygonal pruritic red–purple papules, primarily affecting the extremities, wrists, ankles and lumbar region [1,2]. When oral lesions occur together with skin lesions, diagnosis is relatively straightforward, but in up to 25% of cases, the oral cavity is the only site of involvement—oral lichen planus

(OLP) [1]. OLP has a global prevalence of 1.01% and usually affects women aged 30 to 60 years [3]. Although enormous efforts have been invested in research, there are still many unanswered questions regarding the etiology, pathogenesis and malignant potential of the disease. Clinically, OLP can manifest in six different forms—reticular, papular, plaque-like, atrophic, erosive or bullous [4]. Keratotic forms (reticular, papular, plaque-like) appear as white lesions that can not be rubbed off, while non-keratotic forms present either as red areas of thinned mucosa, erosions or blisters. Wickham striae, representing slightly raised gray–white lines in a net-like configuration, are considered a pathognomonic sign of the disease and should usually be present elsewhere in the oral cavity. Subjective symptoms range from mild discomfort to excruciating pain.

Cases of OLP often present difficulties in terms of differential diagnostic analysis. Due to the wide variety of clinical manifestations, OLP must be distinguished from a number of other white, red, red-white, ulcerative, and bullous lesions of the oral mucosa that may resemble OLP both clinically and histopathologically—the so-called oral lichenoid lesions (OLLs) [5]. On the gingiva, OLP often manifests as desquamative gingivitis—a situation in which it is clinically indistinguishable from some OLP mimics, such as mucous membrane pemphigoid (MMP), pemphigus vulgaris, etc. The following diagnostic criteria have been proposed as an attempt to increase the accuracy of the clinical diagnosis of OLP: detection of multiple lesions with bilateral symmetric distribution; erosive, atrophic, bullous and plaque-type lesions are only accepted as a subtype in the presence of reticular lesions elsewhere in the oral mucosa [6]; lesions are not localized exclusively in contact with dental restorations or in sites of smokeless tobacco placement; lesion onset does not correlate with the start of a medication or the use of cinnamon-containing products [5].

However, due to the high clinical mimicry with other conditions, histological analysis of suspected OLP lesions is generally advised. Moreover, OLP is defined as an oral potentially malignant disorder (OPMD) [7]. Histologically, OLP demonstrates typical but non-pathognomonic features. Therefore, the pathoanatomical diagnosis of the disease is not definitive but should be considered in correlation with the clinical diagnosis and accepted only when the two coincide. Making an accurate histological diagnosis is challenging due to the following factors: 1. The histological finding may vary depending on the clinical form of OLP, the biopsy area, the activity of the condition and the administration of immunosuppressive therapy; 2. No unified diagnostic criteria for the disease have been adopted; 3. There seems to be a low correlation in the diagnosis of oral lichen planus among examiners regardless of the set of histopathological diagnostic criteria used; 4. Many microscopic features of OLP are not specific to OLP and can be found in other diseases [5].

The histological definition of OLP was first formulated by the WHO in 1978. The proposed set of diagnostic criteria includes hyperortho- or hyperparakeratosis; acanthosis or epithelial atrophy; Civatte bodies in the basal layer of the epithelium or superficial lamina propria; liquefaction degeneration in the basal cell layer, eosinophilic material in the basement membrane, saw-tooth rete ridges and a well-defined band-like zone of inflammatory cells (mainly lymphocytes) confined to the superficial lamina propria [8]. A limitation of the WHO diagnostic set is that no criteria were specified to exclude epithelial dysplasia from the diagnosis of OLP. For this reason, according to Ismail SB et al., a significant percentage of patients who developed carcinoma from oral lichen planus were actually misdiagnosed cases of other lichenoid lesions with higher malignant potential [9]. In addition, a distinction between idiopathic OLP and other OLLs, such as contact or drug-induced lichenoid reactions, cannot be made based on these criteria. Furthermore, studies have found that application of the WHO criteria was associated with the highest rate of clinicopathological discrepancy [6] and inter- and intraobserver variability in the histological assessment of oral lichen planus [10].

In 2003, Van der Meij and van der Waal proposed some modifications to the WHO criteria for OLP [6]. The authors retained some of the WHO criteria, namely liquefaction degeneration of the basal cells and a dense band-like inflammatory infiltrate composed mainly of lymphocytes and confined to the superficial lamina propria. The novelty of this modified diagnostic set is the inclusion of an additional criterion to confirm the absence of epithelial dysplasia. Along with this, the authors introduced the term "histopathologically compatible with OLP" for all cases that do not meet all of the listed criteria. This definition points to an oral lichenoid lesion other than OLP. Later, Rad M. et al. found increased clinicopathological agreement in the diagnosis of OLP when applying van der Meij's modified criteria compared to those of the WHO [11]. However, some of the typical features of OLP that stem from important mechanisms of disease pathogenesis, such as lymphocyte migration into the epithelium, were not addressed in the modified 2003 WHO criteria.

The most recent update to the diagnostic criteria for OLP was made by the American Academy of Oral and Maxillofacial Pathology (AAOMP) in 2016 and includes a set of clinical and histological criteria [5]. Lymphocyte exocytosis and lack of verrucous epithelium architectural change are the new criteria added to those cited by Van der Meij and van der Waal. The authors stated that the diagnosis of OLP requires fulfillment of all proposed clinical and histopathological criteria.

The aim of the study was to assess the reliability of the AAOMP histological criteria in diagnosing OLP.

## 2. Materials and Methods

Research Focus Questions

- What is the reproducibility of the histological diagnoses of OLP when applying the different sets of diagnostic criteria?
- Do histological sections, once diagnosed as OLP, meet all diagnostic criteria proposed by the American Academy of Oral and Maxillofacial Pathology?

And if not,

- Which features of OLP are found consistently in all histological sections?

Study Design

This was a retrospective study that analyzed data obtained from histological reports and histological sections from patients with OLP who were diagnosed and biopsied at the Department of Periodontology and Oral Mucosal Diseases, Faculty of Dental Medicine, MU-Plovdiv between 1 January 2013 and 30 June 2016. The initial histological examination that confirmed the diagnosis of OLP was performed at the Department of General and Clinical Pathology of MU-Plovdiv. The study was conducted in accordance with the Declaration of Helsinki and was approved by the Ethics Committee of the Medical University of Plovdiv (R3716/7 October 2014). Histopathological reports were used to extract information regarding the following variables: biopsy site, clinical form of OLP and demographic characteristics of the patients included in the study. Existing hematoxylin and eosin (H&E)-stained histological slides, stored in the pathology laboratory, were revised by a single experienced pathologist who was blinded to the evaluation done retrospectively for this study in order to determine the interobserver variability in the histological diagnosis of OLP. Because the criteria used by the first evaluator were not stated in the histopathology reports, no requirements were placed on the pathologist assigned to the present study regarding the set of diagnostic criteria during this second revision of the diagnosis. After completion of the histological examination, the pathologist was asked to specify the criteria used. The same evaluator was then asked to utilize the newly proposed diagnostic set of the AAOMP while assessing slides, categorizing each criterion listed there as present (P) or absent (A).

Research Materials

- Archived histopathological reports of patients with OLP, biopsied at the Department of Periodontology and Oral Mucosal Diseases, Faculty of Dental Medicine, MU-Plovdiv, between 2013 and 2016. Only patients for whom the clinical diagnosis of OLP was confirmed by the histological examination were included in the study.
- Corresponding hematoxylin and eosin (H&E)-stained histological slides of the included patients.

Histological Analysis

All histological slides selected for revision were analyzed by light microscopy (Leica DM 2000 LED, Leica Microsystems, Wetzlar, Germany). The diagnoses made by the pathologist during this second revision were categorized as "evident OLP", "compatible with OLP" or "other mucosal lesion" and compared with the original. The criteria used by the pathologist correspond to the WHO criteria. The same evaluator was then asked to score all histological slides for the presence (P) or absence (A) of the following morphological parameters: predominantly lymphocytic infiltrate confined to the epithelium–lamina propria interface; basal cell liquefactive (hydropic) degeneration; lymphocytic exocytosis; epithelial dysplasia; verrucous epithelial architectural change. Based on the results obtained, the number of cases that fulfill the criteria proposed by the American Academy of Oral and Maxillofacial Pathology was calculated.

## 3. Results

Over a period of 4 years (2013–2016), a total of 43 patients with a clinically suspected diagnosis of OLP were biopsied at the Department of Periodontology and Oral Mucosal Diseases. In 34 of them, the diagnosis was histologically confirmed. According to the data filled in the histopathological reports, the male to female ratio was 6:28, and age ranged 23–78 years old. The age distribution was as follows: <30 years (2); 31–40 (2); 41–50 (11); 51–60 (7); and >61 (12). The buccal mucosa was the most common site for biopsy (25), followed by gingiva (7) and tongue (2). Diagnoses included 14 patients with reticular form, 1 with papular, 2 with plaque-like, 7 with atrophic, 9 with erosive and 1 with bullous form of OLP.

Of the 34 histological slides initially (at the first histological evaluation) diagnosed with OLP, 31 were categorized as "evident OLP" and another 3 as "compatible with OLP" by the second pathologist. No slides were diagnosed as "other mucosal lesion". The criteria used by the pathologist correspond to the WHO criteria and were as follows: presence of hyperkeratosis and a band-like inflammatory infiltrate consisting predominantly of lymphocytes, presence or absence of acanthosis, epithelial atrophy, Civatte bodies or basal cell liquefaction degeneration. Agreement between the first and second evaluators regarding the diagnosis of OLP was found in 91.1% of the samples.

The morphological findings observed in the studied samples are shown in Table 1. From the diagnostic criteria proposed by the American Academy of Oral and Maxillofacial Pathology, basal cell liquefactive (hydropic) degeneration was found in 35.2% ($n$ = 12), lymphocytic exocytosis in 32.3% ($n$ = 11) and mild epithelial dysplasia in 2.9% ($n$ = 1) of the samples. A band-like predominantly lymphocytic infiltrate, confined to the epithelium–

lamina propria interface, was present in 55.8% ($n = 19$) of the sections, and in another 26.4% ($n = 9$), the infiltrate was polymorphic, composed of lymphocytes and plasma cells (with or without some neutrophils and eosinophils). In 29.4% ($n = 10$) of the samples, deep/perivascular infiltrate was demonstrated. There were no cases of verrucous epithelial architectural change. None of the histological features of OLP were consistently found in all histological sections.

**Table 1.** Frequency of observation of the different histological variables of OLP.

| Variable | Total Sample ($n$ = 34) Frequency (%) | ($n$) |
|---|---|---|
| Hyperkeratosis | 91.1% | 31 |
| Acanthosis | 85.2% | 29 |
| Epithelial atrophy | 17.6% | 6 |
| Erosion | 2.9% | 1 |
| Epidermo-dermal detachment | 23.5% | 8 |
| Basal layer hydropic degeneration | 35.2% | 12 |
| Lymphocytic exocytosis | 32.3% | 11 |
| Epithelial dysplasia | 2.9% | 1 |
| Verrucous epithelialarchitectural change | 0% | 0 |
| Civatte bodies | 8.8% | 3 |
| Saw-tooth rete ridges | 35.2% | 12 |
| Inflammatory infiltrate | 100% | 34 |
| • band-like, lymphocytic infiltrate confined only to the epithelium–lamina propria interface | 55.8% | 19 |
| • polymorphic inflammation (Ly, plasma cells, Eo, Neu) | 26.4% | 9 |
| • deep/perivascular | 29.4% | 10 |
| • dense lymphocytic infiltrate forming tertiary follicles | 2.9% | 1 |

Analysis of the aforementioned data showed that only 17.6% ($n = 6$) of the samples fulfill all histological diagnostic criteria proposed by the American Academy of Oral and Maxillofacial Pathology (simultaneous presence of predominantly lymphocytic infiltrate confined to the epithelium-lamina propria interface; basal cell liquefactive (hydropic) degeneration; lymphocytic exocytosis; absence of epithelial dysplasia; absence of verrucous epithelial architectural change) (Figure 1).

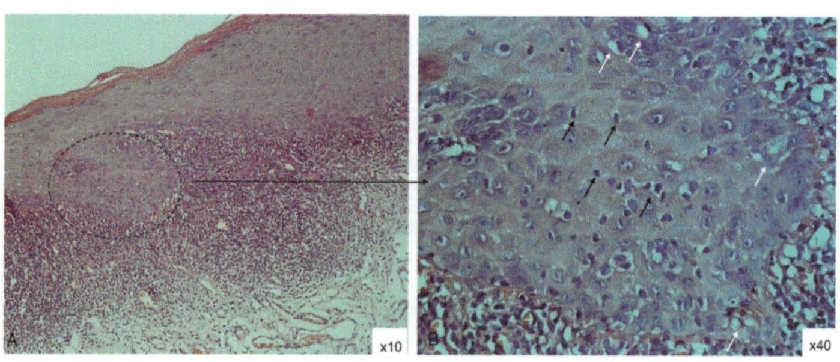


**Figure 1.** Tissue section diagnosed as OLP based on the AAOMP histological criteria, H&E staining: (**A**): $\times 10$ magnification, epithelial hyperkeratosis and acanthosis and dense band-like inflammatory infiltrate of lymphocytes in the superficial lamina propria; (**B**): same specimen $\times 40$ magnification, hydropic degeneration (white arrows), lymphocytic exocytosis (black arrows) and absence of epithelial dysplasia.

Reproducibility of the histological diagnosis of OLP was achieved in only 19.3% of the cases when applying the 1978 WHO criteria versus the newly proposed AAOMP criteria. Figure 2 illustrates a case of discrepancy in the diagnoses of oral lichen planus as a result of the different diagnostic sets used.

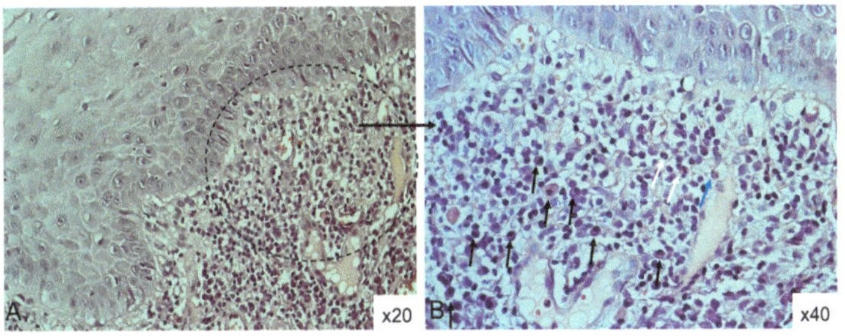


**Figure 2.** Histological section (H&E staining) diagnosed as OLP based on the 1978 WHO criteria, which does not meet the AAOMP diagnostic criteria, due to (**A**): absence of hydropic degeneration and lymphocytic exocytosis in the epithelium (×20 magnification) and (**B**): presence of polymorphic inflammatory infiltrate in the lamina propria; plasma cells (black arrows), eosinophils (white arrows), neutrophil (blue arrow); (×40 magnification).

## 4. Discussion

Oral lichen planus is considered a clinico-pathological diagnosis [6]. Therefore, biopsy should be taken from all patients with clinical manifestations suggestive of OLP, not only to confirm the diagnosis but also to exclude malignancy. However, especially in cases with the classic reticular form of the disease, histological examination is often omitted [3]. This may explain the relatively low number of histological sections from OLP patients over a 4-year period analyzed in the present study. A review of the data from the archive of the Department of Periodontology and Oral Mucosal Diseases showed that out of a total of 81 patients clinically diagnosed with OLP during this period, only 43 had a biopsy performed.

Agreement on the histological diagnosis of OLP between the pathologist who had performed the initial examination and the second pathologist who was asked to review the same tissue sections for the purposes of the present study was achieved in 91.1% of cases. WHO criteria were used by the second observer. The criteria applied during the first examination were not reported in the histopathology reports we reviewed. However, since we intentionally limited the observation period to before 30 June 2016, it is unlikely that the pathologist used AAOMP criteria, as these were first introduced in September 2016. Therefore, we believe that the initial and second revised diagnoses of OLP were made based on the same criteria.

In 1978, the WHO Collaborating Centre for Oral Precancerous Lesions published a number of histological features commonly observed in tissue sections from patients with OLP to be used as diagnostic criteria [8]. However, no requirement was made to fulfill all these criteria. Thus, OLP specimens demonstrating all the typical features of the disease are relatively easy to diagnose, but in cases covering part of the criteria, the diagnosis is made based on the subjective judgment of the pathologist. The difficulty comes from the fact that most of the listed histological features are not specific to OLP but can also be found in other diseases. For example, interface mucositis (band-like chiefly lymphocytic infiltrate in superficial lamina propria) is also present in lupus erythematosus, drug-induced and contact lichenoid reactions, in some cases of proliferative verrucous leukoplakia, oral epithelial dysplasia and squamous cell carcinoma. Liquefaction degeneration of basal keratinocytes could be seen in graft-versus-host disease (GVHD), contact and drug-induced lichenoid reactions and lupus erythematosus. Civatte bodies are a characteristic finding in chronic ulcerative stomatitis (CUS), lupus erythematosus (LE), GVHD, drug-induced lichenoid reactions, etc. [5,12,13]. Another disadvantage of the WHO diagnostic set is that the presence of epithelial dysplasia is not listed as an exclusion criterion. In 1985, Krutchkoff and Eisenberg introduced the term "lichenoid dysplasia" for lesions that histologically demonstrate epithelial dysplasia in combination with band-like chronic inflammatory infiltrate in the superficial lamina propria and/or other lichenoid features (saw-tooth rete pegs, Civatte bodies and basal cell degeneration) [14,15]. In a study by Fitzpatrick et al., band-like inflammatory infiltrate and basal cell degeneration (lichenoid features) were found in 74% and 30% of oral epithelial dysplasia (OED) specimens, respectively [16]. Thus, dysplastic lesions are often diagnosed as OLP. According to current understanding, the use of the term "lichenoid dysplasia" is the main reason for the misdiagnosis of OED (being a separate entity) as OLP. Therefore, the workgroup from the international workshop on nomenclature and classification convened by the WHO Collaborating Centre for Oral Cancer (2020) [7] recommended that the term "lichenoid dysplasia" be removed and stated that if dysplasia is present, the diagnosis should be oral epithelial dysplasia with lichenoid features. In the present study, epithelial dysplasia was found in one specimen (Table 1). However, both the first and second pathologists diagnosed the case as oral lichen planus, which again confirms the assumption that both used the WHO criteria.

The newly proposed diagnostic set of the American Academy of Oral and Maxillofacial Pathology is based on the knowledge accumulated over the years regarding the distinguishing characteristics of some of the most common "OLP mimics" [5]. According to the authors, the use of the listed criteria will make the OLP patient group a more homogeneous population of idiopathic OLP for future research, which would increase the validity of any statements regarding the pathogenesis and malignant potential of the disease.

Liquefaction, also known as hydropic degeneration of the basal cells, is a pathological edema of the keratinocytes due to an increased membrane permeability of the damaged cell. The influx of water in hydropic degeneration dilutes the cytoplasm, separates cell organelles and stretches the cell [17]. Microscopically, the affected keratinocytes appear greatly enlarged with pale and homogenized cytoplasm, creating in places the impression of optically empty cells (Figure 1). In the present study, hydropic degeneration was found in only 35.2% ($n$ = 12) of the OLP tissue sections. Similar results were reported by Sanches et al., who observed basal layer degeneration in 39.6% ($n$ = 19) of the specimens ($n$ = 48) from OLP lesions analyzed in their study [3].

Migration of lymphocytes into the overlying epithelium, known as lymphocytic exocytosis, is a newly added criterion for the diagnosis of OLP by the AAOMP [5]. The general consensus regarding the pathogenesis of the disease is that it is an immune-mediated condition in which CD8+ T-lymphocytes destroy basal keratinocytes by activating the cell death program (apoptosis). Jungell et al. conducted an immunoelectron microscopic study to demonstrate that most of the CD8+ cells were located intraepithelially, adjacent to apoptotic keratinocytes [18]. Therefore, the AAMOP working group considered it justified to observe lymphocyte exocytosis in all cases of OLP and to include it as a mandatory diagnostic criterion. In addition, according to the authors, this finding may help distinguish OLP from other oral lichenoid conditions, such as MMP, because the immune aggression there is directed against adhesion molecules in the basement membrane zone and lymphocytes are not usually seen in the epithelium. However, lymphocyte exocytosis was not a consistent finding among the specimens we analyzed. In particular, it was detected in only 32.3% ($n$ = 11) of them (Figure 1).

The detection of Civatte bodies in the basal layer is not listed as a criterion in the newly proposed AAOMP diagnostic set. Civatte (also known as colloid or hyaline) bodies represent anucleated remnants of epithelial cells formed as a result of an activated process of programmed cell death (apoptosis). In recent years, the thesis of pathologically enhanced apoptosis being present in OLP has been disputed [19]. One of the reasons for this is the reported low number of Civatte bodies [19]. Of note, in our study, colloid bodies were found in only three cases (8.8%).

The absence of verrucous epithelial architectural change was added by the AAOMP as a diagnostic criterion in an attempt to differentiate OLP and proliferative verrucous leukoplakia (PVL), as these two entities share similar clinical and histopathological features [5]. Verrucous architecture is identified by a papillary configuration of the spinous cell layer accompanied by variable levels of mucosal surface corrugation [5]. Such changes were not observed in any of the samples we analyzed.

According to the AAOMP working group, the presence of epithelial dysplasia in the specimen excludes the diagnosis of oral lichen planus [5]. Therefore, "OLP with dysplasia" cannot be the pathologist's conclusion at the first histological examination of a patient. This diagnosis can be made during a follow-up histological examination if signs of malignancy have appeared in the evolution of the initially non-malignant OLP lesion. In the present study, epithelial dysplasia was observed in one specimen. Applying the AAOMP diagnostic criteria, the latter cannot be diagnosed as oral lichen planus.

Last but not least, the mononuclear, predominantly lymphocytic, band-like infiltrate in the superficial lamina propria (interface mucositis), being one of the most characteristic microscopic findings of OLP, is also listed as a mandatory diagnostic criterion by the AAOMP. However, Sanches et al. reported an absent/mild inflammatory infiltrate in 25% of the OLP samples ($n$ = 48) they analyzed [3]. In the present study, inflammatory infiltrate in the epithelium–lamina propria interface was found in all cases. However, in 26.4% ($n$ = 9) of them, the infiltrate was polymorphic (composed of lymphocytes, plasma cells, eosinophils and/or neutrophils) (Figure 2), and in 29.4% ($n$ = 10), a deep/perivascular infiltrate was additionally observed. A dense lymphocytic infiltrate forming tertiary follicles was found in one specimen. All of these findings—diffuse lymphocytic infiltrate mixed with plasma cells and eosinophils extending deeper into the lamina propria, focal perivascular infiltrate and tertiary lymphoid follicles—have been repeatedly highlighted in the literature as distinguishing features of oral lichenoid reactions (OLRs) [12,20]. The latter term refers to lesions that are clinically and histologically similar to those of OLP but have an identifiable causative factor (contact OLR, drug-induced OLR and GVHD-associated OLR), the removal of which results in regression of the lesions. Differentiating OLR from idiopathic OLP is a diagnostic challenge. Unfortunately, even this set of strict criteria may not be helpful in distinguishing these two entities, as OLRs often show microscopic features that fulfill all of the histopathological criteria proposed by the AAOMP. However, the authors recommend pathologists refrain from diagnosing OLP if eosinophils or a perivascular lymphoplasmacytic infiltrate in the deep lamina propria are present, although these findings are not formally listed as exclusion criteria in their diagnostic set (Figure 2) [5]. In the present study, one of the six specimens meeting all AAOMP diagnostic criteria demonstrated a mixed (lymphocyte and plasma cell) infiltrate, and another one demonstrated additional deep/perivascular inflammation. It is worth noting that the clinical type (reticular vs. erosive) and anatomical site (buccal mucosa vs. gingiva) should also be considered when making a histological diagnosis, as both may influence the subsets of inflammatory cells in the infiltrate [5]. For example, areas of erosion and ulceration typically demonstrate superimposed inflammation, resulting in a mixed inflammatory infiltrate rich in neutrophils, and in gingival OLP lesions, the infiltrate is often mixed with plasma cells due to concomitant gingivitis or periodontitis [5,12]. Of note, none of the tissue sections demonstrating a mixed with plasma cell and/or neutrophils infiltrate in the present study were taken from gingiva, and erosion was not found in any of them.

In summary, the results obtained in the present study raised the following concerns: 1. Nine years after the introduction of the AAOMP diagnostic criteria for OLP, their validity has not been confirmed by serious randomized trials, and they have not been adopted by the WHO, which is why a proportion of pathologists (as demonstrated in the present study) still use the WHO criteria from 1978. 2. Strict adherence to the proposed diagnostic set excludes a large number of patients who would otherwise be diagnosed as OLP cases. In the present study, only 6 of 31 specimens, for which two independent pathologists agreed on the diagnosis of OLP, fulfilled all AAOMP histological criteria. These results question the reliability of the proposed diagnostic set. 3. Further studies with an increased number of OLP cases are needed to assess the frequency of observation of the different histological variables to confirm their significance for the diagnosis of the disease. If the results we presented are confirmed by studies with an increased sample size, it would mean that none of the AAOMP histological criteria can be defined as mandatory for the diagnosis of OLP. In this case, a proposal for a new diagnostic set that distinguishes essential (mandatory) versus desirable criteria would be necessary. 4. To date, regardless of the set of diagnostic criteria used, the diagnosis of OLP cannot be made solely on the basis of histological examination. Cases with a histological diagnosis "compatible with OLP" and those with clinic–pathological discordance require monitoring of the evolution of the condition and therapeutic response, control biopsy examination and the implementation of additional diagnostic methods such as direct immunofluorescence, allergic (Patch) test, etc.

The small sample size and single observer assessment of the AAOMP criteria should be noted as limitations of the present study.

## 5. Conclusions

In the present study, a discrepancy was found in the histological diagnoses of oral lichen planus based on the WHO criteria versus the newly proposed AAOMP diagnostic set. The reason for this was that strict adherence to the AAOMP guidelines excluded a large number of OLP cases. The histological features listed by the Academy as mandatory diagnostic criteria were observed in a relatively low percentage of the OLP tissue sections we analyzed, and none of them were consistently found in all histological sections. Further studies are needed to assess the validity of the AAOMP diagnostic criteria.

**Author Contributions:** Conceptualization, M.Z.M.; methodology, M.Z.M.; formal analysis, M.Z.M.; investigation, M.Z.M. and D.A.T.; data curation, M.Z.M.; writing—original draft preparation, M.Z.M.; writing—review and editing, M.Z.M.; visualization, M.Z.M.; funding acquisition, D.A.T. and M.Z.M. All authors have read and agreed to the published version of the manuscript.

**Funding:** This work was funded by the Medical University of Plovdiv.

**Institutional Review Board Statement:** The study was conducted in accordance with the Declaration of Helsinki and approved by the Ethics Committee of Medical University Plovdiv (R3716/7 October 2014).

**Informed Consent Statement:** Informed consent was obtained from all subjects involved in the study.

**Data Availability Statement:** The data that support the findings of this study are available from the corresponding author, [M.Z.M.], upon reasonable request.

**Conflicts of Interest:** The authors have no relevant financial or non-financial interests to disclose.

## References

1. Manchanda, Y.; Rathi, S.K.; Joshi, A.; Das, S. Oral Lichen Planus: An Updated review of etiopathogenesis, clinical presentation, and management. *Indian. Dermatol. Online J.* **2023**, *15*, 8–23. [CrossRef]
2. Vičić, M.; Hlača, N.; Kaštelan, M.; Brajac, I.; Sotošek, V.; Massari, L.P. Comprehensive Insight into Lichen Planus Immunopathogenesis. *Int. J. Mol. Sci.* **2023**, *24*, 3038. [CrossRef]
3. Sanches, A.C.B.; Pires, A.L.P.V.; Medrado, A.R.A.P.; De Almeida Reis, S.R.; Freitas, V.S.; Martins, G.B. Oral Lichen planus: Associations between histomorphometric characteristics and white and red lesions. *Head Neck Pathol.* **2022**, *16*, 969–979. [CrossRef] [PubMed]
4. Mutafchieva, M.Z.; Draganova-Filipova, M.N.; Zagorchev, P.I.; Tomov, G.T. Oral Lichen Planus—Known and Unknown: A Review. *Folia Med.* **2018**, *60*, 528–535. [CrossRef] [PubMed]
5. Cheng, Y.-S.L.; Gould, A.; Kurago, Z.; Fantasia, J.; Muller, S. Diagnosis of oral lichen planus: A position paper of the American Academy of Oral and Maxillofacial Pathology. *Oral Surg. Oral Med. Oral Pathol. Oral Radiol.* **2016**, *122*, 332–354. [CrossRef] [PubMed]
6. Van Der Meij, E.H.; Van Der Waal, I. Lack of clinicopathologic correlation in the diagnosis of oral lichen planus based on the presently available diagnostic criteria and suggestions for modifications. *J. Oral Pathol. Med.* **2003**, *32*, 507–512. [CrossRef] [PubMed]
7. Warnakulasuriya, S.; Kujan, O.; Aguirre-Urizar, J.M.; Bagan, J.V.; González-Moles, M.Á.; Kerr, A.R.; Lodi, G.; Mello, F.W.; Monteiro, L.; Ogden, G.R.; et al. Oral potentially malignant disorders: A consensus report from an international seminar on nomenclature and classification, convened by the WHO Collaborating Centre for Oral Cancer. *Oral Dis.* **2020**, *27*, 1862–1880. [CrossRef] [PubMed]
8. Kramer, I.R.; Lucas, R.B.; Pindborg, J.J.; Sobin, L.H. Definition of leukoplakia and related lesions: An aid to studies on oral precancer. *Oral Surg. Oral Med. Oral Pathol.* **1978**, *46*, 518–539. [PubMed]
9. Ismail, S.B.; Kumar, S.K.S.; Zain, R.B. Oral lichen planus and lichenoid reactions: Etiopathogenesis, diagnosis, management and malignant transformation. *J. Oral Sci.* **2007**, *49*, 89–106. [CrossRef] [PubMed]
10. Van Der Meij, E.H.; Reibel, J.; Slootweg, P.J.; Van Der Wal, J.E.; De Jong, W.F.B.; Van Der Waal, I. Interobserver and intraobserver variability in the histologic assessment of oral lichen planus. *J. Oral Pathol. Med.* **1999**, *28*, 274–277. [CrossRef] [PubMed]
11. Rad, M.; Hashemipoor, M.A.; Mojtahedi, A.; Zarei, M.R.; Chamani, G.; Kakoei, S.; Izadi, N. Correlation between clinical and histopathologic diagnoses of oral lichen planus based on modified WHO diagnostic criteria. *Oral Surg. Oral Med. Oral Pathol. Oral Radiol. Endod.* **2009**, *107*, 796–800. [CrossRef] [PubMed]
12. Müller, S. Oral lichenoid lesions: Distinguishing the benign from the deadly. *Mod. Pathol.* **2017**, *30*, S54–S67. [CrossRef] [PubMed]
13. Müller, S. Oral Manifestations of Dermatologic Disease: A focus on lichenoid lesions. *Head Neck Pathol.* **2011**, *5*, 36–40. [CrossRef] [PubMed]
14. Krutchkoff, D.J.; Eisenberg, E. Lichenoid dysplasia: A distinct histopathologic entity. *Oral Surg. Oral Med. Oral Pathol.* **1985**, *60*, 308–315. [CrossRef] [PubMed]
15. Speight, P.M.; Khurram, S.A.; Kujan, O. Oral potentially malignant disorders: Risk of progression to malignancy. *Oral Surg. Oral Med. Oral Pathol. Oral Radiol.* **2017**, *125*, 612–627. [CrossRef] [PubMed]
16. Fitzpatrick, S.G.; Honda, K.S.; Sattar, A.; Hirsch, S.A. Histologic lichenoid features in oral dysplasia and squamous cell carcinoma. *Oral Surg. Oral Med. Oral Pathol. Oral Radiol.* **2014**, *117*, 511–520. [CrossRef] [PubMed]
17. Miller, M.A.; Zachary, J.F. Mechanisms and morphology of cellular injury, adaptation, and death. In *Elsevier eBooks;* Elsevier: Amsterdam, The Netherlands, 2017; pp. 2–43.e19. [CrossRef]
18. Jungell, P.; Konttinen, Y.T.; Nortamo, P.; Malmström, M. Immunoelectron microscopic study of distribution of T cell subsets in oral lichen planus. *Scand. J. Dent. Res.* **1989**, *97*, 361–367. [CrossRef] [PubMed]
19. Bascones, C.; Gonzalez-Moles, M.A.; Esparza, G.; Bravo, M.; Acevedo, A.; Gil-Montoya, J.A.; Bascones, A. Apoptosis and cell cycle arrest in oral lichen planus. *Arch. Oral Biol.* **2005**, *50*, 873–881. [CrossRef] [PubMed]
20. Kalele, K.; Sarode, S.C.; Sarode, G.S. Oral Lichenoid Reaction: A Review. *Internat J. Oral Maxillofac. Pathol.* **2012**, *3*, 11–20.

diagnostics

MDPI

Article

# Comparative Clinical and Histopathological Study of Oral Leukoplakia in Smokers and Non-Smokers

Andrei-Eduard Șerban [1], Ioanina Părlătescu [2,*], Elena Milanesi [3,4], Iulia Andreea Pelisenco [4], Maria Dobre [4], Mariana Costache [3], Șerban Țovaru [2] and Paula Perlea [2]

1 Doctoral School, Carol Davila University of Medicine and Pharmacy, 050474 Bucharest, Romania; andrei-eduard.serban@drd.umfcd.ro
2 Faculty of Dentistry, Carol Davila University of Medicine and Pharmacy, 050474 Bucharest, Romania; serban.tovaru@gmail.com (Ș.Ț.); paula.perlea@umfcd.ro (P.P.)
3 Faculty of Medicine, Carol Davila University of Medicine and Pharmacy, 050474 Bucharest, Romania; elena.milanesi@umfcd.ro (E.M.); mariana.costache@umfcd.ro (M.C.)
4 Victor Babeș National Institute of Pathology, 050096 Bucharest, Romania; pelisenco.iulia@gmail.com (I.A.P.); maria.dobre@ivb.ro (M.D.)
* Correspondence: ioanina.parlatescu@umfcd.ro

**Abstract: Background/Objectives:** Oral leukoplakia (OLK) is an oral mucosal lesion classified in the oral potentially malignant disorder group and is associated with an increased risk of malignant transformation (MT). The aim of this study was to compare the clinical and histopathological features of two OLK groups, a group of smokers and a group of non-smokers. **Methods:** In this retrospective study, a cohort of 154 patients with OLK was divided into two groups based on the presence of smoking as a major risk factor. OLK diagnoses were established via clinical and histopathological examination. **Results:** Females were more abundant in the non-smoking group than in the smoking group, where males were more abundant ($p < 0.001$). The average age of the smokers was lower than that of the non-smokers ($p = 0.003$). In the smokers, the buccal mucosa was most frequently affected, while in the non-smokers, the gums and the tongue were primarily involved ($p = 0.016$). In female smokers, involvement of the buccal area and multiple-site involvement were statistically significantly more frequently observed compared to that in female non-smokers ($p = 0.006$). Non-dysplastic lesions were predominant in both groups, with severe dysplasia observed more frequently in the non-smokers than in the smokers. MT was higher in the non-smoker group compared to that in the smoker group. **Conclusions:** OLK in smokers is different from OLK in non-smokers concerning female gender involvement, site location, the number of lesions, and the MT rate.

**Keywords:** oral leukoplakia; oral medicine; smoker; oral potentially malignant disorder

## 1. Introduction

Oral leukoplakia (OLK) is an oral mucosa lesion that is part of a large subgroup of diseases described by the WHO (World Health Organization) as oral potentially malignant disorders (OPMDs) that carry a high risk of malignant transformation. The OPMD group includes oral leukoplakia, erythroplakia, proliferative verrucous leukoplakia, oral submucous fibrosis, oral lichen planus, actinic cheilitis, palatal lesions in reverse smokers, oral lupus erythematosus, dyskeratosis congenita, oral lichenoid lesions, and oral graft-versus-host disease [1]. Of all the members of the OPMD group, OLK is one of the most common and extensively researched. Over time, OLK has been defined in a variety of ways, and the up-to-date definition is a "white plaque of questionable risk having excluded (other) known diseases or disorders that carry no increased risk for cancer" [2]. The prevalence of this disease varies according to different authors. Zhang et al. described an overall prevalence of 1.39% based on 69 studies with 17,524 participants, a prevalence of 1.82% for Europe in population-based studies, and a prevalence of 4.85% for specific population studies [3], while Mello et al. reported a prevalence of 4.11% for OLK (95% CI = 1.98–6.97) [4]. The most frequent oral mucosa sites affected by OLK are the buccal mucosa, the floor of the mouth, and the tongue, but all areas of the oral mucosa can be involved [5]. The most common clinical classification of OLK divides it into a homogeneous form and a nonhomogeneous form, with verrucous, speckled, and nodular subtypes [6].

The OLK risk factors are well known and consist of smoking, alcohol consumption, and betel nut chewing [5]. The European Commission reported in 2023 that 19% of the adult population of Romania had a smoking habit, the same as the European average, with one out of five adults smoking [7]. EUROSTAT reported that 11.8% of individuals smoke fewer than 20 cigarettes/day, and 3.8% smoke more than 20 cigarettes/day [8]. Regarding alcohol consumption, the European Commission reported that 35% of Romanians consumed alcohol in excessive amounts at least once per month in 2019, a figure above the European average of 19% [7]. Local additional factors such as frictional trauma and the presence of a candida infection may exacerbate the lesions, and their removal from the initial evaluation of OLK lesions has been recommended [1].

The main concern of researchers and clinicians is the malignant transformation (MT) risk of OLK lesions, which varies greatly depending on different factors. The most reliable predictors for MT are an advanced age (50+ years), female gender, tongue location, non-homogenous clinical type, and the presence of epithelial dysplasia [9].

Malignant transformation rates vary per author and meta-analysis, from 6.64% to 9.8% [9–11]. Bhattarai et al. reported a 7.39 times higher risk of MT in recurrent OLK compared to the non-recurrent form, and a pooled proportion of recurrence at 22% for different surgical interventions [12]. MT is more likely to occur in patients with moderate or severe epithelial dysplasia than in those with mild or no dysplasia [5].

Treatment selection for OLK is an ongoing discussion in oral medicine research, with some authors debating whether surgical treatment may increase the risk of MT [13]. $CO_2$ laser treatment is effective, reliable, and associated with a low recurrence rate [12,14], while non-surgical treatments like photodynamic therapy seem to show great prospects [15,16].

Our research supports the continuous debate in the scientific literature regarding the onset of oral squamous cell carcinoma (OSCC), particularly in the absence of identified risk factors [17–19]. The development of OSCC may be related to a number of genetic factors or different epigenetic subtypes and mutations [20,21], or to a compromised immune system [22]. Research on oral leukoplakia in individuals with unknown risk factors may provide insights into OSCC development.

The aim of this study was to assess the clinical and histopathological features and MT risk differences between smoker and non-smoker OLK groups in our cohort from Bucharest, Romania.

## 2. Materials and Methods

The present study is an analytic retrospective cohort study that presents a thorough analysis of oral leukoplakia. The differences between patients divided into two subgroups, smokers and non-smokers, were investigated. Participants in the study were identified from the Oral Medicine Department of the Faculty of Dentistry of the Carol Davila University of

Medicine and Pharmacy in Bucharest and our private practice. The patients were consulted between 1996 and 2024. The selection criteria included detailed demographic and clinical data as well as a histopathological confirmation of oral leukoplakia diagnosis. The cases with inconclusive clinical and histopathological information or missing informed consent were excluded from this analysis (exclusion criteria). The dysplasia grades were assessed by the same pathologist (C.M.). The demographic data recorded were gender, age, and smoking status. The clinical form of the OLK lesions was classified, as recommended by van der Waal, 2015 [6], as homogenous or non-homogenous (further categorized as verrucous, speckled, or nodular). We also recorded the number of lesions (single or multiple lesions) and the size of the lesions: smaller than 2 $cm^2$, between 2 and 4 $cm^2$, and larger than 4 $cm^2$. The initial lesion location classification used the WHO topography for oral cancer [23], but it included a large number of sites. Thus, we reduced it to 6 anatomical locations as follows: buccal mucosa, tongue, gums, the floor of the mouth, other sites, and multiple sites. For a more efficient approach, as recommended by Zhang et al. [24], we divided the oral mucosa into high-risk sites, which included the tongue mucosa, the floor of the mouth, the soft palate, and low-risk sites, the remaining oral mucosa. The grading of epithelial dysplasia was carried out in accordance with the WHO standards [25]: no dysplasia, mild dysplasia, moderate dysplasia, and severe dysplasia. The result of the candida mycological examination was recorded, as well as the follow-up period and whether malignant transformation occurred. The treatment selection was individualized for each patient, local irritative factors were removed, and smoking reduction or cessation was recommended. The histopathological result was the deciding factor for subsequent treatment, which ranged from clinical and histopathological monitoring to surgical excision depending on the lesion site, dimension, and patient's general health state.

The ethical approval and the acceptance of the study protocol were obtained from the Ethics Committee of Carol Davila University of Medicine and Pharmacy Bucharest Romania cod PO-35-F-03 number 1139/13.01.2023. This study was performed according to the recommendations of the Declaration of Helsinki. Written informed consent was obtained from all the patients.

Statistical Package for the Social Sciences (SPSS version 17.0) was used to conduct the statistical analysis. Differences in age between the two groups were assessed using the *t*-test, while for categorical variables, statistical significance was evaluated using the chi-square test or Fisher's exact test.

## 3. Results

We analyzed the clinical and histopathological data of 154 OLK patients to better comprehend the distinctions attributable to smoking in the present study. The cohort included 88 females (57.1%) and 66 males (42.9%) with an overall mean age of 55.16 $\pm$ 12.45 (min 26–max 86 years). The cohort was divided into two groups: 108 smokers (including 23 ex-smokers at the time of diagnosis—patients who had quit smoking for at least 1 year) and 46 non-smokers. Table 1 presents data on the demographic and clinical features of OLK lesions in both groups of patients. The average age of the smokers was significantly lower than that of the non-smokers (53.22 years vs. 59.67 years) ($p = 0.003$). Of the 108 smokers, $n = 58$ (53.70%) were male and $n = 50$ (46.30%) were female. In the non-smoker group, there were more females ($n = 38$; 82.61%) compared to males ($n = 8$; 17.39) ($p < 0.001$, $\chi^2 = 17.369$). We detected that single lesions were more frequent in the non-smoker group (76.09%) compared to (51.85%) the smokers ($p = 0.005$, $\chi^2 = 7.838$).

**Table 1.** Demographic and clinical characteristics: comparison between smokers and non-smokers.

| Variable | Smokers ($n$ = 108) | Non-Smokers ($n$ = 46) | $p$-Value |
|---|---|---|---|
| **Age** | 53.22 ± 11.27 | 59.67 ± 13.96 | ***0.003*** |
| **Gender** | | | |
| *Male* | 58 (53.70%) | 8 (17.39%) | ***<0.001*** $\chi^2$ = 17.369 |
| *Female* | 50 (46.30%) | 38 (82.61%) | |
| **Clinical form** | | | |
| *Homogeneous* | 67 (62.04%) | 32 (69.57%) | 0.372 $\chi^2$ = 0.79 |
| *Non-homogeneous* | 41 (37.96%) | 14 (30.43%) | |
| **Site of OLK lesion** | | | |
| *Buccal* | 31 (28.70%) | 7 (15.22%) | ***0.016*** (Fisher Test) |
| *Tongue* | 7 (6.48%) | 10 (21.74%) | |
| *Gums* | 29 (26.85%) | 14 (30.43%) | |
| *Floor of mouth* | 8 (7.41%) | 1 (2.17%) | |
| *Other sites* | 4 (3.71%) | 5 (10.87%) | |
| *Multiple sites* | 29 (26.85%) | 9 (19.57%) | |
| **Number of lesions** | | | |
| *Single* | 56 (51.85%) | 35 (76.09%) | ***0.005*** $\chi^2$ = 7.838 |
| *Multiple* | 52 (48.15%) | 11 (23.91%) | |
| **Location by risk** | | | |
| *High risk* | 38 (35.29%) | 13 (28.26%) | 0.403 $\chi^2$ = 0.698 |
| *Low risk* | 70 (64.81%) | 33 (71.74%) | |
| **Size** | | | |
| <2 cm$^2$ | 55 (50.93%) | 21 (45.65%) | 0.278 $\chi^2$ = 2.562 |
| 2–4 cm$^2$ | 29 (26.85%) | 18 (39.13%) | |
| >4 cm$^2$ | 24 (22.22%) | 7 (15.22%) | |
| **Candida infection *** | | | |
| *Negative* | 26 (49.06%) | 10 (58.82%) | 0.483 $\chi^2$ = 0.492 |
| *Positive* | 27 (50.94%) | 7 (41.18%) | |

* Available for 53 smokers and 17 non-smokers.

Comparing the lesion sites of smokers vs. non-smokers, we found an overall significant difference ($p$ = 0.016): in smokers, the buccal mucosa was more frequently involved (28.70%) than in non-smokers (15.22%), along with the floor of the mouth (7.41% vs. 2.17%). In the non-smoker group, the tongue and the gums were more frequently involved compared to the smoker group (for the tongue 21.74% vs. 6.48%, and for gums 30.43% vs. 26.85%). No statistical difference was found regarding the high-risk and low-risk sites. In the smoker group, the high-risk sites were more involved compared to the non-smoker group (35.29% vs. 28.26%). Meanwhile, in the non-smoker group, the low-risk sites were more involved (71.74% vs. 64.81%).

OLK clinical forms showed no significant differences between the two groups, with a similar frequency of homogenous forms in the non-smokers (69.57%) and in the smokers 62.04%. The non-homogenous form was more frequently encountered in smokers (37.96%) than in the non-smoker group (30.43%), without a significant difference.

Comparing the two groups, there was no significant difference in terms of lesion size, with the most lesions being under 2 cm$^2$ in both groups, followed by 2–4 cm$^2$ and larger than 4 cm$^2$.

Candida examination was performed in 70 patients (53 smokers and 17 non-smokers) and was found to be positive in 50.94% of smokers and 41.18% of non-smokers.

Two separate analyses stratifying the cohort by sex were conducted to assess whether there was a significant association between the smoker status and the following variables: clinical form, site of the OLK lesion, number of lesions, location by risk, size, and presence of candida infection. When considering the female group ($n$ = 88), a significant association between the site of the OLK lesion and smoker status was found ($p$ = 0.006): the buccal area was affected in 28% of the smokers, while in the non-smokers, the buccal area was affected only in 15.22% of the cases. Moreover, multiple site lesions were found in 30% of female smokers and in 21.5% of non-smokers. Another significant association between female smokers and non-smokers was found considering the number of lesions ($p$ = 0.02). The same analysis was conducted on the male group, and no significant associations were found for all the tested variables considering smoker status (Table 2).

**Table 2.** Clinical characteristics by gender groups: comparison between smokers and non-smokers.

| **Female Group ($n$ = 88)** | | | |
|---|---|---|---|
| **Variable** | **Smokers ($n$ = 50)** | **Non-Smokers ($n$ = 38)** | ***p*-Value** |
| **Site of OLK lesion** | | | |
| *Buccal* | 14 (28.00%) | 4 (10.53%) | ***0.006*** (Fisher Test) |
| *Tongue* | 3 (6.00%) | 10 (26.32%) | |
| *Gums* | 15 (30.00%) | 11 (28.94%) | |
| *Floor of mouth* | 3 (6.00%) | 1 (2.63%) | |
| *Other sites* | 0 (0%) | 4 (10.53%) | |
| *Multiple sites* | 15 (30.00%) | 8 (21.05%) | |
| **Number of lesions** | | | |
| *Single* | 26 (52%) | 29 (76.32%) | ***0.02*** $\chi^2$ = 5.447 |
| *Multiple* | 24 (48%) | 9 (23.68%) | |
| **Male group ($n$ = 88)** | | | |
| **Variable** | Smokers ($n$ = 58) | Non-Smokers ($n$ = 8) | *p*-value |
| **Site of OLK lesion** | | | |
| ***Buccal*** | 17 (29.31%) | 3 (37.50%) | 0.856 (Fisher Test) |
| ***Tongue*** | 4 (6.90%) | 0 (0%) | |
| ***Gums*** | 14 (24.13%) | 3 (37.50%) | |
| ***Floor of mouth*** | 5 (8.63%) | 0 (0%) | |
| ***Other sites*** | 4 (6.90%) | 1 (12.50%) | |
| ***Multiple sites*** | 14 (24.13%) | 1 (12.50%) | |
| **Number of lesions** | | | |
| ***Single*** | 30 (51.72%) | 6 (75.00%) | 0.275 (Fisher Test) |
| ***Multiple*** | 28 (48.28%) | 2 (25.00%) | |

No significant associations in the female group were found for the other variables considering smoker status.

*Histopathological Results*

The histopathological data are reported in Table 3. The analysis revealed a similar frequency of the non-dysplastic lesions in both groups (56.48% smokers vs. 60.87% in non-smokers). Mild dysplasia was found in 37.04% of patients in the smoker group and

26.09% of patients in the non-smoker group. Severe dysplasia was found more frequently in non-smokers (8.70% vs. 3.70% in smokers), without reaching statistical significance.

**Table 3.** Histopathological evaluation, follow-up, and outcome.

| Variable | Smokers ($n$ = 108) | Non-Smokers ($n$ = 46) | $p$-Value |
|---|---|---|---|
| **Histopathological evaluation** | | | |
| *No dysplasia* | 61 (56.48%) | 28 (60.87%) | 0.071 (Fisher Test) |
| *Mild dysplasia* | 40 (37.04%) | 12 (26.09%) | |
| ***Moderate dysplasia*** | 4 (3.70%) | 4 (8.70%) | |
| ***Severe dysplasia*** | 3 (2.78%) | 2 (4.34%) | |
| **Presence of dysplasia** | | | |
| ***No dysplasia*** | 61 (56.48%) | 28 (60.87%) | 0.255 $\chi^2$ = 0.492 |
| ***Dysplasia*** | 47 (43.52%) | 18 (39.13%) | |
| **Mean period of follow-up** * | 36.40 months | 35.05 months | |
| **Outcome** ** | | | |
| ***Malignant transformation*** | 8 (9.88%) | 7 (18.92%) | 0.171 $\chi^2$ = 1.872 |
| ***Non-malignancy*** | 73 (90.12%) | 30 (81.08%) | |

* Available for 86 smokers and 39 non-smokers; ** available for 81 smokers and 37 non-smokers.

The mean period of follow-up for the cohort was 35.98 (1–228) months, 36.40 months for the smokers and 35.05 months for non-smokers.

During follow-up, malignant transformation occurred in 15 patients (12.71%), 8 smokers (8.99%), and 7 non-smokers (18.92%). Although this event was more frequent in the non-smokers, statistical significance was not reached. The MT rate per year for the entire cohort was 4.23%, while that in the smoker group was 2.63% and that in the non-smoker group was 2.39%.

## 4. Discussion

Since the World Health Organization's initial definition of OLK in 1978 [26], smoking has been acknowledged as a significant factor in the etiology of OLK; however, there is a scarcity of research evaluating the clinical and histopathological characteristics that differentiate OLK according to smoking status in the literature [27–34]. Thus, we investigated the clinical and histopathological differences in OLK in smokers and non-smokers. There is a large variation regarding the clinical features of OLK, based mainly on geographic distribution and in close connection with population habits.

Our cohort included 154 cases of oral leukoplakia, divided into two groups as follows: 108 cases of OLK in smokers (70.12%) and 46 cases of OLK in non-smoker patients (29.88%). The present findings reveal that OLK was diagnosed more frequently in women than in males (57.10% vs. 42.90%) in the whole cohort. This result is consistent with reports from Holland [27] that found 140 OLK cases, 69% in women, and a study from Beijing [28] on 875 OLK cases that reported 57.3% to be female patients. Conversely, Kusiak et al. [29] reported a study of 416 OLK cases where 52.9% of patients were male. A population-based cohort study evaluating 1888 histopathologically confirmed OLK cases in Northern California found that 57.36% of patients were male [30], and a single-center study of 676 cases in Japan [31] reported more men than females (53.7% vs. 46.3%).

We observed that the non-smoking group had a predominance of females (82.61%), and there was a higher proportion of men (53.39%) in the smoking group ($p < 0.001$, $\chi^2 = 17.369$). This is comparable to a previous study conducted in Spain [32] on 52 OLK cases, which found that 82% of non-smokers were female, and 78% of smokers were male. This result is consistent with a 2012 Brazilian study [33] that found that the smoker group was dominated by men, and the non-smoker group was dominated by women. On the other hand, Schepman et al. [34] report that women are predominant in both in the non-smoker cohort and the entire cohort.

The mean age was higher in the non-smoker group than in the smoker group, similar to Freitas et al. [32]. This is similar to the mean age described in OLK in a study by Kokubun et al., where in 676 OLK cases, the onset age was >50 years [31]. However, as stated by the researchers, the data sheets of the patients in the Japanese cohort did not include information regarding smoking habits or alcohol intake.

The homogeneous clinical form of OLK was most frequently encountered in all patients, unrelated to smoking habits—62.04% in smokers, and 69.57% in non-smokers. This result is consistent with the reports of Evren et al. [27], which found no correlation between tobacco usage and the clinical form of OLK, and is different from previous reports that found a strong relationship between homogenous OLK and smoking [29] or detected a higher frequency in smokers. In our observations, in the smoker group, the most frequently affected site was the buccal mucosa followed by gums and multiple sites, and in non-smokers the gums were followed by multiple sites. The majority of OLK lesions were less than 2 $cm^2$ in size. Kokubun et al. [31] found the tongue and the gums to be the primary sites of involvement in their OLK cohort, differentiating them only by sex and not by other criteria.

Dysplasia was identified in 65 cases (42.20%) in all OLK patients. The percentages of smokers and non-smokers were slightly different (43.52% vs. 39.13%). This outcome is different from other studies: Chaturvedi et al. [30] reported 15% dysplasia, Pentenero et al. [34] reported 15.8%, and Evren et al. [27] reported 60%. Consistent with the findings of Evren et al. [27], in our study, smoking did not correlate with the histopathological categories.

Regarding the MT rate, in 15 of our cohort cases, MT occurred. The percentage was 12.71% for the entire cohort, with an average of 4.23% per year. In a previous study [35] on a smaller series of OLK patients, we reported an MT rate of 7.5%. The outcome of the present study is higher than average, as Aguire-Urizar et al. [9] report an OLK MT rate of 9.8% for 5 years (2015–2020) (95% CI: 7.9–11.7), and Pimenta-Barros et al. [11] found a pooled MT rate of 6.64% (95% CI: 5.21–8.21) in a meta-analysis with 55 studies including 41,231 OLK cases published before June 2024. Guan et al. [10] reported an MT pooled MT rate of 7.20% (95% CI: 5.40–9.10) for 26 OLK studies published in the last 20 years (2000–2022). We also observed that the non-smokers' group had almost twice the MT rate compared to the smokers' group, with 9.88% for the smokers (8 out of 108) and 18.92% for the non-smoker group (7 out of 46). Also, we observed that all seven cases from the non-smokers' group with MT were in female subjects. The predominance of malignant transformation in females is well established, even though to our knowledge no previous research has provided the rate of malignant transformation for distinct non-smoking OLK groups [5,10,34]. This is in agreement with Pentenero et al. [36], who report that DNA ploidy might identify a subset OLK with higher epithelial dysplasia manifestation and higher malignant transformation risk, even though its value in predicting MT is limited and further studies are needed. Treatment for oral leukoplakia is an ongoing discussion; in a systematic review, Lodi et al. [37] found that there is no evidence of a treatment that is effective in preventing the development of oral cancer, with some being effective in healing oral lesions but not preventing relapse and side effects. Oral malignancy remains one of the most aggressive cancers in humans, with mortality rates of 13.6% reported for Europe in 2020 [38].

The current study has some limitations. The study group size was constrained and contingent upon patient accessibility, needs, and compliance with follow-up appointments. The methodology used was not identical to that used in previously published research. We did not consider alcohol consumption, as it is challenging to accurately estimate the specific amount of alcohol intake in current clinical practice. In the Introduction, we detailed alcohol intake as reported by the EUROSTAT in the general population, considering it a major risk factor for malignant transformation. A further disadvantage, mostly attributable to the study's retrospective design, was the absence of current data concerning emerging smoking modalities (such as vaping, e-cigarettes, and nicotine pouches) and other novel potential risk factors. Therefore, we emphasize the need for new prospective research regarding the impact of new risk factors on oral mucosal lesions.

The strengths and novelty of this research lie in our aim to differentiate and compare oral leukoplakia lesions in patients exposed to smoking as a primary risk factor. We found few studies that reported oral leukoplakia from this point of view, and those we found used other methodologies and different types of analysis.

As we observed that patients with unknown risk factors usually progress with a worse clinical outcome, we consider that there is a need for genetic testing and immunohistochemistry tests to select the most appropriate individualized treatment approach. We recommend histopathological examination in all oral leukoplakia lesions, as it remains the most reliable method for evaluating the malignant transformation potential. Subsequently, biopsies should be performed during follow-up, along with other tests in case of clinical changes in the lesions or the onset of clinical symptoms.

## 5. Conclusions

Our study revealed statistical differences between OLK in smokers and non-smokers concerning gender—with a higher proportion of females in the non-smoker group. The most commonly affected areas were smokers' buccal mucosa and non-smokers' gums. The homogeneous type was the most encountered clinical form of OLK in all patients and was unrelated to smoking behavior. The presence of dysplasia did not significantly differ between smokers and non-smokers.

We report that the non-smokers had an almost twofold higher rate of malignant transformation than the smokers, and that all of the non-smokers' malignant transformation cases were in women.

**Author Contributions:** Conceptualization, A.-E.Ș., I.P. and Ș.Ț.; methodology, A.-E.Ș. and P.P.; software, E.M.; validation, I.A.P., M.D. and M.C.; formal analysis, E.M.; investigation, P.P. and M.C.; resources, I.P. and Ș.Ț.; data curation, A.-E.Ș. and I.A.P.; writing—original draft preparation, A.-E.Ș. and I.P.; writing—review and editing, A.-E.Ș., E.M. and I.P.; visualization, P.P.; supervision, Ș.Ț.; project administration, A.-E.Ș.; funding acquisition, I.P. All authors have read and agreed to the published version of the manuscript.

**Funding:** The publication of this paper was supported by the University of Medicine and Pharmacy Carol Davila through the institutional program Publish not Perish.

**Institutional Review Board Statement:** The study was conducted in accordance with the Declaration of Helsinki and approved by the Ethics Committee of Carol Davila University of Medicine and Pharmacy Bucharest, PO-35-F-03 number 1139/13.01.2023.

**Informed Consent Statement:** Informed consent was obtained from all subjects involved in the study.

**Data Availability Statement:** The data presented in this study are available on reasonable request from the corresponding author.

**Conflicts of Interest:** The authors declare no conflicts of interest.

## Abbreviations

The following abbreviations are used in this manuscript:

| | |
|---|---|
| OLK | Oral leukoplakia |
| OPMD | Oral potentially malignant disorders |
| MT | Malignant transformation |
| WHO | World Health Organization |

## References


1. Warnakulasuriya, S.; Kujan, O.; Aguirre-Urizar, J.M.; Bagan, J.V.; González-Moles, M.Á.; Kerr, A.R.; Lodi, G.; Mello, F.W.; Monteiro, L.; Ogden, G.R.; et al. Oral potentially malignant disorders: A consensus report from an international seminar on nomenclature and classification, convened by the WHO Collaborating Centre for Oral Cancer. *Oral Dis.* **2021**, *27*, 1862–1880. [CrossRef] [PubMed]
2. Warnakulasuriya, S.; Johnson, N.W.; van der Waal, I. Nomenclature and classification of potentially malignant disorders of the oral mucosa. *J. Oral Pathol. Med.* **2007**, *36*, 575–580. [CrossRef] [PubMed]
3. Zhang, C.; Li, B.; Zeng, X.; Hu, X.; Hua, H. The global prevalence of oral leukoplakia: A systematic review and meta-analysis from 1996 to 2022. *BMC Oral Health* **2023**, *23*, 645. [CrossRef] [PubMed] [PubMed Central]
4. Mello, F.W.; Miguel, A.F.P.; Dutra, K.L.; Porporatti, A.L.; Warnakulasuriya, S.; Guerra, E.N.S.; Rivero, E.R.C. Prevalence of oral potentially malignant disorders: A systematic review and meta-analysis. *J. Oral Pathol. Med.* **2018**, *47*, 633–640. [CrossRef] [PubMed]
5. Warnakulasuriya, S. Clinical features and presentation of oral potentially malignant disorders. *Oral Surg. Oral Med. Oral Pathol. Oral Radiol.* **2018**, *125*, 582–590. [CrossRef] [PubMed]
6. van der Waal, I. Oral leukoplakia, the ongoing discussion on definition and terminology. *Med. Oral Patol. Oral Cir. Bucal* **2015**, *20*, e685–e692. [CrossRef] [PubMed] [PubMed Central]
7. OECD/European Union. *Health at a Glance: Europe 2022: State of Health in the EU Cycle*; OECD Publishing: Paris, France, 2022. [CrossRef]
8. EUROSTAT, Data Browser. Available online: https://ec.europa.eu/eurostat/databrowser/view/hlth_ehis_sk3e$defaultview/default/table?lang=en (accessed on 1 December 2024).
9. Aguirre-Urizar, J.M.; Lafuente-Ibáñez de Mendoza, I.; Warnakulasuriya, S. Malignant transformation of oral leukoplakia: Systematic review and meta-analysis of the last 5 years. *Oral Dis.* **2021**, *27*, 1881–1895. [CrossRef] [PubMed]
10. Guan, J.Y.; Luo, Y.H.; Lin, Y.Y.; Wu, Z.Y.; Ye, J.Y.; Xie, S.M.; Li, J. Malignant transformation rate of oral leukoplakia in the past 20 years: A systematic review and meta-analysis. *J. Oral Pathol. Med.* **2023**, *52*, 691–700. [CrossRef] [PubMed]
11. Pimenta-Barros, L.A.; Ramos-García, P.; González-Moles, M.Á.; Aguirre-Urizar, J.M.; Warnakulasuriya, S. Malignant transformation of oral leukoplakia: Systematic review and comprehensive meta-analysis. *Oral Dis.* **2024**, *31*, 69–80. [CrossRef] [PubMed]
12. Bhattarai, B.P.; Singh, A.K.; Singh, R.P.; Chaulagain, R.; Søland, T.M.; Hasséus, B.; Sapkota, D. Recurrence in Oral Leukoplakia: A Systematic Review and Meta-analysis. *J. Dent. Res.* **2024**, *103*, 1066–1075. [CrossRef] [PubMed] [PubMed Central]
13. Holmstrup, P.; Dabelsteen, E. Oral leukoplakia-to treat or not to treat. *Oral Dis.* **2016**, *22*, 494–497. [CrossRef] [PubMed]
14. Mogedas-Vegara, A.; Hueto-Madrid, J.A.; Chimenos-Küstner, E.; Bescós-Atín, C. Oral leukoplakia treatment with the carbon dioxide laser: A systematic review of the literature. *J. Cranio-Maxillofac. Surg.* **2016**, *44*, 331–336. [CrossRef] [PubMed]
15. Li, Y.; Wang, B.; Zheng, S.; He, Y. Photodynamic therapy in the treatment of oral leukoplakia: A systematic review. *Photodiagnosis Photodyn. Ther.* **2019**, *25*, 17–22. [CrossRef] [PubMed]
16. Angjelova, A.; Jovanova, E.; Polizzi, A.; Santonocito, S.; Lo Giudice, A.; Isola, G. The Potential of Nano-Based Photodynamic Treatment as a Therapy against Oral Leukoplakia: A Narrative Review. *J. Clin. Med.* **2023**, *12*, 6819. [CrossRef] [PubMed] [PubMed Central]
17. Kolegova, E.S.; Patysheva, M.R.; Larionova, I.V.; Fedorova, I.K.; Kulbakin, D.E.; Choinzonov, E.L.; Denisov, E.V. Early-onset oral cancer as a clinical entity: Aetiology and pathogenesis. *Int. J. Oral Maxillofac. Surg.* **2022**, *51*, 1497–1509. [CrossRef] [PubMed]
18. Tran, Q.; Maddineni, S.; Arnaud, E.H.; Divi, V.; Megwalu, U.C.; Topf, M.C.; Sunwoo, J.B. Oral cavity cancer in young, non-smoking, and non-drinking patients: A contemporary review. *Crit. Rev. Oncol. Hematol.* **2023**, *190*, 104112. [CrossRef] [PubMed] [PubMed Central]
19. Heller, M.A.; Nyirjesy, S.C.; Balsiger, R.; Talbot, N.; VanKoevering, K.K.; Haring, C.T.; Old, M.O.; Kang, S.Y.; Seim, N.B. Modifiable risk factors for oral cavity cancer in non-smokers: A systematic review and meta-analysis. *Oral Oncol.* **2023**, *137*, 106300. [CrossRef] [PubMed]

20. Adorno-Farias, D.; Morales-Pisón, S.; Gischkow-Rucatti, G.; Margarit, S.; Fernández-Ramires, R. Genetic and epigenetic landscape of early-onset oral squamous cell carcinoma: Insights of genomic underserved and underrepresented populations. *Genet. Mol. Biol.* **2024**, *47* (Suppl. S1), e20240036. [CrossRef] [PubMed] [PubMed Central]
21. Campbell, B.R.; Chen, Z.; Faden, D.L.; Agrawal, N.; Li, R.J.; Hanna, G.J.; Iyer, N.G.; Boot, A.; Rozen, S.G.; Vettore, A.L.; et al. The mutational landscape of early- and typical-onset oral tongue squamous cell carcinoma. *Cancer* **2021**, *127*, 544–553. [CrossRef] [PubMed] [PubMed Central]
22. Valero, C.; Yuan, A.; Zanoni, D.K.; Lei, E.; Dogan, S.; Shah, J.P.; Morris, L.G.T.; Wong, R.J.; Mizrachi, A.; Patel, S.G.; et al. Young non-smokers with oral cancer: What are we missing and why? *Oral Oncol.* **2022**, *127*, 105803. [CrossRef] [PubMed] [PubMed Central]
23. Available online: https://icd.who.int/browse10/2016/en#/C00-C14 (accessed on 1 December 2024).
24. Zhang, L.; Cheung, K.-J.; Lam, W.L.; Cheng, X.; Poh, C.; Priddy, R.; Epstein, J.; Le, N.D.; Rosin, M.P. Increased genetic damage in oral leukoplakia from high-risk sites: Potential impact on staging and clinical management. *Cancer* **2001**, *91*, 2148–2155. [CrossRef] [PubMed]
25. *Head and Neck Tumors, WHO Classification of Tumors*, 5th ed.; International Agency for Research on Cancer: Lyon, France, 2024; Volume 9, ISBN 13 978-92-832-4514-8.
26. World Health Organization Collaborating Center for Oral Precancerous Lesions. Definition of leukoplakia and related lesions: An aid to studies on oral precancer. *Oral Surg. Oral.Med. Oral Pathol.* **1978**, *46*, 518–553. [CrossRef]
27. Evren, I.; Brouns, E.R.; Poell, J.B.; Wils, L.J.; Brakenhoff, R.H.; Bloemena, E.; de Visscher, J.G.A.M. Associations between clinical and histopathological characteristics in oral leukoplakia. *Oral Dis.* **2023**, *29*, 696–706. [CrossRef] [PubMed] [PubMed Central]
28. Wang, T.; Wang, L.; Yang, H.; Lu, H.; Zhang, J.; Li, N.; Guo, C.B. Development and validation of nomogram for prediction of malignant transformation in oral leukoplakia: A large-scale cohort study. *J. Oral Pathol. Med.* **2019**, *48*, 491–498. [CrossRef] [PubMed]
29. Kusiak, A.; Maj, A.; Cichońska, D.; Kochańska, B.; Cydejko, A.; Świetlik, D. The Analysis of the Frequency of Leukoplakia in Reference of Tobacco Smoking among Northern Polish Population. *Int. J. Environ. Res. Public Health* **2020**, *17*, 6919. [CrossRef] [PubMed] [PubMed Central]
30. Chaturvedi, A.K.; Udaltsova, N.; Engels, E.A.; Katzel, J.A.; Yanik, E.L.; Katki, H.A.; Lingen, M.W.; Silverberg, M.J. Oral Leukoplakia and Risk of Progression to Oral Cancer: A Population-Based Cohort Study. *J. Natl. Cancer Inst.* **2020**, *112*, 1047–1054. [CrossRef] [PubMed] [PubMed Central]
31. Kokubun, K.; Nakajima, K.; Akashi, Y.; Yamamoto, K.; Katakura, A.; Matsuzaka, K. Clinicopathological evaluation of oral leukoplakia: A single-center study of 676 cases in Japan. *Oral Surg. Oral Med. Oral Pathol. Oral Radiol.* **2024**, *137*, 529–536. [CrossRef]
32. Freitas, M.D.; Blanco-Carrión, A.; Gándara-Vila, P.; Antúnez-López, J.; García-García, A.; Gándara Rey, J.M. Clinicopathologic aspects of oral leukoplakia in smokers and nonsmokers. *Oral Surg. Oral Med. Oral Pathol. Oral Radiol. Endod.* **2006**, *102*, 199–203. [CrossRef] [PubMed]
33. Lima, J.S.; dos Santos Pinto, D., Jr.; de Sousa, S.O.M.; Corrêa, L. Oral leukoplakia manifests differently in smokers and non-smokers. *Braz. Oral Res.* **2012**, *26*, 543–549. [CrossRef] [PubMed]
34. Schepman, K.P.; van der Meij, E.H.; Smeele, L.E.; van der Waal, I. Malignant transformation of oral leukoplakia: A follow-up study of a hospital-based population of 166 patients with oral leukoplakia from The Netherlands. *Oral Oncol.* **1998**, *34*, 270–275. [CrossRef] [PubMed]
35. Tovaru, S.; Costache, M.; Perlea, P.; Caramida, M.; Totan, C.; Warnakulasuriya, S.; Parlatescu, I. Oral leukoplakia: A clinicopathological study and malignant transformation. *Oral Dis.* **2023**, *29*, 1454–1463. [CrossRef] [PubMed]
36. Pentenero, M.; Castagnola, P.; Castillo, F.V.; Isaevska, E.; Sutera, S.; Gandolfo, S. Predictors of malignant transformation in oral leukoplakia and proliferative verrucous leukoplakia: An observational prospective study including the DNA ploidy status. *Head Neck* **2023**, *45*, 2589–2604. [CrossRef] [PubMed]
37. Lodi, G.; Franchini, R.; Warnakulasuriya, S.; Varoni, E.M.; Sardella, A.; Kerr, A.R.; Carrassi, A.; MacDonald, L.C.; Worthington, H.V. Interventions for treating oral leukoplakia to prevent oral cancer. *Cochrane Database Syst. Rev.* **2016**, *7*, CD001829. [CrossRef] [PubMed] [PubMed Central]
38. Sarode, G.; Maniyar, N.; Sarode, S.C.; Jafer, M.; Patil, S.; Awan, K.H. Epidemiologic aspects of oral cancer. *Dis. Mon.* **2020**, *66*, 100988. [CrossRef] [PubMed]

*diagnostics* MDPI

*Article*

# Assessment of a Bioimpedance-Based Method for the Diagnosis of Oral Cancer

**Kristina Horvat Šikonja [1,*], Ivica Richter [1], Marko Velimir Grgić [2], Krešimir Gršić [3], Dinko Leović [3], Lovorka Batelja Vuletić [4] and Vlaho Brailo [1,5]**

1 Department of Oral Medicine, School of Dental Medicine, University of Zagreb, 10000 Zagreb, Croatia; ivica.richter@ri.t-com.hr (I.R.); brailo@sfzg.unizg.hr (V.B.)
2 Clinic for Otolaryngology and Head and Neck Surgery, Clinical Hospital Centre "Sestre Milosrdnice", 10000 Zagreb, Croatia; marko_grgic@yahoo.com
3 Clinic for Otolaryngology and Head and Neck Surgery, University Clinical Hospital Centre Zagreb, 10000 Zagreb, Croatia; kresimir.grsic@gmail.com (K.G.); dinko.leovic@gmail.com (D.L.)
4 Department of Pathology, School of Medicine, University of Zagreb, 10000 Zagreb, Croatia; lovorka.batelja.vuletic@mef.hr
5 Clinic for Dentistry, University Clinical Hospital Centre Zagreb, 10000 Zagreb, Croatia
* Correspondence: dr.kristina.horvat@gmail.com

**Abstract: Background/Objectives:** Oral cancer (OC) is a disease with poor prognosis mainly due to late diagnosis. There is considerable interest in the use and development of rapid, point of care (POC) non-invasive methods that can accelerate the diagnostic process. Bioimpedance (BI) is resistance to the passage of electric currents through tissue that reflects structural changes in the tissue. The aim of this study was to determine the spectrum of BI values in patients with oral cancer, to compare them with other oral lesions and healthy controls, and to determine the diagnostic value of the BI-based method for diagnosis of OC. **Methods:** Ninety-three participants divided into three groups participated in this study. The first group (31 participants) consisted of patients with histologically confirmed OC, the second group (31 participants) consisted of patients with an active reticular form of oral lichen planus (positive controls; OLP) and the third group (31 participants) consisted of healthy controls. In OC and OLP patients, BI was measured at three points (non-ulcerated lesional mucosa, clinically unaffected perilesional mucosa and unaffected mucosa on the contralateral side). In healthy controls, BI was measured on a healthy mucosa in the corresponding anatomical region. Measurements were performed at nine frequencies (1, 2, 5, 7, 10, 20, 70 and 100 kHz). **Results**: In OC patients, BI values in the lesion were significantly lower than BI values in clinically intact perilesional mucosa and the unaffected contralateral side at all frequencies. Furthermore, BI values of the clinically intact perilesional mucosa were significantly lower than the BI values of the healthy contralateral mucosa at frequencies of 1 kHz, 2 kHz, 5 kHz, 7 kHz and 10 kHz. Patients with OC had significantly lower BI values compared to patients with OLP and individuals with healthy oral mucosa at all frequencies. **Conclusions**: This study demonstrated the very good to excellent ability of this method to detect OC lesions, which needs to be confirmed by further studies on a larger number of participants.

**Keywords:** oral cancer; bioimpedance; oral mucosa; diagnostics

## 1. Introduction

Oral cancer (OC), a disease which accounts for 3.5% of all cancer diagnoses, belongs to a group of diseases with high morbidity and mortality [1]. The largest share of OC is diagnosed in Asia (64.2%), followed by Europe (17.4%), North America (7.6%), South America (5.6%), Africa (3.8%) and Oceania (1.3%) [2,3]. Based on gender stratification, the incidence rate is significantly higher in men (13.1/100,000) than in women (5/100,000), and the risk of the disease increases with age [1].

The main risk factors for the development of OC are tobacco and alcohol use, with an exponential increase in risk in the presence of both factors. Approximately 70% of cancers in this region can be explained by exposure to one or both of the aforementioned risk factors [4]. The most common localizations of OC are the ventral and lateral tongue and the floor of the mouth (over 50% of cases), mostly in Western countries [5–9]. Other localizations are the buccal mucosa, retromolar area, maxillary and mandibular gingiva, soft palate and, less frequently, hard palate.

Pain is not a common symptom in patients with OC; it occurs in 30–40% of cases, and it usually appears when the lesions reach the advanced stage [10]. In later and larger lesions, symptoms can vary from mild discomfort to severe pain, especially in the tongue. Other symptoms include ear pain, bleeding, loose teeth, difficulty speaking, dysphagia, trismus, paraesthesia and difficulty using dentures [11].

Due to the advanced stage at the time of diagnosis, the disease has a poor prognosis, with an overall five-year survival rate of less than 55%. Treatment often includes surgical interventions, radiotherapy or chemotherapy, which significantly impairs the quality of life. Prognosis and survival rates undoubtedly depend on the stage of the lesion at the time of diagnosis and the rapid and adequate therapeutic response. Five-year survival rates drop significantly in patients with locally and regionally advanced disease, emphasizing the importance of early diagnosis [12].

Early diagnosis significantly improves prognosis and outcomes, reaching a 5-year survival rate of up to 90% [13]. Traditionally, the gold standard of screening for OC is a conventional examination of the oral cavity, and a definitive diagnosis is made on the basis of a lesion biopsy [5,14]. Biopsy, however, has several limitations. It is an invasive procedure that some patients may be reluctant to undertake. Next, it is usually performed in specialist institutions, and waiting for the procedure can cause additional stress for the patient. The biopsy should be performed by a specialist with experience in the management of oral mucosal lesions in order to avoid taking an unrepresentative sample. Because of its invasiveness, biopsy requires specific infection control precautions that require trained personnel and additional resources. Accordingly, there is considerable interest in the use and development of new, rapid, non-invasive methods for the assessment of lesions, which can be used at the point of care (POC) and which are not so dependent on subjective assessment, like, for example, an assessment of epithelial dysplasia [15–18]. The use of POC testing brings multiple benefits, both clinical and economic. Clinically, it enables faster diagnosis, immediate administration of therapy, better patient cooperation and a reduction in complications and administrative burdens, which lead to greater patient satisfaction. Economic benefits include a reduction in the number of clinical examinations, a shorter stay in health facilities, targeted interventions and a reduction in the loss of working days, which positively affect productive years and general economic indicators [15–18].

Bioimpedance (BI) is a measure that expresses resistance to the passage of electric current through tissue. BI is a characteristic of all living tissues and changes depending on the structure and chemical composition of the tissue [19]. Changes in structure and/or chemical composition result in changed electrical resistance of tissues. The application of BI for diagnostic purposes in medicine and dentistry is based on this principle. Due to their non-invasiveness, BI-based methods have certain advantages over invasive methods—they are simpler to perform, are more comfortable for the patient and present less of a problem in terms of disinfection, sterilization and infection control. The application of BI-based methods in medicine and dentistry is very diverse, from the examination of pathological changes in the tissue to the determination of the length of the root canal [20–22].

Due to the fact that different structural alterations in tissue facilitate the flow of electric current, i.e., lower tissue resistance, BI-based methods able to register these alterations are studied as a non-invasive method for the diagnosis of oral cancer (and other cancers as well). A recent systematic review identified five such studies [23]. All of the studies reported significantly lower BI values in OC compared to healthy tissue. The review concluded that due to its non-invasiveness, reliability and immediate results, BI appears to be a promising tool for oral cancer screening [24–28].

The aim of this study was to determine the spectrum of BI values in patients with oral cancer, to compare them with the values of other oral lesions and healthy subjects, and to determine the diagnostic value of the BI-based method for the diagnosis of OC.

## 2. Materials and Methods

This study was approved by the ethics committee of the University of Zagreb School of Dental Medicine (No. 05-PA-30-VIII-6/2019) and University Clinical Hospital Zagreb (No. 02/21 AG). Ninety-three participants divided into three groups participated in the study. Before the enrolment, all participants signed informed consent according to the Declaration of Helsinki.

The first group (31 participants) consisted of patients with histologically confirmed OC from the Department of Maxillofacial Surgery University Clinical Hospital Zagreb and University Clinical Hospital "Sestre Milosrdnice". Patients with another type of cancer, patients with localization not suitable for the placement of the measuring electrode (oropharynx, gingiva and hard palate) and patients who were not able to comprehend the informed consent were excluded.

The second group (31 participants) consisted of patients from the University of Zagreb, School of Dental Medicine, Department of Oral Medicine with an active reticular form of oral lichen planus (positive controls; OLP). The diagnosis of OLP was established based on clinical and histological characteristics of the lesions. Exclusion criteria were similar to the ones applied in the OC group.

The third group (31 participants) consisted of patients from other departments of the University of Zagreb, School of Dental Medicine, with clinically normal oral mucosa, which was confirmed by an experienced oral medicine specialist (healthy controls; HC).

The intraoral sensor consisted of three concentric electrodes made of sintered aluminium alloys of high conductivity, coated with an insulating layer of Teflon, with a total diameter of 8 mm. In order to ensure stable contact and uniform pressure of the sensor on the oral mucosa, the sensor was connected to a dental suction unit which produced a constant negative pressure of 250 mBar, thus ensuring its stability during the measurement. The sensor was connected to the measuring device NI USB-6251 (National Instruments®, Austin, TX, USA) via electrical conductors, and the measuring device was connected to the laptop via the USB port. Measuring software, developed using the Lab View 8.5.1 software package (National Instruments®, Austin, TX, USA), converted electrical signals into digital records and stored them in a database. A schematic diagram of the measuring system is displayed in Figure 1. The measurement was simple and non-invasive—the electrode was placed on the selected place on the oral mucosa, and the system registered the measurement. After placing the sensor on the oral mucosa, an alternate current at 9 different frequencies passed between the electrodes through the tissue, and the voltage between the electrodes was measured. Measurements were performed at 9 frequencies (1, 2, 5, 7, 10, 20, 70 and 100 kHz). The device permits users to set the frequency range manually through the software from 0 to 100 kHz. Since there is no standard frequency range universally accepted for BI measurements of oral mucosa, the aforementioned frequencies were determined arbitrarily in order to assess which frequency yields the best discriminative ability to identify OC lesions.

In OC patients, BI was measured at 3 reference points:

1. Morphologically changed but non-ulcerated mucosa of the OC lesion;
2. Clinically intact mucosa in the immediate vicinity of the tumour, i.e., 5 mm away from the tumour border;
3. Healthy oral mucosa of the corresponding anatomical region on the contralateral/unaffected side. Measurements on healthy contralateral mucosa were always performed in the same region as the tumour, but on the unaffected side.

The measurement was repeated in the same way in the group of positive controls, while in the group of negative controls BI was measured on a healthy mucosa in the corresponding anatomical region. Each measurement was repeated three times, and the mean value of the three measurements was used in further calculations.

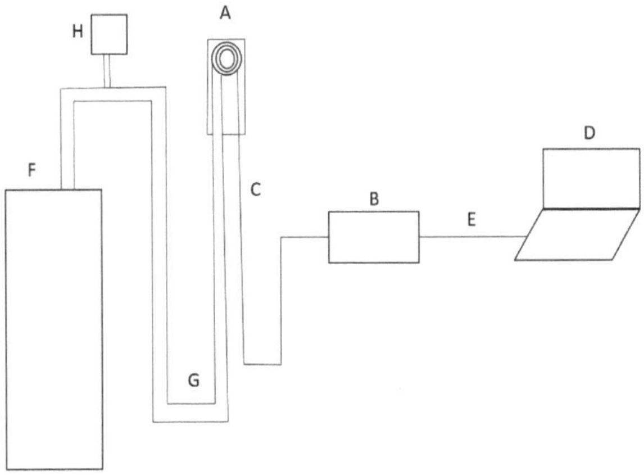


**Figure 1.** Schematic diagram of the measuring system. The intraoral sensor (A) was connected to the measuring device (B) with an electric conductor (C). The measuring device (B) registered resistance to the flow of the electric current. The device (B) was connected to the laptop (D) by a USB cable (E). Analytical software stored on the laptop (D) converted the electrical signal from the device (B) into digital data. To maintain the constant pressure of the sensor (A) on the oral mucosa, the intraoral sensor was connected to the dental suction unit (F) by a rubber tube (G). A constant pressure of 250 mBar was maintained and controlled with a manometer (H).

Normality of distribution was assessed by the Shapiro–Wilk test. Since all variables (except age) deviated from a normal distribution, the median and interquartile range (IQR) were used to display BI values, while the mean value ± standard deviation was used to present age. Within-group differences in BI were assessed by Friedman's analysis of variance of followed by the Dunn–Bonferroni post hoc test. BI differences between groups were assessed by the Kruskal–Wallis test followed by Dunn's post hoc. The discriminative ability of the method for the identification of oral cancer was tested by receiver operating characteristic (ROC) curve analysis and classified according to the area under the curve (AUC) size as follows: >0.9, excellent; 0.8–0.9, very good; 0.7–0.8, good; 0.6–0.7, satisfactory. $p$ values less than 0.05 ($p < 0.05$) were considered statistically significant.

## 3. Results

A total of 93 participants (53 women and 40 men) with an average age of 62.0 ± 11.5 years participated in this study. Demographic and clinical data on the participants are presented in Table 1. No statistically significant difference in age and gender between the participants was found ($p = 0.713$; $p = 0.102$). A statistically significant difference was found in the localization of the lesion/measurement point between the groups ($p < 0.0001$).

**Table 1.** Demographic and clinical characteristics of the participants.

| | Oral Cancer | Positive Controls | Healthy Controls | $p$ |
|---|---|---|---|---|
| Sex, N (%) | | | | |
| Male | 21 (67.7) | 13 (41.9) | 19 (61.3) | 0.102 |
| Female | 10 (31.3) | 18 (58.1) | 12 (38.7) | |
| Age (mean ± SD) | 62.1 ± 12.8 | 63.2 ± 11.2 | 60.8 ± 10.7 | 0.713 |
| Localization of the lesion, N (%) | | | | |
| Buccal mucosa | 10 (32.3) | 28 (90.3) | Not applicable | $p < 0.0001$ * |
| Tongue border | 12 (38.7) | 3 (9.7) | | |
| Floor of the mouth | 9 (29) | 0 | | |

**Table 1.** *Cont.*

| | Oral Cancer | Positive Controls | Healthy Controls | *p* |
|---|---|---|---|---|
| TNM stage | | | | |
| 1 | 4 | Not applicable | Not applicable | Not applicable |
| 2 | 4 | | | |
| 3 | 11 | | | |
| 4 | 12 | | | |
| Tumour differentiation, N (%) | | | | |
| Well differentiated | 27 (87.1) | Not applicable | Not applicable | Not applicable |
| Poorly differentiated | 4 (12.9) | | | |

* $p < 0.05$.

### 3.1. *Bioimpedance Spectra in Patients with Oral Cancer*

Figure 2 displays the results of BI measurements in the group of patients with OC. The BI values of the lesion were significantly lower than the BI values of the clinically intact perilesional mucosa and the BI values of healthy mucosa contralaterally at all frequencies ($p < 0.05$). Furthermore, the BI values of the clinically intact perilesional mucosa were significantly lower than the BI values of the healthy contralateral mucosa at frequencies of 1 kHz, 2 kHz, 5 kHz, 7 kHz and 10 kHz ($p < 0.05$) (Figure 2).

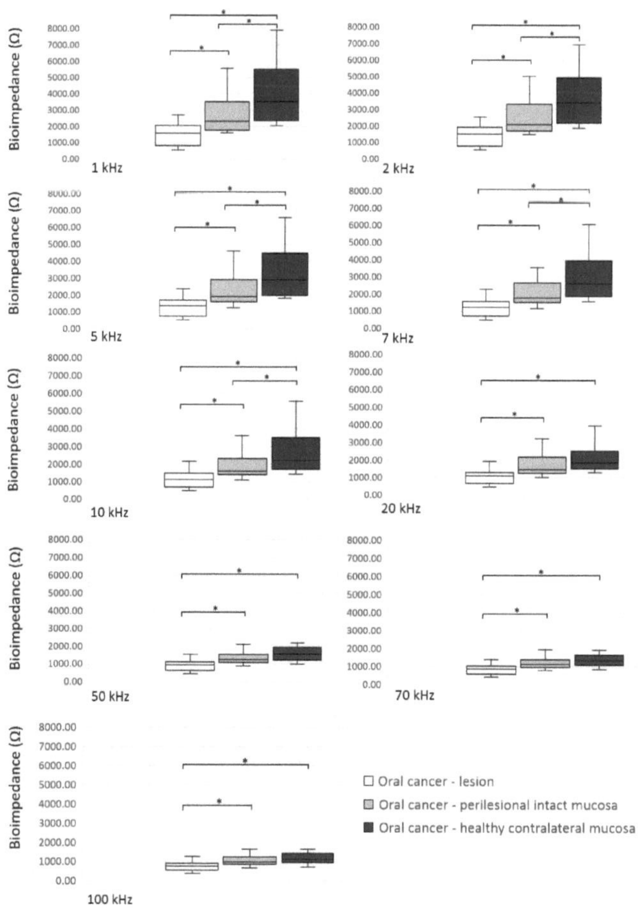


**Figure 2.** Bioimpedance measurements in a group of patients with oral cancer. Significant differences ($p < 0.05$) are marked with an asterisk (*).

### 3.2. Comparison of Bioimpedance Values in the Lesion Between Oral Cancer Patients and Controls

Figure 3 displays a comparison of BI values in the lesion between the three groups of participants. Patients with OC had significantly lower BI values in the lesional tissue compared to lesional tissue in positive controls and healthy controls at all measured frequencies ($p < 0.05$), except at the frequency of 100 Hz. At the frequency of 100 Hz, BI values in the OC lesion were significantly lower than BI values of the lesional tissue in positive controls ($p < 0.0001$) and lower but not significantly different than BI values in healthy controls ($p = 0.064$) (Figure 3).

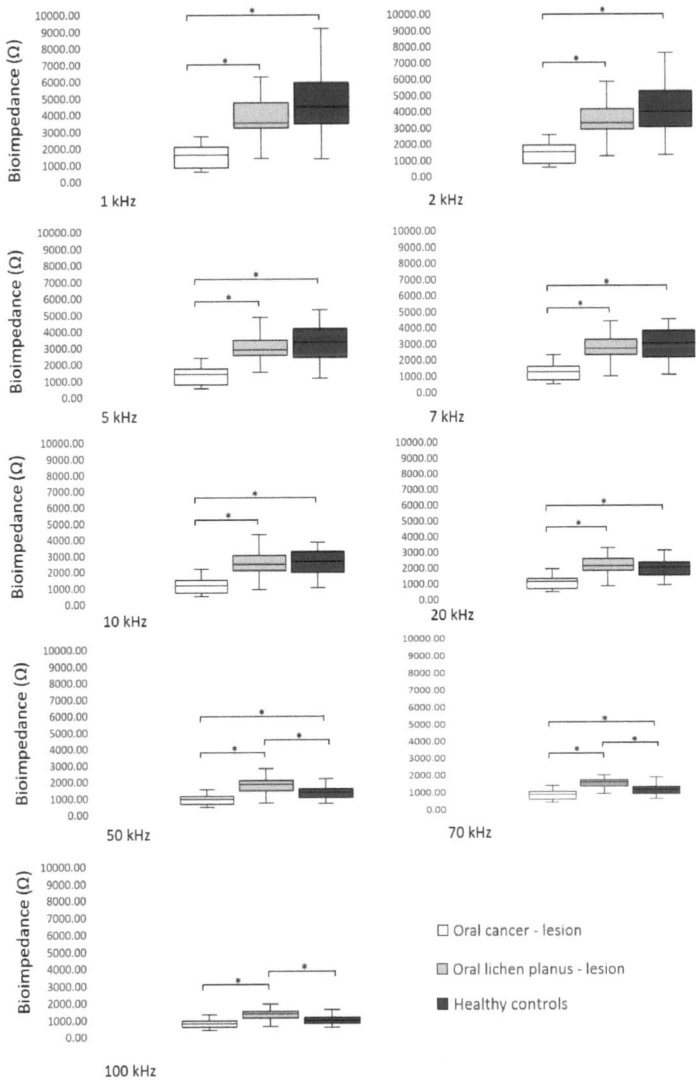


**Figure 3.** Comparison of bioimpedance values of the lesion between three groups of participants. Significant differences ($p < 0.05$) are marked with an asterisk (*).

### 3.3. Comparison of Bioimpedance Values in the Clinically Intact Perilesional Mucosa Between Oral Cancer Patients and Controls

Figure 4 displays a comparison of BI values on the clinically intact perilesional mucosa between three groups of participants. The BI values of the clinically intact perilesional mucosa in OC patients were lower than the BI values of the clinically intact perilesional mucosa in positive controls and the BI values in healthy controls at the frequencies of 1 kHz, 2 kHz, 5 kHz, 7 kHz and 10 kHz ($p < 0.05$). At higher frequencies (20 Hz, 50 Hz, 70 Hz and 100 Hz), the BI values of the clinically intact perilesional mucosa in OC patients were significantly lower than the BI values of the clinically intact perilesional mucosa in positive controls but not significantly different from the BI values in healthy controls (Figure 4).

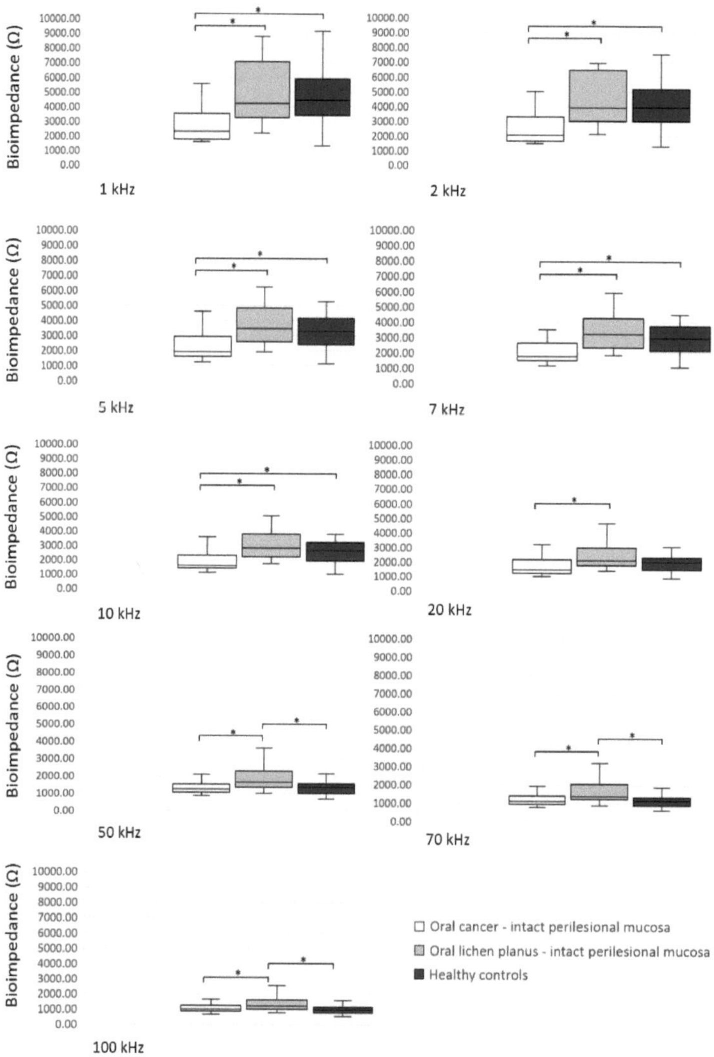


**Figure 4.** Comparison of bioimpedance values of the clinically intact perilesional mucosa between three groups of participants. Significant differences ($p < 0.05$) are marked with an asterisk (*).

### *3.4. Assessment of the Ability of the Bioimpedance-Based Method to Identify Oral Cancer Lesions*

Assessment of the ability of the BI-based method to identify oral cancer lesions was performed by ROC curve analysis. The analysis showed the excellent to very good discriminating ability of the method, with AUC values from 0.958 to 0.792, depending on the measurement frequency. The AUC decreased with the increase in measurement frequency (Figure 5).

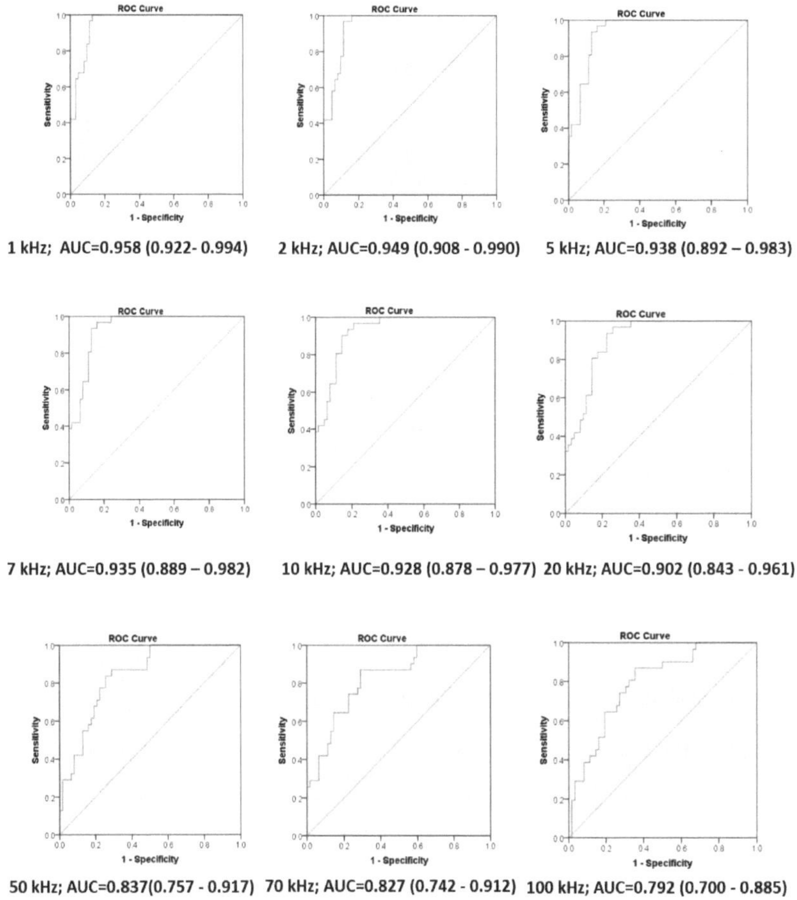


**Figure 5.** Analysis of the discriminatory ability of the method for the detection of oral cancer on frequencies from 1 kHz to 100 kHz. The area under the curve (AUC) and 95% confidence intervals (95% CI) at corresponding frequencies are displayed below each graph. The AUC was highest at the frequency of 1 kHz and decreased as the frequency increased.

## 4. Discussion

The results of this study demonstrated that OC lesions have lower BI values compared to the surrounding healthy tissue. The EI values of the OC and surrounding healthy tissue decreased as the frequency of measurement increased, and the differences with regard to the type of tissue were less pronounced. Lower BI values in OC lesions compared to healthy tissue are a result of changes in the electrical properties of cancer tissue. At low frequencies, electric current moves through intercellular spaces without the possibility of penetrating cells, and the BI values are dominated by the results from the most superficial layer of the oral mucosa [20]. In healthy tissue, the cells are densely packed and tightly connected to each other. The intercellular space is very narrow and provides higher resistance to the low-frequency current. On the other hand, tumour tissue has a larger extracellular space due to the loss of intercellular connections, more extracellular matrix, the altered permeability of the cell membrane, the reduced cell density and the different cell orientation, resulting in a drop in resistance and easier penetration of current into the intercellular space [21,22]. Similar results were reported in the studies of Sun et al. [24], Ching et al. [25], Sarode et al. [26] and Murdoch et al. [27]. The authors explained the obtained differences in EI values between tumour tissue and healthy mucosa with ultrastructural changes in the tumour tissue and the consequent changes in the electrical properties of tissues and cells described earlier. This is further supported by the study by Sarode et al., who reported statistically significant differences between well- and poorly differentiated carcinomas of the oral cavity [26]. It is known that poorly differentiated cancers have a more altered tissue architecture and more intercellular space compared to well-differentiated cancers, which is why the resistance to the flow of electric current is lower. In this study, it was not possible to determine the difference between poorly and well-differentiated cancers, because the number of well-differentiated cancers was several times greater than that of poorly differentiated cancers (27 vs. 4) among our patients.

Regarding the differences between the intact perilesional mucosa and the healthy contralateral mucosa, the EI values at frequencies from 1 kHz to 10 kHz were significantly lower than the EI values on the healthy contralateral mucosa. At higher frequencies (20–100 kHz), the impedance of the intact perilesional mucosa was lower than that of the contralateral healthy mucosa, but not enough to achieve a statistically significant difference. Perilesional tissue, up to 1 cm from the edge of the malignant lesion, although it may appear macroscopically healthy, may show changes compared to normal oral tissue [29]. EI values of perilesional tissue may be higher than in cancer lesions, but lower than in completely healthy tissue due to the presence of subclinical changes or initial stages of malignant tissue transformation that are not yet clinically visible. The obtained results could not be compared with the results of other studies, because there were no studies in the available literature that compared EI values on perilesional clinically unchanged mucosa and healthy mucosa in patients with OC.

A comparison between the groups revealed that the EI values measured on OC lesions were significantly lower compared to the EI values of healthy controls at all frequencies, except for the frequency of 100 kHz, where the values were lower, but the difference was not statistically significant. Furthermore, the values of EI in OC lesions were significantly lower at all frequencies than positive controls, i.e., of EI values on lesions in patients with OLP. This finding is not surprising because patients with OLP, despite subepithelial inflammation and degeneration of basal cells, have preserved epithelial stratification and proper cell orientation, which is not the case with the cancer tissue. In addition, patients with OLP have hyperkeratosis as an additional factor that negatively affects electrical conductivity even in healthy tissue. A study by Richter et al. reported the highest EI values in healthy participants on the hard palate, a region that has the thickest corneal layer in the entire oral cavity [30].

Regarding the comparison of EI values on perilesional mucosa, it was found that EI values on clinically intact perilesional mucosa in patients with OC were lower than EI values on clinically unaffected mucosa of patients with OLP and healthy controls at lower frequencies (1 kHz, 2 kHz, 5 kHz, 7 kHz and 10 kHz). At higher frequencies (20 kHz, 50 kHz, 70 kHz and 100 kHz), significant differences were found only between clinically intact perilesional mucosa in patients with OC and patients with OLP. The results cannot be compared with the results of other studies because to our knowledge no studies in the available literature measured EI on the clinically intact perilesional mucosa in OC patients. This result can be explained by the fact that the low-frequency current passes through the intercellular space in contrast to the high-frequency current that passes through the cells [22]. Measuring EI values at low frequencies could possibly detect more subtle changes in the tissue that are not yet clinically visible. This needs to be confirmed by further studies, and if found to be correct, could represent a potential method for preoperative assessment of tumour margins. The distance of the tumour from the resection margin is a factor known to significantly influence local disease control and patient survival [31–33].

The results showed a good to excellent ability of the method to identify OC lesions (AUC 0.792–0.958). AUC values were highest at the frequency of 1 Hz and gradually decreased with the increase in frequency. This is not surprising considering the previously mentioned property of the lower-frequency electric current that passes through the intercellular spaces and thus better reflects changes in the tissue structure, in contrast to the higher-frequency current that passes through the cells [22]. In patients with OC, however, changes also exist at the cellular level, which is why measurements at higher frequencies were able to identify OC lesions as well. However, the best diagnostic performance (sensitivity of 96.8% and specificity of 87.1%) was achieved at the lowest frequency, i.e., 1 Hz.

The above results are in agreement with studies of other authors that also reported the very good ability of EI-based methods to identify OSCC. In an in vitro study by Carobbio et al., EI values were determined on samples of different tissues affected by OSCC at frequencies of 10–100 kHz [34]. On 384 mucosal samples, the device achieved very good discriminatory ability with an AUC value of 0.81, a sensitivity of 87% and a specificity of 76%. In the study by Murdoch et al. [27], which tested a commercially available device (ZedScan®, Zilico Ltd., Manchester, UK) intended to aid in the diagnosis of cervical lesions, the AUC value was 0.776, sensitivity 65.2% and specificity 91%. The device used a frequency range of 0.076–625 kHz, and 10 subjects with OC, 37 positive controls (patients with dysplastic lesions of varying degrees) and 51 healthy subjects participated in the study. Tatullo et al. reported the very good ability of an EI-based device to detect OLP lesions by measuring EI at a frequency of 50 kHz in 52 OLP patients and 11 control subjects [28]. The AUC value in the mentioned study was 0.89. The differences between the results of this study and the results in the literature can be explained by the different constructions of the devices, different measurement frequencies and different numbers of participants.

This study has several limitations that need to be mentioned. It was conducted on a relatively small number of respondents (31), and based on that number it is not possible to draw definitive conclusions about the effectiveness of the method/device. The number of participants in our study was not significantly different from the number of participants in the other studies—5 participants with OC in the study by Ching et al., 12 participants with OC in the study by Sun et al., and 10 participants with OC and 37 subjects with different dysplastic lesions of the oral mucosa in the study by Murdoch et al. [24,25,27]. A study by Sarode et.al. involved 50 patients with OC, and the study by Tatullo et al. involved 52 participants with OLP [26,28]. Regardless of the number of participants, the trend of decreased BI values in OC patients is obvious and needs to be further evaluated in larger studies.

One might note a slight male predominance in the OC group and a slight female predominance in the OLP group, which was a consequence of the disease epidemiology (i.e., higher prevalence of OC in males compared to females and vice versa for OLP). This predominance, however, did not reach statistical significance. Even though females are reported to have higher BI values of oral mucosa compared to males [30,35], we believe that the difference between the groups was not caused by different prevalences of males and females in both groups but by structural changes in tissue architecture caused by tumour formation. This is supported by significant differences in the BI values of the OC lesions and contralateral healthy mucosa in OC patients, as BI values are more affected by local changes in tissue than factors such as age and sex.

As for the selection of participants, patients with OC all had histologically confirmed disease that also had a clear clinical presentation, for which an experienced clinician did not need any auxiliary diagnostic tool. However, the purpose of this study was to evaluate a method that can differentiate a suspicious lesion well, and it was necessary to test it precisely on histologically confirmed OC lesions. A diagnostic device based on this method could, at the level of a general dentist, accelerate the decision to refer patients to specialist treatment and potentially shorten the "second lost time" in the process of OC diagnosis [36]. In specialist practice, such a device could speed up the decision on biopsy of a suspicious lesion. As for the control group, patients with active reticular OLP were selected as a positive control because the lesions of active reticular OLP have a marked red and white component, elements that are also visible in erythroleukoplakia, a lesion that most often represents the early stage of OC [37,38]. We wanted to have a group of positive controls that would resemble the early stage of OC as much as possible. Therefore, patients with ulcerations of other aetiologies were not included as positive controls, as ulceration represents a more advanced stage of OC. This was also not the case in other studies on BI and oral cancer [23–28]. There are no data in the literature about the BI values of oral ulcerations of other aetiologies, so one can only speculate about the differences between such lesions and OC. However, it is unlikely that the inflammatory infiltrate underlying such lesions would affect the electrical resistance of the tissue in the same way as the altered tissue architecture present in OC lesions does.

## 5. Conclusions

In conclusion, the results of this study demonstrated that OC lesions have a lower spectrum of BI values compared to OLP lesions and healthy oral mucosa. The study demonstrated the very good to excellent ability of this method to detect OC lesions, which needs to be confirmed by further studies on a larger number of participants.

**Author Contributions:** Conceptualization: K.H.Š., M.V.G. and V.B.; methodology: K.H.Š., I.R., M.V.G. and V.B.; validation: V.B. and I.R.; formal analysis: V.B.; investigation: K.H.Š., K.G. and D.L.; data curation: K.H.Š., K.G. and D.L.; writing—original draft preparation: K.H.Š.; writing—review and editing: K.H.Š., V.B., M.V.G. and L.B.V.; supervision: M.V.G. and V.B. All authors have read and agreed to the published version of the manuscript.

**Funding:** This research received no external funding.

**Institutional Review Board Statement:** This study was approved by the ethics committee of the University of Zagreb School of Dental Medicine (No. 05-PA-30-VIII-6/2019; 13 June 2019) and University Clinical Hospital Zagreb (No. 02/21 AG; 20 December 2019). Before the enrolment, all participants signed informed consent forms according to the Declaration of Helsinki.

**Informed Consent Statement:** Informed consent was obtained from all subjects involved in this study.

**Data Availability Statement:** The data presented in this study are available on request from the corresponding author.

**Acknowledgments:** We would like to thank the head nurse of the oncology department of the Clinic for Otolaryngology and Head and Neck Surgery, University Clinical Hospital Centre Zagreb, Marina Hršak, for her help in enrolment of the patients.

**Conflicts of Interest:** The authors declare no conflicts of interest.

## References

1. WHO. *Global Oral Health Status Report: Towards Universal Health Coverage for Oral Health by 2030*; World Health Organization: Geneva, Switzerland, 2022; pp. 45–52. Available online: https://www.who.int/publications/i/item/9789240061484 (accessed on 1 September 2024).
2. Sarode, G.; Maniyar, N.; Sarode, S.C.; Jafer, M.; Patil, S.; Awan, K.H. Epidemiologic aspects of oral cancer. *Disease-a-Month* **2020**, *66*, 100988. [CrossRef] [PubMed]
3. Cheong, S.C.; Vatanasapt, P.; Yi-Hsin, Y.; Zain, R.B.; Kerr, A.R.; Johnson, N.W. Oral cancer in South East Asia: Current status and future directions. *Transl. Res. Oral Oncol.* **2017**, *2*, 2057178X17702921. [CrossRef]
4. Ustrell-Borràs, M.; Traboulsi-Garet, B.; Gay-Escoda, C. Alcohol-based mouthwash as a risk factor of oral cancer: A systematic review. *Med. Oral Patol. Oral Cir. Bucal* **2020**, *25*, e1. [CrossRef]
5. Rivera, C. Essentials of oral cancer. *Int. J. Clin. Exp. Pathol.* **2015**, *8*, 11884–11894.
6. Tan, Y.; Wang, Z.; Xu, M.; Li, B.; Huang, Z.; Qin, S.; Nice, E.C.; Tang, J.; Huang, C. Oral squamous cell carcinomas: State of the field and emerging directions. *Int. J. Oral Sci.* **2023**, *15*, 44. [CrossRef]

7. Bahadur, S. Guidelines in Management of Carcinoma of the Tongue and Floor of Mouth. In *Management of Oral Cancers*; Springer Singapore: Singapore, 2021; pp. 133–147.
8. Albuquerque, R.; López-López, J.; Marí-Roig, A.; Jané-Salas, E.; Roselló-Llabrés, X.; Santos, J.R. Oral tongue squamous cell carcinoma (OTSCC): Alcohol and tobacco consumption versus non-consumption. A study in a Portuguese population. *Braz. Dent. J.* **2011**, *22*, 517–521. [CrossRef]
9. Dhanuthai, K.; Rojanawatsirivej, S.; Thosaporn, W.; Kintarak, S.; Subarnbhesaj, A.; Darling, M.; Kryshtalskyj, E.; Chiang, C.-P.; Shin, H.-I.; Choi, S.-Y.; et al. Oral cancer: A multicenter study. *Med. Oral Patol. Oral Cir. Bucal* **2017**, *23*, e23–e29. [CrossRef]
10. Yang, Y.; Zhang, P.; Li, W. Comparison of orofacial pain of patients with different stages of precancer and oral cancer. *Sci. Rep.* **2017**, *7*, 203. [CrossRef]
11. Bradley, P.T.; Lee, Y.K.; Albutt, A.; Hardman, J.; Kellar, I.; Odo, C.; Randell, R.; Rousseau, N.; Tikka, T.; Patterson, J.M.; et al. Nomenclature of the symptoms of head and neck cancer: A systematic scoping review. *Front. Oncol.* **2024**, *14*, 1404860. [CrossRef]
12. Chakravarthy, H.; Manoharan, S.; Damodaran, D.; Shamsudeen, S.; Lavanya, S. Assessment of Pattern of Cervical Lymph Node Metastasis in Squamous Cell Carcinoma of Oral Cavity. *Asian Pac. J. Cancer Care* **2024**, *9*, 417–423. [CrossRef]
13. Yang, J.; Guo, K.; Zhang, A.; Zhu, Y.; Li, W.; Yu, J.; Wang, P. Survival analysis of age-related oral squamous cell carcinoma: A population study based on SEER. *Eur. J. Med. Res.* **2023**, *28*, 413. [CrossRef] [PubMed]
14. Jeng, P.Y.; Chang, M.C.; Chiang, C.P.; Lee, C.F.; Chen, C.F.; Jeng, J.H. Oral soft tissue biopsy surgery: Current principles and key tissue stabilization techniques. *J. Dent. Sci.* **2024**, *19*, 11–20. [CrossRef] [PubMed]
15. Vibhute, N.; Jagtap, S.; Patil, S. Velscope guided oral cancer screening: A ray of hope in early oral cancer diagnosis. *J. Oral Maxillofac. Pathol.* **2021**, *25*, 548. [CrossRef] [PubMed]
16. Ilhan, B.; Lin, K.; Guneri, P.; Wilder-Smith, P. Improving Oral Cancer Outcomes with Imaging and Artificial Intelligence. *J. Dent. Res.* **2020**, *99*, 241–248. [CrossRef]
17. Price, C.P. Regular review: Point of care testing. *BMJ* **2001**, *322*, 1285–1288. [CrossRef]
18. Loubiere, S.; Moatti, J.P. Economic evaluation of point-of-care diagnostic technologies for infectious diseases. *Clin. Microbiol. Infect.* **2010**, *16*, 1070–1076. [CrossRef]
19. Scholz, B.; Anderson, R. On Electrical Impedance Scanning—Principles and Simulations. *Electromedica* **2000**, *68*, 35–44.
20. Åberg, P. Electronic Biopsies—Applications and Data Analysis. Ph.D. Thesis, Kongl Karolinska Medico Chirurgico Institutet, Stockholm, Sweden, 2002.
21. Nicander, I.; Rundquist, L.; Ollmar, S. Electric Impedance Measurements at Six Different Anatomic Locations of Macroscopically Normal Human Oral Mucosa. *Acta Odontol. Scand.* **1997**, *55*, 88–93. [CrossRef]
22. Birgersson, U. Electrical Impedance of Human Skin and Tissue Alterations Mathematical Modeling and Measurements. Ph.D. Thesis, Karolinska Institutet, Stockholm, Sweden, 2012.
23. Gupta, V.; Agrawal, U.; Goel, P. Bioimpedance: A Tool for Screening Oral Cancer—A Systematic Review. *Contemp. Clin. Dent.* **2023**, *14*, 91–97. [CrossRef]
24. Sun, T.P.; Ching, C.T.S.; Cheng, C.S.; Huang, S.H.; Chen, Y.J.; Hsiao, C.S.; Chang, C.H.; Huang, S.Y.; Shieh, H.L.; Liu, W.H.; et al. The use of bioimpedance in the detection/screening of tongue cancer. *Cancer Epidemiol.* **2010**, *34*, 207–211. [CrossRef]
25. Congo, T.S.C.; Ching, C.T.S.; Sun, T.P.; Huang, S.H.; Hsiao, C.S.; Chang, C.H.; Huang, S.Y.; Chen, Y.J.; Cheng, C.S.; Shieh, H.L.; et al. A preliminary study of the use of bioimpedance in the screening of squamous tongue cancer. *Int. J. Nanomed.* **2010**, *5*, 213–220.
26. Sarode, G.S.; Sarode, S.C.; Kulkarni, M.; Karmarkar, S.; Patll, S.; Auciustine, D. Bioimpedance Assessment of Oral Squamous Cell Carcinoma with Clinicopathological Correlation. *J. Contemp. Dent. Pract.* **2015**, *16*, 715–722. [PubMed]
27. Murdoch, C.; D'Apice, K.; Thornhill, M.H.; Brown, B.H.; Hearnden, V.; Speight, P.M.; Hegarty, A.M.; Healey, J.; Highfield, P.; Tidy, J. Use of electrical impedance spectroscopy to detect malignant and potentially malignant oral lesions. *Int. J. Nanomed.* **2014**, *9*, 4521–4532. [CrossRef] [PubMed]
28. Tatullo, M.; Marrelli, M.; Amantea, M.; Paduano, F.; Santacroce, L.; Gentile, S.; Scacco, S. Bioimpedance Detection of Oral Lichen Planus Used as Preneoplastic Model. *J. Cancer* **2015**, *6*, 976–983. [CrossRef] [PubMed]
29. Singhal, M.; Tandon, A.; Juneja, S.; Shetty, D.C.; Kumar, S.; Jain, A. Molecular Analysis as a Guide to Determining the Extent and Pathophysiology of Perilesional Tissues in Oral Epithelial Dysplasias. *J. Maxillofac. Oral Surg.* **2020**, *19*, 447–455. [CrossRef]
30. Richter, I.; Alajbeg, I.; Vučićević Boras, V.; Andabak Rogulj, A.; Brailo, V. Mapping Electrical Impedance Spectra of the Healthy Oral Mucosa: A Pilot Study. *Acta Stomatol. Croat.* **2015**, *49*, 331–339. [CrossRef]
31. Lang, K.; Held, T.; Freudlsperger, C.; Plath, K.; Hoffmann, J.; Plinkert, P.K.; Debus, J.; Adeberg, S. Oral Cavity Squamous Cell Carcinoma: Impact of Clear Margin Distance on Locoregional Control in Patients Undergoing Postoperative Radiotherapy. *Technol. Cancer Res. Treat.* **2024**, *23*, 15330338241258596. [CrossRef]
32. Sunkara, P.R.; Graff, J.T.; Cramer, J.D. Association of Surgical Margin Distance with Survival in Patients with Resected Head and Neck Squamous Cell Carcinoma. *JAMA Otolaryngol.–Head Neck Surg.* **2023**, *149*, 317. [CrossRef]
33. Kanatas, A.; Walshaw, E.G.; Wu, J.; Fabbroni, G.; Chengot, P. Prognostic factors in oral cancer surgery—Results from a UK tertiary centre. *Eur. J. Surg. Oncol.* **2023**, *49*, 755–759. [CrossRef]
34. Carobbio, A.L.C.; Cheng, Z.; Gianiorio, T.; Missale, F.; Africano, S.; Ascoli, A.; Fragale, M.; Filauro, M.; Marchi, F.; Guastini, L.; et al. Electric Bioimpedance Sensing for the Detection of Head and Neck Squamous Cell Carcinoma. *Diagnostics* **2023**, *13*, 2453. [CrossRef]

35. Horvat, K.; Richter, I.; Vucelić, V.; Gršić, K.; Leović, D.; Škrinjar, I.; Andabak Rogulj, A.; Velimir Grgić, M.; Brailo, V. Impact of Age and Sex on Electrical Impedance Values in Healthy Oral Mucosa. *Bioengineering* **2022**, *9*, 592. [CrossRef] [PubMed]
36. Lima, A.M.; Meira, I.A.; Soares, M.S.; Bonan, P.R.; Mélo, C.B.; Piagge, C.S. Delay in diagnosis of oral cancer: A systematic review. *Med. Oral Patol. Oral Cir. Bucal* **2021**, *26*, e815–e824. [CrossRef] [PubMed]
37. Lorenzo-Pouso, A.I.; Lafuente-Ibáñez de Mendoza, I.; Pérez-Sayáns, M.; Pérez-Jardón, A.; Chamorro-Petronacci, C.M.; Blanco-Carrión, A.; Aguirre-Urízar, J.M. Critical update, systematic review, and meta-analysis of oral erythroplakia as an oral potentially malignant disorder. *J. Oral Pathol. Med.* **2022**, *51*, 585–593. [CrossRef] [PubMed]
38. Brailo, V. Dentist and early detection of oral carcinoma. *Acta Med. Croat.* **2015**, *69*, 45–48.

diagnostics

MDPI

Article

# Quantitative Evaluation of Enamel Thickness in Maxillary Central Incisors in Different Age Groups Utilizing Cone Beam Computed Tomography a Retrospective Analysis

Kinga Mária Jánosi [1], Diana Cerghizan [1,*], Izabella Éva Mureșan [1], Alpár Kovács [2], Andrea Szász [2], Emese Rita Markovics [1], Krisztina Ildikó Mártha [1] and Silvia Izabella Pop [1]

1 Faculty of Dental Medicine, George Emil Palade University of Medicine, Pharmacy, Science and Technology of Târgu Mureș, 38 Gh. Marinescu Str., 540139 Târgu Mureș, Romania; kinga.janosi@umfst.ro (K.M.J.); izabella-eva.muresan@umfst.ro (I.É.M.); emese.markovics@umfst.ro (E.R.M.); krisztina.martha@umfst.ro (K.I.M.)

2 Private Practice, 540501 Târgu Mureș, Romania; alparko@yahoo.com (A.K.); andiiszasz@gmail.com (A.S.)

* Correspondence: diana.cerghizan@umfst.ro; Tel.: +40-740076876

**Abstract: Background/Objectives:** The presence of enamel on the tooth surface is crucial for the long-term success of minimally invasive adhesive restorations such as dental veneers. Our study aims to evaluate the enamel thickness in the incisal, middle, and cervical portions of the labial surface of the upper central incisors using cone beam computed tomography (CBCT). This imaging method provides detailed and accurate three-dimensional images with a low radiation dose, allowing an accurate assessment of enamel thickness. The analysis aims to identify variations in enamel thickness depending on the age and different levels of the labial tooth surface. **Methods:** 800 CBCT scans performed for diagnostic or therapeutic purposes on patients aged 18–60 years were analyzed. The data were gathered from the imaging archives of private practitioners from Targu Mures and the "George Emil Palade" University of Medicine, Pharmacy, Science, and Technology of Targu Mures. Enamel thickness measurements were conducted using the OnDemand3D Communicator CBCT evaluation program, with subsequent statistical analysis performed using GraphPad Instat Prism software. **Results:** Results showed significant variation in enamel thickness between the incisal, middle, and cervical segments of the labial surface of the upper central incisors. A decrease in enamel thickness with age has been observed. In patients aged 18–40, mean values of enamel thickness 1 mm and 3 mm above the cementoenamel junction (CEJ) were 0.48 ± 0.092, respectively, 0.819 ± 0.158. In patients over 40, the mean values were 0.454 ± 0.116 and 0.751 ± 0.067 at 1 mm, respectively, 3 mm above the CEJ. Statistically significant differences were found between the two age groups at 1 mm and 3 mm above the CEJ, with $p < 0.0001$ and $p = 0.0214$. **Conclusions:** A statistically significant decrease can be observed in enamel thickness in almost the entire labial surface of the upper central incisors with aging. The varied thickness of the enamel at different tooth levels requires individualized planning for each patient to maximize the long-term aesthetic and functional results.

**Keywords:** cone beam computed tomography (CBCT); dental enamel; dental imaging; enamel thickness; prosthodontics

## 1. Introduction

Society considers a perfect smile a sign of beauty, health, and success. Nowadays, patients desire to improve phonetic and masticatory functions and achieve "perfect" aesthetics. Physical appearance has become crucial in defining a person's identity, and a beautiful smile is essential [1,2]. Modern dentistry is characterized by using minimally invasive tooth preparation with maximum dental hard tissue preservation [3]. The presence of enamel plays an essential role in the long-term success of minimally invasive prosthetic restorations such as dental veneers, ensuring high-quality adhesive cementation [4,5], restoration durability, and accurate tooth shade [6–8]. Laminate veneers are commonly used to restore aesthetics and function [9], especially in the frontal area of the dental arches [10,11].

Any deviation from the prescribed protocol could lead to failure and compromise the integrity of the restorations [12,13].

Precisely measuring enamel thickness is essential in avoiding treatment setbacks before tooth preparation or orthodontic stripping procedures.

In a research study focused on porcelain laminate veneer preparation, investigators analyzed the enamel thickness in different sections of the labial surface of maxillary central and lateral incisors. The study demonstrated a significant variation in enamel thickness across different tooth surface regions, with the labial gingival third being the most vital area. These findings highlight the essentiality of careful enamel preservation during tooth preparation for adhesive restorations, especially laminate veneers [14].

Numerous techniques are utilized to measure enamel thickness accurately. A range of traditional and digital tools and techniques are employed for this purpose. Conventional techniques include physical sections and radiographic methods, while digital radiographs, computer-generated micro-CT sections [15,16], Optical Coherence Tomography (OCT) [17], and cone beam computed tomography (CBCT) [18] are examples of digital techniques. These tools and techniques can measure enamel thickness with high precision [19–21].

Grine et al. found that measuring enamel thickness using the lateral flat plane radiograph method had limitations [22]. Other studies have suggested an alternative, non-invasive, and potentially reliable method for measuring enamel thickness using CBCT. CBCT can offer a significant advantage over conventional radiography because it provides detailed and accurate three-dimensional (3D) images of dental structures. However, more research is needed to determine the level of precision and reliability of this method [23–25]. This technology is commonly used in dentistry, providing high-quality 3D images of anatomical structures with a relatively low radiation dose. It is useful in dental and maxillofacial imaging, allowing clinicians to visualize the teeth, jaws, and surrounding structures in a non-invasive manner. The cone-shaped X-ray beam allows for a more focused and precise image than traditional CT scans, making it a valuable tool for accurate diagnosis and treatment planning [26,27]. It uses multiplanar images, so it is possible to magnify the image, fix certain landmarks, and measure distances between specific anatomical structures. The user-friendly interface of the OnDemand3D software is popular among dental professionals. It is an advanced tool for processing, analyzing, and visualizing 3D images, performing cephalometric analysis, dental measurements, and assessment of facial structures to aid diagnosis and treatment planning. Quality assurance features (tools for image calibration, artifact detection, and image standardization) can help clinicians obtain high-quality diagnostic information. The Dental Volume Reformat—Dental Volume Reformatter (DVR) is the main module of the OnDemand 3D App that provides various formats of 3D images such as axial, panoramic, sagittal section, TMJ, and others [28].

The benefits of CBCT include its ability to produce more explicit images even in the presence of metal restorations or implants, fast processing and viewing of images, and significantly lower radiation doses (up to 96% lower) compared to conventional CT scans. CBCT produces sections of 0.1 mm, whereas CT produces sections with a thickness of 1 mm [29]. Additionally, CBCT is safe for repeated imaging [27] and reliable for measuring accurately the enamel thickness on different tooth surfaces, providing detailed and accurate images that different authors demonstrated in their studies [30–32]. Several studies have evaluated the enamel thickness on different portions of the vestibular surface of the maxillary incisors, concluding that there are variations in thickness at different levels related to the patient's age. However, few studies utilize CBCT examinations for this purpose.

This study aimed to assess the enamel thickness at various segments of the labial surface of the maxillary central incisors and explore potential associations with the age of participants using cone beam computed tomography (CBCT) scans. The null hypothesis was that there is no statistically significant difference in enamel thickness at the entire labial surface of the maxillary central incisors with aging.

## 2. Materials and Methods

### 2.1. Study Design

This retrospective study was conducted at the Faculty of Dental Medicine of the University of Medicine, Pharmacy, Science, and Technology "George Emil Palade" from Targu Mures. This study was designed to evaluate the enamel thickness of patients who had undergone diagnostic or therapeutic procedures at the university and at private dental offices in Targu Mures. This study was carried out in compliance with the Declaration of Helsinki and was approved by the Ethics Committee of the University (3084/22.04.2024). All participants provided written informed consent.

Following the anonymization of data, a single individual with expertise in dental radiology examined standardized CBCT scans of patients aged between 18 and 60. The data were obtained from the university's imaging archive as well as from various dentists in Targu Mures. The examined records were taken as part of the patients' diagnostic examinations or for therapeutic purposes, and as such, the patients were not unnecessarily exposed to additional radiation.

### 2.2. Sample Size

The sample size for this study was determined using the G*Power version 3.1.9.6. software (Franz Faul, Universität Kiel, Kiel, Germany) based on a pilot study performed prior. The calculations indicated that a minimum of 359 CBCT scans for each study group (total sample size of 718) would be necessary; this size would provide greater than 95% power to detect significant differences, with an effect size of 0.80 at a significance level of $\alpha = 0.05$. Thus, 800 CBCT full arch scans were included in this study according to the inclusion and exclusion criteria (Table 1), resulting in a total of 1600 examined maxillary central incisors. Two same-size groups were formed according to age: patients aged 18–40 years and those aged over 40 years.

**Table 1.** Inclusion and exclusion criteria for the CBCT records.

| Inclusion Criteria | Exclusion Criteria |
|---|---|
| Patients over 18 years | Patients younger than 18 years |
| Permanent dentition | Mixed/deciduous dentition |
| Presence of both maxillary central incisors | Malaligned maxillary central incisors |
| Sound permanent maxillary central incisors (no caries, endodontic treatments, or restorations) | Supernumerary teeth |
| | No shape or structural abnormalities |
| Completely erupted maxillary central incisors | Orthodontic treatment in progress |
| Full arch scans | Poor technical quality of the scans |

### 2.3. Imaging Methods Used

During this study, cone beam computed tomography (CBCT) was used as the imaging method. The CBCT scans were taken using a KaVo OP 3D imaging system (KaVo Ltd., Charlotte, NC, USA). The following scanning parameters were used for optimal image quality: 6 milliamperes of tube current (mA), 90 kilovolts (kV) of tube voltage, and a field of view (FOV) of 8 × 15 cm. The scans had a resolution set to a voxel size of 200 μm, considered a standard resolution allowing detailed examination of the anatomical structures. Each patient should be seated with teeth in maximum intercuspation position during the scanning process. The Frankfurt plane must align parallel to the floor; the mid-sagittal plane must remain perpendicular to the ground for accurate and consistent imaging.

### 2.4. Data Collection

The measurements were taken using OnDemand3D Communicator specialized software, version 1.0 (Cybermed, Daejeon, Republic of Korea) using the Dental module.

The enamel thickness of 1600 maxillary central incisors was recorded in the sagittal profile section of the midline. Four landmarks were selected on the median longitudinal axis of the tooth: (a) 1 mm incisally from cemento-enamel junction (CEJ); (b) 3 mm incisally from CEJ; (c) 5 mm incisally from CEJ; (d) 1 mm apically from the incisal edge (IE). (Figure 1). The tools used ("Taper, Ruler") were selected from the "Measure" menu.

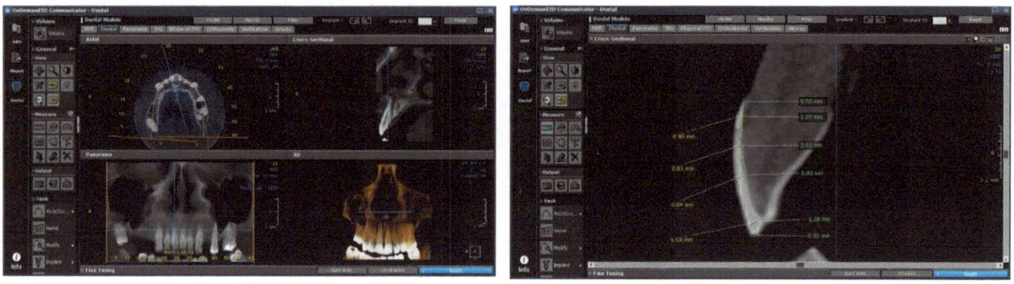

(**a**) (**b**)

**Figure 1.** The visualization of the CBCT images: (**a**) the Dental module of the OnDemand3D communicator software version 1.0 (Cybermed, Daejeon, Republic of Korea); (**b**) the landmarks used for the measurements.

The enamel thickness was measured by the same operator three times at each landmark. The arithmetic mean of these measurements was obtained, thus determining the result of the measurements. The data obtained were recorded in a database for later analysis.

The standard values were established based on the measurements taken by several authors on the labial surface of the central incisor:

- 1 mm above the cemento–enamel junction (CEJ), enamel thickness ranges from 0.17 mm to 0.52 mm, with a mean thickness of 0.31 mm.
- on the middle third of the surface, 5 mm from the CEJ, ranges from 0.45 mm to 0.93 mm, with a mean thickness of 0.75 mm [19,33,34].

### 2.5. Test–Retest Reliability

The interclass correlation coefficient (ICC) was calculated to determine the reliability of the measurements. The results showed an ICC over 0.75 for all the measurements performed, representing good to excellent reliability. The analysis of the standard error of the measurement showed a variability between 0.023 and 0.035, which demonstrates minimal variation between the measurements.

### 2.6. Statistical Analysis

The resulting data were analyzed using the GraphPad Prism 8 program for macOS (version 10.3.1 (464)). The mean (M), median (Me), and standard deviation (SD) were calculated. The statistical significance was set at $p < 0.05$. Given the non-normal distribution of the data, as confirmed using the Shapiro–Wilk test and the heterogeneity of variances indicated using Levene's test, we employed the Mann–Whitney test to explore the differences between the enamel thickness related to age and gender. This choice was guided by the test's suitability for non-parametric data. The Wilcoxon test explored the differences between the values obtained from the performed measurements and the standard values.

### 2.7. Abbreviations

- For the group aged between 18 and 40 years:

11g: right central incisor, 1 mm incisally from CEJ
11c: right central incisor, 3 mm incisally from CEJ
11m: right central incisor, 5 mm incisally from CEJ
11i: right central incisor, 1 mm apically from the IE
21g: left central incisor, 1 mm incisally from CEJ
21c: left central incisor, 3 mm incisally from CEJ
21m: left central incisor, 5 mm incisally from CEJ
21i: left central incisor, 1 mm apically from the IE

- For the group aged over 40 years:

11G: right central incisor, 1 mm incisally from CEJ
11C: right central incisor, 3 mm incisally from CEJ
11M: right central incisor, 5 mm incisally from CEJ
11I: right central incisor, 1 mm apically from the IE
21G: left central incisor, 1 mm incisally from CEJ
21C: left central incisor, 3 mm incisally from CEJ
21M: left central incisor, 5 mm incisally from CEJ
21I: left central incisor, 1 mm apically from the IE

## 3. Results

The mean age of the patients was 41.86 (SD = 11.63), 32.43 (SD = 7.892) for the 18–40 years group, respectively, and 51.30 (SD = 5.360) for patients over 40 years.

The results of the descriptive analysis conducted on the values obtained in the two groups included in the study are presented in Tables 2 and 3.

**Table 2.** Descriptive statistics for the group aged between 18 and 40 years.

| | Mean (m) | Median (M) | Minimum (min) | Maximum (Max) | Std. Deviation (SD) | Std. Error of Mean | Lower 95% CI of Mean | Upper 95% CI of Mean |
|---|---|---|---|---|---|---|---|---|
| 11g | 0.48 | 0.48 | 0.28 | 0.61 | 0.092 | 0.005 | 0.471 | 0.489 |
| 11c | 0.819 | 0.835 | 0.49 | 1.06 | 0.158 | 0.008 | 0.803 | 0.834 |
| 11m | 0.964 | 0.955 | 0.6 | 1.19 | 0.151 | 0.008 | 0.95 | 0.979 |
| 11i | 1.106 | 1.1 | 0.81 | 1.43 | 0.146 | 0.007 | 1.092 | 1.121 |
| 21g | 0.498 | 0.48 | 0.28 | 0.78 | 0.136 | 0.007 | 0.485 | 0.511 |
| 21c | 0.806 | 0.79 | 0.53 | 1.08 | 0.162 | 0.008 | 0.79 | 0.822 |
| 21m | 0.936 | 0.925 | 0.63 | 1.18 | 0.143 | 0.007 | 0.922 | 0.95 |
| 21i | 1.078 | 1.105 | 0.73 | 1.27 | 0.138 | 0.007 | 1.065 | 1.092 |

**Table 3.** Descriptive statistics for the group aged over 40 years.

| | Mean (m) | Median (M) | Minimum (min) | Maximum (Max) | Std. Deviation (SD) | Std. Error of Mean | Lower 95% CI of Mean | Upper 95% CI of Mean |
|---|---|---|---|---|---|---|---|---|
| 11G | 0.454 | 0.455 | 0.3 | 0.72 | 0.116 | 0.006 | 0.442 | 0.465 |
| 11C | 0.751 | 0.73 | 0.67 | 0.9 | 0.067 | 0.003 | 0.745 | 0.758 |
| 11M | 0.959 | 1.01 | 0.75 | 1.1 | 0.13 | 0.007 | 0.946 | 0.972 |
| 11I | 1.095 | 1.11 | 0.79 | 1.57 | 0.232 | 0.012 | 1.072 | 1.118 |
| 21G | 0.46 | 0.46 | 0.36 | 0.55 | 0.059 | 0.003 | 0.454 | 0.466 |
| 21C | 0.776 | 0.795 | 0.65 | 0.89 | 0.081 | 0.004 | 0.768 | 0.784 |
| 21M | 0.964 | 0.975 | 0.8 | 1.09 | 0.097 | 0.005 | 0.954 | 0.973 |
| 21I | 1.09 | 1.085 | 0.77 | 1.35 | 0.21 | 0.01 | 1.069 | 1.111 |

By comparing the values measured at the level of the right central incisor within the two groups included in the study, using the Mann–Whitney test, no statistically significant differences were found at the landmarks placed 1 mm apically from the IE and at 5 mm incisally from CEJ (Table 4, Figure 2).

**Table 4.** Mann–Whitney test results for the median values of the right central incisors related to the different age groups.

| Selected Landmarks | Difference Between Medians | *p*-Value |
|---|---|---|
| 1mm incisally from CEJ | 0.0250 | <0.0001 |
| 1 mm apically from the IE | 0.010 | 0.1797 |
| 5 mm incisally from CEJ | 0.055 | 0.7017 |
| 3 mm incisally from CEJ | −0.105 | <0.0001 |

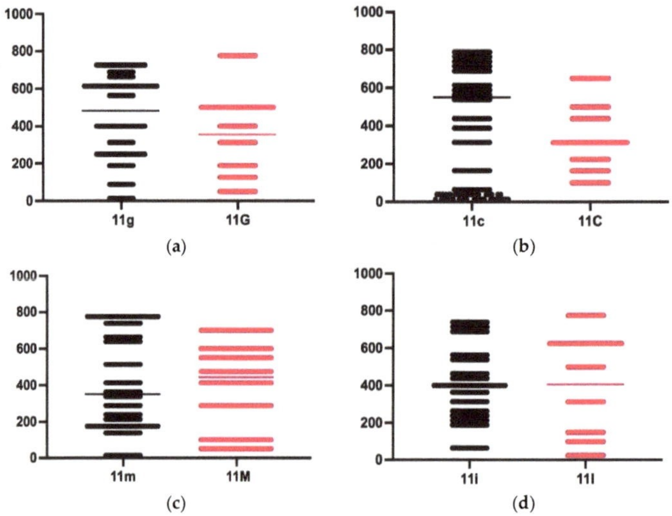


**Figure 2.** The differences between the values recorded by measuring the thickness of the enamel at the level of the right central incisor in the two groups studied: (**a**) difference at the landmark placed 1 mm incisally from CEJ; (**b**) difference at the landmark placed 3 mm incisally from CEJ; (**c**) difference at the landmark placed 5 mm incisally from CEJ; (**d**) difference at the landmark placed 1 mm apically from the IE.

At the level of the left central incisor, by comparing the measurements made at the selected landmarks within the two groups included in the study, it was found that there is no statistical difference at the landmark positioned 1 mm incisal from the CEJ and that located 1 mm apically from the IE (Table 5, Figure 3).

**Table 5.** Mann–Whitney test results for the median values of the left central incisors, related to the different age groups.

| Selected Landmarks | Difference Between Medians | *p*-Value |
|---|---|---|
| 1mm incisally from CEJ | −0.020 | 0.0845 |
| 1 mm apically from the IE | 0.005 | 0.7739 |
| 3 mm incisally from CEJ | 0.050 | 0.0214 |
| 5 mm incisally from CEJ | 0.005 | 0.0214 |

The values obtained in our study were compared with the mean values from the literature as well as with the maximum values that we considered as standard values. The results are presented in Tables 6–9.

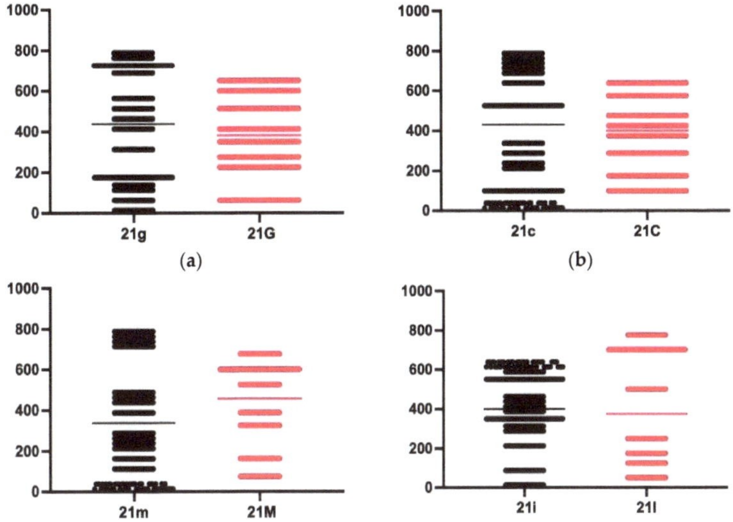


**Figure 3.** The differences between the values recorded by measuring the thickness of the enamel at the level of the left central incisor in the two groups studied: (**a**) difference at the landmark placed 1 mm incisally from CEJ; (**b**) difference at the landmark placed 3 mm incisally from CEJ; (**c**) difference at the landmark placed 5 mm incisally from CEJ; (**d**) difference at the landmark placed 1 mm apically from the IE.

**Table 6.** The discrepancies recorded between the values measured at 1 mm above the CEJ obtained within the study groups and the mean of the standard values.

| | Discrepancy | Mean of the Standard Values | *p*-Value |
|---|---|---|---|
| 11g | 0.170 | 0.31 | <0.0001 |
| 11G | 0.145 | | |
| 21g | 0.170 | | |
| 21G | 0.150 | | |

**Table 7.** The discrepancies recorded between the values measured at 1 mm above the CEJ obtained within the study groups and the maximum standard values.

| | Discrepancy | Mean of the Standard Values | *p*-Value |
|---|---|---|---|
| 11g | −0.04 | 0.52 | <0.0001 |
| 11G | −0.065 | | |
| 21g | −0.04 | | |
| 21G | −0.060 | | |

**Table 8.** The discrepancies recorded between the values measured at 5 mm incisally from CEJ obtained within the study groups and the mean of the standard values.

| | Discrepancy | Mean of the Standard Values | *p*-Value |
|---|---|---|---|
| 11m | 0.205 | 0.75 | <0.0001 |
| 11M | 0.260 | | |
| 21m | 0.175 | | |
| 21M | 0.225 | | |

**Table 9.** The discrepancies recorded between the values measured at 5 mm incisally from CEJ obtained within the study groups and the maximum standard values.

| | Discrepancy | Mean of the Standard Values | *p*-Value |
|---|---|---|---|
| 11m | 0.025 | 0.93 | <0.0001 |
| 11M | 0.080 | | 0.0293 |
| 21m | −0.005 | | 0.9998 |
| 21M | 0.045 | | <0.0001 |

## 4. Discussion

This study evaluates the enamel thickness at various levels of the labial surface of the upper incisors and explores potential associations with tooth age using CBCT scans.

Several authors have explored enamel thickness using different measurement methods. Ferrari et al. utilized a laboratory caliper with a millimeter scale to measure the enamel thickness of ten maxillary anterior teeth designated for ceramic veneers without considering the patient's age. Different enamel thicknesses were recorded at different levels of the labial surface: 0.4 mm gingivally, 0.9 mm in the middle third, and 1.0 mm at the incisal third [35]. Others [19,36,37] evaluated the labial enamel thickness of upper incisors by scanning electron microscope (SEM) or CBCT at 1, 3, and 5 mm distances from the CEJ to analyze the correlation between chronological age and enamel thickness in a population aged between 35 and 70 years, with 0.28 mm, 0.50 mm, and 0.73 mm thicknesses, and an inverse correlation between age and enamel thickness (1 mm = 0.31 ± 0.01; 3 mm = 0.54 ± 0.01; 5 mm = 0.75 ± 0.02/0.4 mm, 0.6 mm, 0.9 mm average values). Huysmans et al. proved the applicability of ultrasonic measurements for determining enamel thickness. At the same time, Louwerse pointed out the method's limitations, such as the inability to detect thickness changes of less than 0.33 mm [38,39]. Smith et al. used an invasive method to examine enamel thickness on the bucolingual cross-section of extracted molars on micrographs related to population and sex [40]. There have also been reported attempts to determine enamel thickness using lateral radiographs with a parallel film technique. The measurements obtained on the radiographs were compared with those from the longitudinal cross-section of the molars. This method has proven unprecise [22]. In other studies, without sex and age references, micro-CT or periapical radiographs were used to determine the enamel thickness on maxillary premolars and canines, proving the reliability and high accuracy of the method [32,41].

We can find similar studies about enamel thickness evaluation based on CBCT measurements in the literature. Brokos et al. demonstrated by CBCT measurements that the enamel thickness of the upper incisors decreases with age. The examined teeth were divided into three groups according to age. The obtained average values were young (846 μm), middle (758 μm), and aged (705 μm), with higher values in females. The location of the teeth did not influence the values; central and lateral incisors showed similar mean values [25].

The statistical analysis of our values obtained after the measurements showed no differences between the two age groups studied in most enamel thickness landmarks. Small but statistically significant differences were observed 1 mm above the CEJ. A similar study by Kunin et al. [42] revealed reduced enamel thickness in older people, especially in the gingival area. By comparing the values obtained through the measurements with the standard values selected from several studies, it was demonstrated that the values obtained in this study are lower, especially in the group over 40 years old. Our mean values recorded at the level of the incisal area and the middle third of the labial surface, regardless of age, are higher than those at the cervical level. Our findings follow those obtained by Mohamed, who concluded that dentin exposure must be avoided during tooth preparation, critically at the cervical level [6]. The reduced enamel thickness at this level, especially in older people, as observed in our study, requires rigorous treatment planning with the help of minimally invasive restorations to avoid compromising them. The same results were reported in a study conducted by Pahlevan et al., who performed measurements after tooth preparation for veneers and emphasized the importance of hard dental tissue preservation, especially at the cervical level [14]. The central incisors on both sides of the dental arch exhibit approximately equal enamel thickness, similar within each age category. By understanding these mean values, practitioners with varying experience levels can easily apply a standardized approach to minimally invasive preparation. Considering these values obtained using depth guidance techniques, primarily through mock-up preparation, excessive preparation, and the occurrence of dentin islands, which could compromise the longevity of the restoration, it can be avoided. Combining various magnification techniques with the mock-up preparation technique can significantly reduce excessive tooth structure removal, preserving hard dental tissues. In the case of preparation for veneers, the correct choice of bur size depends on the enamel thickness and the material from which the future restoration will be fabricated.

This study uses CBCT imaging to provide information about enamel thickness variations of upper central incisors. The findings may enhance dental treatment planning and prosthetic interventions in minimally invasive clinical practice. The quantity and quality of the remaining enamel after preparation can significantly influence the durability of the restoration from the cementation process onwards. The thicker the layer of remaining enamel and enamel–ceramic is, the more resistant the veneer is to the forces that can cause its fracture [12]. According to Yāgci et al., obtaining a maximal shear bond strength and optimal marginal sealing is necessary to maintain tooth preparation only in the enamel [43]. The statistical analysis of our values obtained after the measurements showed no differences between the two age groups studied at most enamel thickness landmarks. Small but statistically significant differences were observed 1 mm above the CEJ. A similar study by Kunin et al. [42] revealed reduced enamel thickness in older people, especially in the gingival area.

Limitations of the study: As this was a retrospective study, the factors influencing the quality and uniformity of the data recorded (ex., patient positioning) through CBCT could not be controlled. The measurements were made only at the level of the labial surface of the central incisors. Factors that could influence enamel thickness, such as previous orthodontic treatments, the level of dental wear, and the patients' sex, were not considered. The study groups were limited to a specific geographical location, which may affect the generalization of the results. These limitations underscore the need for further research to enhance the applicability of the findings, making the research more inclusive and impactful. Future studies should be extended to other dental groups and a more diverse population by considering a broader range of factors influencing enamel thickness, such as diet, dental hygiene, genetic aspects, and patients' gender, which will lead to a more comprehensive individualization of treatment planning, especially in minimally invasive dentistry.

## 5. Conclusions

Based on the findings of this study, the following conclusions were drawn:

The null hypothesis is rejected. A statistically significant decrease can be observed in enamel thickness in almost the entire labial surface of the upper central incisors with aging. The precise evaluation of enamel thickness is essential during the treatment planning for minimally invasive prosthetic rehabilitation with dental veneers. The enamel thickness variations at different levels of the tooth surface require individualized planning for each patient to maximize the long-term success of aesthetic and functional adhesive restorations.

**Author Contributions:** Conceptualization, K.M.J.; data curation, I.É.M.; formal analysis, A.K. and A.S.; investigation, K.M.J.; methodology, D.C.; resources, E.R.M.; supervision, S.I.P.; visualization, K.I.M.; writing—original draft preparation, K.M.J.; writing—review and editing, D.C. and S.I.P. All authors have read and agreed to the published version of the manuscript.

**Funding:** This research received no external funding.

**Institutional Review Board Statement:** This study was conducted in accordance with the Declaration of Helsinki on experimentation involving human subjects, as revised in 2013, and approved by the Ethical Committee of the University of Medicine, Pharmacy, Science, and Technology "G. E. Palade" of Târgu Mureș, Romania (3084/22.04.2024).

**Informed Consent Statement:** Written informed consent was obtained from all subjects involved in the study, including consent to publish the findings.

**Data Availability Statement:** The datasets analyzed during this study are available from the first author on request.

**Conflicts of Interest:** The authors declare no conflicts of interest.

## References

1. AlSagob, E.I.; Alkeait, F.; Alhaimy, L.; Alqahtani, M.; Hebbal, M.; Ben Gassem, A.A. Impact of Self-Perceived Dental Esthetic on Psycho-Social Well-Being and Dental Self Confidence: A Cross-Sectional Study Among Female Students in Riyadh City. *Patient Prefer. Adherence* **2021**, *15*, 919–926. [CrossRef] [PubMed] [PubMed Central]
2. Aishwarya, A.; Aiswarya, D.S.; Sasi, A.I.; Akshaya, V.S.; Subodh, A.; Praveen, D. Dental Aesthetics and Its Impact on Psychosocial Wellbeing among Students of Dental Colleges in South Kerala. *Int. J. Dent. Med. Sci. Res.* **2023**, *5*, 378–388. [CrossRef]
3. Yu, H.; Zhao, Y.; Li, J.; Luo, T.; Gao, J.; Liu, H.; Liu, W.; Liu, F.; Zhao, K.; Liu, F.; et al. Minimal Invasive Microscopic Tooth Preparation in Aesthetic Restoration: A Specialist Consensus. *J. Esthet. Restor. Dent.* **2019**, *11*, 31. [CrossRef]
4. Aminian, A.; Brunton, P.A. A Comparison of the Depths Produced Using Three Different Tooth Preparation Techniques. *J. Prosthet. Dent.* **2003**, *89*, 19–22. [CrossRef]
5. Öztürk, E.; Bolay, Ş.; Hickel, R.; Ilie, N. Shear Bond Strength of Porcelain Laminate Veneers to Enamel, Dentine and Enamel–Dentine Complex Bonded with Different Adhesive Luting Systems. *J. Dent.* **2013**, *41*, 97–105. [CrossRef]
6. Mohamed, M. Effect of Preparation Depth on the Fracture Resistance of Two Monolithic Ceramic Laminate Veneers. *Egypt. Dent. J.* **2022**, *68*, 2509–2517. [CrossRef]
7. Zhu, J.; Gao, J.; Jia, L.; Tan, X.; Xie, C.; Yu, H. Shear bond strength of ceramic laminate veneers to finishing surfaces with different percentages of preserved enamel under a digital guided method. *BMC Oral Health* **2022**, *22*, 3. [CrossRef]
8. Alavi, A.A.; Behroozi, Z.; Nik Eghbal, F. The shear bond strength of porcelain laminate to prepared and unprepared anterior teeth. *J. Dent.* **2017**, *18*, 50–55.
9. Vanlıoğlu, B.A.; Kulak-Özkan, Y. Minimally invasive veneers: Current state of the art. *Clin. Cosmet. Investig. Dent.* **2014**, *6*, 101–107. [CrossRef]
10. Cherukara, G.; Seymour, K.; Samarawickrama, D. A Study into the Variations in the Labial Reduction of Teeth Prepared to Receive Porcelain Veneers—A Comparison of Three Clinical Techniques. *Br. Dent. J.* **2002**, *192*, 401–404. [CrossRef]
11. Cherukara, G.P.; Seymour, K.G.; Zou, D.Y.D.; Samarawickrama, D.Y.D. Geographic Distribution of Porcelain Veneer Preparation Depth with Various Clinical Techniques. *J. Prosthet. Dent.* **2003**, *89*, 544–550. [CrossRef] [PubMed]
12. Ge, C.; Green, C.C.; Sederstrom, D.; McLaren, E.A.; White, S.N. Effect of porcelain and enamel thickness on porcelain veneer failure loads in vitro. *J. Prosthet. Dent.* **2014**, *111*, 380–387. [CrossRef] [PubMed]
13. Burke, F.T. Survival rates for porcelain laminate veneers with special reference to the effect of preparation in dentin: A literature review. *J. Esthet. Restor. Dent.* **2012**, *24*, 257–265. [CrossRef] [PubMed]
14. Pahlevan, A.; Mirzaee, M.; Yassine, E.; Ranjbar Omrany, L.; Hasani Tabatabaee, M.; Kermanshah, H.; Arami, S.; Abbasi, M. Enamel Thickness After Preparation of Tooth for Porcelain Laminate. *J. Dent.* **2014**, *11*, 428–432.
15. Gaboutchian, A.V.; Knyaz, V.A.; Maschenko, E.N.; Dac, L.X.; Maksimov, A.A.; Emelyanov, A.V.; Korost, D.V.; Stepanov, N.V. Measuring Dental Enamel Thickness: Morphological and Functional Relevance of Topographic Mapping. *J. Imaging* **2023**, *9*, 127. [CrossRef]
16. Bijle, M.N.; Mallineni, S.K.; Tsoi, J. Qualitative and Quantitative Micro-CT Analysis of Natal and Neonatal Teeth. *Children* **2022**, *9*, 560. [CrossRef] [PubMed] [PubMed Central]
17. Miyagi, H.; Oki, K.; Tsukiyama, Y.; Ayukawa, Y.; Koyano, K. Assessment of the Accuracy in Measuring the Enamel Thickness of Maxillary Incisors with Optical Coherence Tomography. *Diagnostics* **2022**, *12*, 1634. [CrossRef]

18. Hakami, Z.; Marghalani, H.Y.; Hedad, I.; Khawaji, M.; Abutaleb, G.; Hakami, A.; Almoammar, S.; Alshehri, A. Comparison of Tooth Color and Enamel and Dentinal Thickness between Orthodontically Treated and Untreated Individuals. *Diagnostics* **2023**, *13*, 2066. [CrossRef]
19. Atsu, S.S.; Aka, P.S.; Kucukesmen, H.C.; Kilicarslan, M.A.; Atakan, C. Age-Related Changes in Tooth Enamel as Measured by Electron Microscopy: Implications for Porcelain Laminate Veneers. *J. Prosthet. Dent.* **2005**, *94*, 336–341. [CrossRef]
20. Trivedi, A.; Trivedi, S.; Chhabra, S.; Bansal, A.; Jain, A.; Kaushal, P.; Sachdeva, S.; Kukreja, N. "It doesn't matter what lost what matter is what remains" R.D.T (Remaining Dentin Thickness): A review. *J. Pharm. Negat. Results* **2022**, *13*, 1004–1014.
21. Olejniczak, A.J.; Grine, F.E. Assessment of the accuracy of dental enamel thickness measurements using microfocal X-ray computed tomography. *Anat. Rec. A Discov. Mol. Cell Evol. Biol.* **2006**, *288A*, 263–275. [CrossRef] [PubMed]
22. Grine, F.E.; Stevens, N.J.; Jungers, W.L. An evaluation of dental radiograph accuracy in the measurement of enamel thickness. *Arch. Oral Biol.* **2001**, *46*, 1117–1125. [CrossRef] [PubMed]
23. Plotino, G.; Grande, N.M.; Pecci, R.; Bedini, R.; Pameijer, C.H.; Somma, F. Three-dimensional imaging using microcomputed tomography for studying tooth macromorphology. *J. Am. Dent. Assoc.* **2006**, *137*, 1555–1561. [CrossRef] [PubMed]
24. Baumgaertel, S.; Palomo, J.M.; Palomo, L.; Hans, M.G. Reliability and accuracy of cone-beam computed tomography dental measurements. *Am. J. Orthod. Dentofac. Orthop.* **2009**, *136*, 19–25. [CrossRef] [PubMed]
25. Brokos, Y.P.; Stavridakis, M.; Bortolotto, T.; Krejci, I. Evaluation of enamel thickness of upper anterior teeth in different age groups by Dental Cone Beam Computed Tomography Scan, in vivo. *Int. J. Adv. Case Rep.* **2015**, *2*, 1396–1409.
26. Pop, S.I.; Cerghizan, D.; Mițariu, L.; Jánosi, K.M.; D'Andrea, A. CBCT Evaluation of Alveolar Bone Change and Root Resorption after Orthodontic Treatment: A Retrospective Study. *Diagnostics* **2024**, *14*, 1757. [CrossRef]
27. Issrani, R.; Issrani, R.; Ganji, K. Cone-Beam Computed Tomography: A New Tool on the Horizon for Forensic Dentistry. *Int. J. Environ. Res. Public Health* **2022**, *19*, 5352. [CrossRef]
28. Băciuţ, M.F. *Implantologie Orală*; Editura Medicală Universitară "Iuliu Haţieganu": Cluj-Napoca, Romania, 2007; pp. 127–152, ISBN (10) 973-693-208-7/(13) 978-973-693-208-3.
29. Khalil, S.K.; Mudhir, A.M.; Sirri, M.R. Accuracy of CBCT and Intraoral Scanner Images for Measuring Tooth Widths and Bolton's Ratio: A Comparative Study with Gold Standard (Plaster Models) in Duhok's Adult Population. *SN Appl. Sci.* **2023**, *5*, 257. [CrossRef]
30. Wang, Y.; He, S.; Yu, L.; Li, J.; Chen, S. Accuracy of Volumetric Measurement of Teeth in Vivo Based on Cone Beam Computer Tomography. *Orthod. Craniofac. Res.* **2011**, *14*, 206–212. [CrossRef]
31. Abulhamael, A.M.; Barayan, M.; Makki, L.M.; Alsharyoufi, S.M.; Albalawi, T.H.S.; Zahran, S.; Alkhattab, O.; Kutbi, A.S.; Alrehili, R.S.; Alzamzami, Z.T. The Accuracy of Cone Beam Computed Tomography Scans in Determining the Working Length in Teeth Requiring Non-surgical Endodontic Treatment: A Retrospective Clinical Study. *Cureus* **2024**, *16*, e59907. [CrossRef] [PubMed] [PubMed Central]
32. Aktuna Belgın, C.; Serindere, G.; Orhan, K. Accuracy and Reliability of Enamel and Dentin Thickness Measurements on Micro-Computed Tomography and Digital Periapical Radiographs. *J. Forensic Radiol. Imaging* **2019**, *18*, 32–36. [CrossRef]
33. Jacobson, N.; Frank, C.A. The Myth of Instant Orthodontics: An Ethical Quandary. *J. Am. Dent. Assoc.* **2008**, *139*, 424–434. [CrossRef] [PubMed]
34. Shillingburg, H.T., Jr.; Grace, C.S. Thickness of Enamel and Dentin. *J. South Calif. Dent. Assoc.* **1973**, *41*, 33–36. [PubMed]
35. Ferrari, M.; Patroni, S.; Balleri, P. Measurement of Enamel Thickness in Relation to Reduction for Etched Laminate Veneers. *Int. J. Periodontics Restor. Dent.* **1992**, *12*, 407–413.
36. Kedici, P.S.; Atsü, S.; Gökdemir, K.; Sarikaya, Y.; Gürbüz, F. Micrometric Measurements by Scanning Electron Microscope (SEM) for Dental Age Estimation in Adults. *J. Forensic Odontostomatol.* **2000**, *18*, 22–26. [PubMed]
37. Al-Zahawi, A.R.; Ibrahim, R.O.; Talabani, R.M.; Dawood, S.N.; Garib DS, H.; Abdalla, A.O. Age and Sex Related Change in Tooth Enamel Thickness of Maxillary Incisors Measured by Cone Beam Computed Tomography. *BMC Oral Health* **2023**, *23*, 971. [CrossRef]
38. Huysmans, M.C.D.N.J.M.; Thijssen, J.M. Ultrasonic Measurement of Enamel Thickness: A Tool for Monitoring Dental Erosion? *J. Dent.* **2000**, *28*, 187–191. [CrossRef]
39. Louwerse, C.; Kjaeldgaard, M.; Huysmans, M.C.D.N.J.M. The Reproducibility of Ultrasonic Enamel Thickness Measurements: An In Vitro Study. *J. Dent.* **2004**, *32*, 83–89. [CrossRef]
40. Smith, T.M.; Olejniczak, A.J.; Reid, D.J.; Ferrell, R.J.; Hublin, J.J. Modern Human Molar End Thickness and Enamel–Dentine Junction Shape. *Arch. Oral Biol.* **2006**, *51*, 974–995. [CrossRef]
41. Akli, E.; Araujo, E.A.; Kim, K.B.; McCray, J.F.; Hudson, M.J. Enamel Thickness of Maxillary Canines Evaluated with Microcomputed Tomography Scans. *Am. J. Orthod. Dentofac. Orthop.* **2020**, *158*, 391–399. [CrossRef]
42. Kunin, A.A.; Evdokimova, A.Y.; Moiseeva, N.S. Age-Related Differences of Tooth Enamel Morphochemistry in Health and Dental Caries. *EPMA J.* **2015**, *6*, 3. [CrossRef]
43. Yağci, F.İ.L.İ.Z.; Türker, G.; Yılancı, H. Determination of the Thickness of the Safe Enamel for Laminate Veneer Preparation and Orthodontic Stripping by CBCT. *Niger. J. Clin. Pract.* **2021**, *24*, 525–533. [CrossRef]

*diagnostics*

MDPI

*Article*

# Application of Targeted Optical Coherence Tomography in Oral Cancer: A Cross-Sectional Preliminary Study

**Vera Panzarella [1,2], Fortunato Buttacavoli [1,3,*], Vito Rodolico [4], Laura Maniscalco [4], Alberto Firenze [2,4], Viviana De Caro [5], Rodolfo Mauceri [1,3], Simona E. Rombo [2,6] and Giuseppina Campisi [3,7]**

1 Department of Precision Medicine in Medical, Surgical and Critical Care (Me.Pre.C.C.), University of Palermo, 90127 Palermo, Italy; vera.panzarella@unipa.it (V.P.); rodolfo.mauceri@unipa.it (R.M.)

2 Center for Sustainability and Ecological Transition (CSTE), University of Palermo, 90127 Palermo, Italy; alberto.firenze@unipa.it (A.F.); simonaester.rombo@unipa.it (S.E.R.)

3 Unit of Oral Medicine and Dentistry for Fragile Patients, Department of Rehabilitation, Fragility, and Continuity of Care, University Hospital "Policlinico Paolo Giaccone" in Palermo, 90127 Palermo, Italy; giuseppina.campisi@policlinico.pa.it

4 Department of Health Promotion, Mother and Child Care, Internal Medicine and Medical Specialties (ProMISE), University of Palermo, 90127 Palermo, Italy; vito.rodolico@unipa.it (V.R.); laura.maniscalco04@unipa.it (L.M.)

5 Department of Biological, Chemical and Pharmaceutical Sciences and Technologies, University of Palermo, 90123 Palermo, Italy; viviana.decaro@unipa.it

6 Department of Mathematics and Computer Science (DMeI), University of Palermo, 90127 Palermo, Italy

7 Department of Biomedicine, Neurosciences and advanced Diagnostics (BIND), University of Palermo, 90127 Palermo, Italy

* Correspondence: fortunato.buttacavoli@unipa.it; Tel.: +39-0916554216

**Abstract:** Background/Objectives: The diagnosis of oral potentially malignant disorders (OPMDs) and oral squamous cell carcinoma (OSCC) represent a significant challenge in oral medicine. Optical coherence tomography (OCT) shows promise for evaluating oral tissue microstructure but lacks standardized diagnostic protocols tailored to the structural variability and lesions of oral mucosa. Methods: This cross-sectional observational study aims to evaluate the diagnostic accuracy of targeted biopsy-based and site-coded OCT protocols for common OPMDs and OSCC. Adult patients clinically diagnosed with OPMDs, including oral leukoplakia (OL), oral lichen planus (OLP), and OSCC were enrolled. Clinical and OCT evaluation before and after punch scalpel-site registration preceding diagnostic biopsy on the target site was performed. Blinded observers analyzed the OCT scans for OCT-based diagnoses. Sensitivity, specificity, and diagnostic accuracy for OCT evaluations before and after punch scalpel-site registration were statistically compared with histological findings. Results: A dataset of 2520 OCT scans and 210 selected images from 21 patients was obtained. Sensitivity and specificity post-target site registration were high for OSCC (98.57%, 100.00%), OL (98.57%, 98.57%), and OLP (97.14%, 98.57%). The positive predictive values ranged from 97.14% to 100.00%, while negative predictive values ranged from 98.57% to 99.29%. Inter-observer agreements were strong for OSCC (0.84) and moderate for OL (0.54) and OLP (0.47–0.49). Targeted OCT scans significantly improved diagnostic accuracy for all conditions ($p < 0.001$). Conclusions: This preliminary study supports using site-targeted OCT scans followed by a site-targeted punch biopsy, enhancing precision in oral diagnostics. This approach is foundational for developing pioneering automated algorithms guiding oral cancer and pre-cancer diagnosis via OCT imaging.

**Keywords:** optical coherence tomography; oral cancer; squamous cell carcinoma of head and neck; oral potentially malignant disorders; precancerous conditions; oral biopsy

## 1. Introduction

Oral carcinogenesis encompasses a multifaceted, multistage process leading to malignant transformation of the normal squamous cells of the oral mucosa. This complex development, influenced by several risk factors [1], is a protracted phenomenon that spans years. During this progression, oral potentially malignant disorders (OPMDs) usually emerge, comprising a diverse spectrum of lesions, each with varying temporal and localized transformation risks, acting as precursors to oral squamous cell carcinoma (OSCC). The critical potential of OPMDs to advance to OSCC underscores the urgency for timely detection and intervention.

The possible adoption by oral health practitioners of a proactive approach to early identification and managing these conditions can reduce the burden of oral cancer, fostering a comprehensive and personalized preventive protocol.

In clinical settings, the diagnosis of oral lesions primarily relies on visual inspection, followed by biopsy and histopathological examination, which remains the gold standard for definitive diagnosis. Additional diagnostic modalities include toluidine blue staining, brush biopsy with cytological analysis, and fluorescence visualization (e.g., VELscope) that can help in identifying suspicious areas [2,3]. Advanced imaging techniques, such as high-resolution micro-endoscopy (HRME) and narrow-band imaging (NBI), offer real-time visualization of mucosal abnormalities but are limited by operator dependency and variable specificity [4]. Cross-sectional imaging methods like MRI and CT scans are used for deeper tissue assessment but lack the resolution to discern superficial epithelial changes crucial for early-stage diagnosis. Despite the availability of several oral screening devices [2–5], the clinical heterogeneity and overlapping features of these disorders pose significant challenges in accurate differentiation between 'abiding' OPMDs and those with dysplasia already in progress.

In this scenario, the diagnostic delay in oral cancer remains paradoxically high, with a late diagnosis rate still high for an anatomical region that is among the easiest to inspect. Consequently, the mortality rate of OSCC patients has remained unchanged over the last 20 years, despite the innovative screening and therapeutic techniques available today [6,7]. Non-invasive, standardized, and easy-to-use strategies remain the key method to promote early diagnosis and improve the prognosis of OPMDs and OSCC. In oral oncology, optical techniques have been used to non-invasively provide information regarding the biological tissue changes in optical characteristics that might result in improved life-saving outcomes for oral cancer patients, from screening and staging to follow-up [8,9].

Among these, Optical Coherence Tomography (OCT) is an emerging technology enabling cross-sectional imaging of biological tissues [10–12], permitting a non-invasive evaluation of ultrastructural characteristics of mucosal organizations. The potential validity of OCT in oral carcinogenesis has been widely investigated since several ex vivo and in vivo studies have compared the OCT images of normal and pathological lesions to histological results [13–17]. OCT proved a potential diagnostic indicator of progressive tissue transformation scans from normal epithelium to early invasive carcinoma in the oral cavity [11,18–22]. Especially in the artificial intelligence (AI) era, these innovative potentials have also been considered for the development of automated diagnostic-based-OCT algorithms, to improve optical interpretation of oral carcinogenesis [23–28].

However, no accurate automated diagnostic tool can be employed without a standardized protocol for the selection and purchase of clinical, digital, optical, and histological images of the oral lesions, which is currently needed, particularly concerning the use of OCT on early oral carcinogenesis [10,29–31]. The lack of procedural standardization and interoperability intervenes in all the operational sequences involved in the development of AI models applied to oral cancer diagnosis, starting from the clinical, histological, and OCT-guided evaluation of the suspected lesion. Moreover, in general, to date, there is no validated operational protocol for the correct OCT interpretations of OPMDs and OSCC, which respects their morphological/chromatic heterogeneity (i.e., ulcerative, hyperkeratotic, vegetating lesions) and variable microstructure of the mucosa in several oral sites. This places very strong limits on the possibility of having correct and reproducible interpretations of these lesions, using OCT, making plans for its use for the non-invasive monitoring of OPMD and the early diagnosis of OSCC useless. Particularly, standardized OCT collection of images is essential to ensure that the datasets obtained are comprehensive, reliable, and accurately representative of the targeted pathologies. This entails meticulous attention to sampling technique, and clinical, optical, and histological image labelling, to improve the overall quality and reproducibility of oral carcinogenesis OCT-based interpretation.

This study introduces the first phase of a multistep project aiming to offer a standardized OCT diagnostic algorithm for the most common OPMDs, comprising oral leukoplakia (OL), oral lichen planus (OLP), and OSCC. Particularly, this preliminary cross-sectional investigation aims to validate a clinical protocol based on the use of structured OCT digital lesion patterns. Through the application of these models to OCT scans of targeted biopsy sites, the aim is to enhance the diagnostic precision of OCT for early oral cancer and precursor oral lesions compared to traditional histopathological examination.

To the best of our knowledge, it is the first time that a standardized clinical, digital-OCT and histological design integrated model for the evaluation of OL, OLP and OSCC, to support the development of targeted diagnostic automatized optical algorithms, has been proposed in the literature.

## 2. Materials and Methods

The study protocol conformed to the ethical guidelines of the 1964 Declaration of Helsinki and its later amendments or comparable ethical standards. It was also approved by the Institutional Review Board of University Hospital "Policlinico Paolo Giaccone" in Palermo (Italy), approval number 11/2016. Adherence to research reporting guidelines, specifically STROCSS for cross-sectional studies, ensures comprehensive and transparent reporting of our research findings [32].

### *2.1. Sample Selection*

All participants, after providing written informed consent, were consecutively recruited at the Oral Medicine Unit of the University Hospital "Policlinico Paolo Giaccone" in Palermo (Italy), between January and March 2024.

The eligibility criteria were the following:

1. Age $\geq$ 18 years;
2. Ability to provide informed consent;
3. Clinical diagnosis strongly suggestive of OPMDs and OSCC, according to WHO classification and consensus for oral cancer and head and neck [33,34].

Patients were screened through a comprehensive conventional oral examination (COE) [35] including OCT scans and biopsy, to ensure a comprehensive understanding of the clinical presentation of eligible oral lesions, providing essential contextual information for the subsequent diagnostic procedures.

A digital photographic set per lesion was made to record the site of future evaluation, by OCT and histology, of the lesions. All photographs were taken using a Nikon D7200 Camera, with a Nikon AF-S DX 105 mm F2.8G Lens and Nikon R1C1 dual flash (Nikon Corporation, Tokyo, Japan).

Demographic data on gender and age were collected. Each lesion was site-coded applying the 2021 NIH/SEER ICD-0-3.2 topographical classification codes (from C02.0 to C02.2 for the mobile tongue, C03.0 and C03.1 for the upper and lower gum, respectively, and C06.0 for cheek mucosa, buccal mucosa, and internal cheek) [36,37].

### *2.2. Phase 1: OCT Evaluation Pre-Target Site Registration*

For this study, we used the device OCT SS-OCT VivoSight®, Michelson Diagnostics Ltd., version 2.0, Orpington, Kent, UK. The system type is a Swept-source Fourier-Domain OCT. The light source of the device is a Santec HSL-2000-12 wide sweep laser with a central wavelength of 1305 $\pm$ 15 nm and a frequency sweep range of $\geq$150 nm. The axial optical resolution in tissues is <10 μm and the lateral resolution is <7.5 μm, with a maximum scan width of 6 mm $\times$ 6 mm to a focal depth of $\approx$2 mm.

The scan obtained was of the "EnFace" type with a default width set to 6 mm with 120 slices, corresponding to a slicing step of 50 µm, for a total scan duration of 12 s.

The preliminary OCT assessment was conducted by the same oral expert (G.C.) on the most clinically suggestive area for each lesion, taking into consideration standardized and histologically compared OCT patterns of OL, OLP and OSCC, validated in the previously published investigations [19,38–45]. In particular, these studies focus on OL, OLP and OSCC, with OCT parameters/patterns evaluating the various mucosal layers (Keratinized Layer (KL), Stratified Epithelial Layer (SEL), Basement Membrane (BM), and Lamina Propria (LP)), compared to healthy mucosa, as detailed in Figure 1.

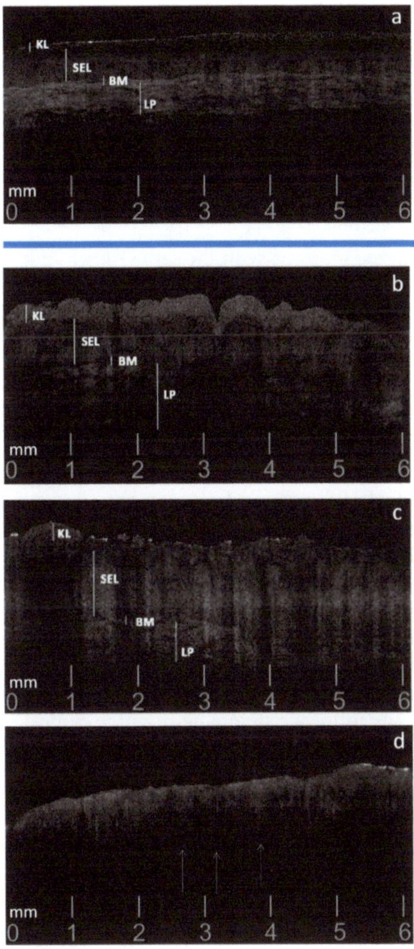


| | OCT – HEALTHY MUCOSA |
|---|---|
| KL | 1) Assessable<br>2) Slightly hyper-reflective<br>3) Thin thickness/distinguishable from SEL |
| SEL | 1) Assessable<br>2) Hypo-reflective<br>3) Distinguishable from KL/LP |
| BM | Continuously assessable |
| LP | 1) Well demarcated<br>2) Hyper-reflective |

| | OCT – OL |
|---|---|
| KL | 1) Assessable<br>2) Strongly hyper-reflective<br>3) Increased thickness/distinguishable from SEL |
| SEL | 1) Assessable<br>2) Hypo-reflective<br>3) Distinguishable from KL/LP |
| BM | Continuously assessable |
| LP | 1) Slightly demarcated<br>2) Discontinuously hyper-reflective |

| | OCT – OLP |
|---|---|
| KL | 1) Discontinuously assessable<br>2) Moderately hyper-reflective<br>3) Discontinuously distinguishable from SEL |
| SEL | 1) Assessable<br>2) Strongly hyper-reflective<br>3) Discontinuously distinguishable from KL/Distinguishable from LP |
| BM | Discontinuously assessable |
| LP | 1) Slightly demarcated<br>2) Hyper-reflective |

| | OCT – OSCC |
|---|---|
| KL | *Not assessable*<br>*Indistinguishable from SEL* |
| SEL | *Not assessable (*)*<br>*Indistinguishable from KL/LP* |
| BM | *Not assessable (*)* |
| LP | *Not assessable (*)* |

**Figure 1.** Guiding pattern criteria for the selection of OCT scans, comparing the patterns observed in healthy oral mucosa (**a**) with those in OL (**b**), OLP (**c**), and OSCC (**d**). OL: Oral Leukoplakia; OLP: Oral Lichen Planus; OSCC: Oral Squamous Cell Carcinoma; KL: Keratinized Layer; SEL: Stratified Epithelial Layer; BM: Basement Membrane; LP: Lamina Propria. (*) Presence of 'icicle-like' structures: hyper-reflective conical configurations that extend from the superficial cellular layers (SEL) to the deeper ones (BM and LP), commonly reported in OSCC, suggestive of neoplastic intra/sub-epithelial infiltration (indicated by white arrows ↑) [19].

For each recruited lesion, 120 OCT scans were obtained. From this set, the 10 most representative scans were meticulously selected, employing rigorous criteria grounded in image definition. Preference was given to scans exhibiting optimal visualization of tissue stratification, clear delineation, and pronounced contrast among epithelial components, selecting OCT images that showcased discernible patterns in the most recognizable manner possible.

### 2.3. Phase 2: OCT Evaluation Post-Target Site Registration

After the OCT preliminary evaluation (Figure 2a–f), the target registration of the most representative site for biopsy was performed (Figure 2g,i,k). Specifically, following topical surface anesthesia with lidocaine 25 mg/g + prilocaine 25 mg/g in a cream formulation, the site was marked by the circular blade of a disposable punch biopsy scalpel, 6 mm in diameter (KAI medical, Gifu, Japan), deepened into the supra-epithelial layers, to avoid bleeding and discomfort (≈0.5 mm). Intra-oral photographs of targeted sites were recorded. On this marked site, the same operator (G.C.) carried out a secondary OCT scan session, as previously detailed, obtaining the 10 most representative OCT scans for each lesion, based on the same selected OCT pattern (Figure 2h,j,l).

### 2.4. Phase 3: Targeted Biopsy and Histological Evaluation

After the OCT evaluation steps, the targeted biopsy, with the same punch biopsy scalpel used in the preliminary step, and in the same pre-registered site, was finalized for each lesion, to provide histological confirmation. The surgical margins of the tissue samples were oriented by sutures and photographed to record the preserved orientation equal to the oral in vivo localization.

A comprehensive histological examination, also including the search for epithelial dysplasia, was performed on all collected samples to definitively confirm the initial clinical suspicions. To ensure precise correspondence between the histological analysis and the OCT scans, for each biopsy specimen, while maintaining the spatial orientation, a surgical marker was employed to draw a line across the diametral line. The biopsy specimens were subjected to routine processing, involving fixation in a 10% formalin solution followed by embedding in paraffin. These formalin-fixed, paraffin-embedded (FFPE) samples were then sectioned to a thickness of 5 μm, specifically oriented to correspond with the OCT imaging. These sections were subsequently stained using standard hematoxylin and eosin (H&E) staining techniques and meticulously examined to validate and establish the final diagnosis. The pathologist (VR), responsible for the dissection of the specimens, undertook an independent and blinded evaluation of the histological images. This approach ensured an impartial assessment, free from any influence stemming from the clinical or OCT-based diagnoses.

### 2.5. Phase 4: Blinded Pre- and Post-Site Registration OCT Inter-Comparison to Histological Diagnosis

To strengthen the diagnostic assessment, two distinct OCT examiners (V.P. and F.B.) independently evaluated the OCT images collected pre- and post-site registration. Their OCT evaluations were blinded to both the clinical diagnosis and the histopathological findings. These examiners were assigned the responsibility of discerning structural alterations, employing the same OCT patterns used in the previous steps. The proposed OCT-based diagnoses were then compared to the confirmatory histopathologic diagnoses by a pathologist (V.R.) for both pre- and post-site registration OCT scanning sessions (Figure 2m–o).

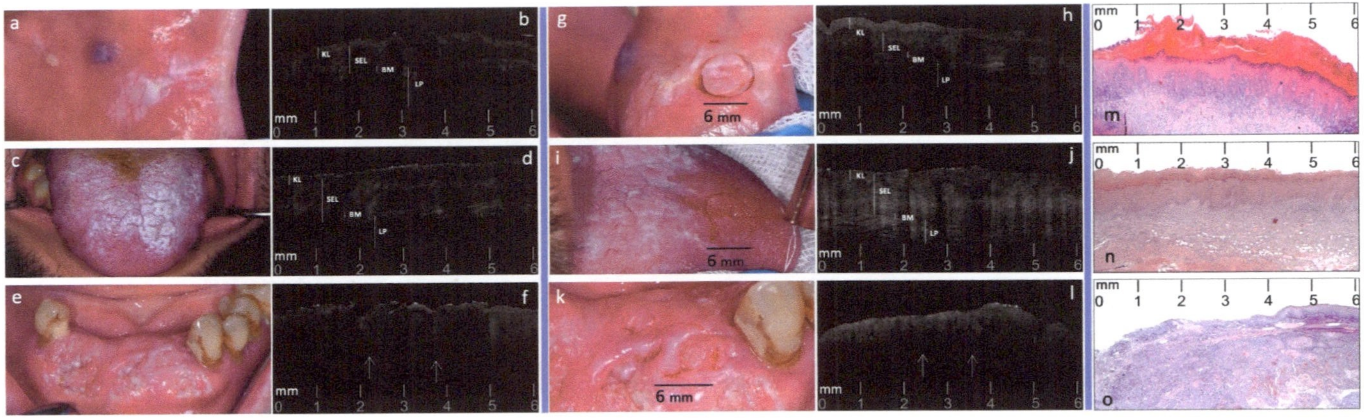


**Figure 2.** Pre- and post-target site registration clinical, and related OCT most representative scans, compared to histopathology confirmatory images of three selected cases of OL, OLP and OSCC (**a**,**b**): pre-site registration clinical image (**a**) and OCT scan (**b**) of a case of homogeneous OL on the left buccal mucosa. (**c**,**d**): pre-site registration clinical image (**c**) and OCT scan (**d**) of a case of reticular OLP on the dorsal surface of the tongue. (**e**,**f**): pre-site registration clinical image (**e**) and OCT scan (**f**) of a case of OSCC on lower anterior alveolar mucosa. (**g**,**h**): post-site registration clinical image (**c**) and OCT scan (**d**) of the previous OL case. (**i**,**j**): post-site registration clinical image (**i**) and OCT scan (**j**) of the previous OLP case. (**k**,**l**): post-site registration clinical image (**k**) and OCT scan (**l**) of the previous OSCC case. (**m**–**o**): histopathology confirmatory images (H&E stain; original magnification ×2.5) of the previous OL, OLP and OSCC cases, ((**m**), (**n**), (**o**) respectively). KL: Keratinized Layer; SEL: Stratified Epithelial Layer; BM: Basement Membrane; LP: Lamina Propria; white arrows (↑): 'icicle-like' structures.

To ensure robustness and consistency in the measurements, a secondary scoring round was conducted after a one-month interval, allowing for the evaluation of intra-observer agreement concerning the two separate OCT scan sessions. Throughout this process, a crucial measure was taken to prevent any bias: OCT images were intentionally randomized to guarantee that the initial recording did not exert any influence on the subsequent evaluations. This rigorous methodology was meticulously employed to ensure the accuracy, reliability, and integrity of the diagnostic comparisons between OCT and histological data.

### 2.6. Statistical Analysis

The continuous variables were summarized as mean and standard deviation, while categorical variables were analyzed as counts and percentages. Sensitivity, specificity, and positive and negative predicted values were computed for OSCC, OL, and OLP on preliminary OCT images and OCT after punch-targeted tissue. 95% confidence intervals (95% CI) for sensitivity and specificity were obtained with the exact Clopper-Pearson method. At the same time, 95% CI for predictive values was computed as suggested by Mercaldo et al., 2007, except in the case of 0 or 100% where the Clopper-Pearson method was used [46]. Cohen's kappa was used to assess the two observers' agreement on preliminary OCT images and OCT after punch-targeted tissue. Furthermore, the McNemar test for paired data was applied to assess, for each observer, whether the differences between pre- and post-site target registration OCT-based diagnosis affect the identification of the specific disease. Statistical analysis was performed with MedCalc, and an alpha value of 0.05 was considered statistically significant.

## 3. Results

According to the 2021 NIH/SEER ICD-O-3.2 topographical classification, 21 suspected lesions were recruited: seven homogeneous OL (three from the buccal mucosa (C06.0, mean age: 68.7 years; SD: 6.65), four from the ventral tongue (C02.2, mean age: 69.5 years; SD: 6.80)); seven reticular/plaque OLP (four from the buccal mucosa (C06.0, mean age: 64.5 years; SD: 7.89), three from the dorsal tongue (C02.0, mean age: 61.3 years; SD: 1.70)); seven OSCC (three from the anterior inferior alveolar mucosa (C03.1, mean age: 70.7 years; SD: 1.70), four from the lateral tongue border (C02.1, mean age: 75.0 years; SD: 0.82)).

For each lesion, a total of 120 OCT scans were acquired in both OCT evaluation sessions (phases 1–2), resulting in a cumulative dataset of 2520 scans per session. After the selection of the 10 most representative OCT images for each lesion, a total of 210 scans per session was finally processed for the next evaluation phases.

In particular, targeted biopsies were performed, and histological diagnosis was confirmed for all 21 recruited lesions: seven OL, seven OLP and seven OSCC (phase 3). For OL and OLP, no dysplasia was detected.

The diagnostic accuracy of pre- and post-site registration OCT-based diagnoses for both operators was evaluated (phase 4), showing increased sensitivity and specificity values with the application of target scanning for all lesions. Notably, post-target scans exhibited a sensitivity of 98.57% for OSCC, with a specificity of 100.00%. For OL, sensitivity reached 98.57% and specificity was 98.57%. Regarding OLP, sensitivity was 97.14% and specificity was 98.57%. Positive predictive values for OSCC were 100.00%, while for OL and OLP they were 97.18% and 97.14%, respectively. Similarly, negative predictive values exceeded 99% for all conditions (Table 1).

The correctness and correspondence between the OCT-based diagnosis proposed by each observer and the histological diagnosis were confirmed by the McNemar test. The percentage of preliminary OCT images, scanned before the target site registration, and interpreted with the correct diagnosis compared to histopathology, reached over 68.6% for both scoring sessions; higher percentages were obtained for OSCC images (82.9%). The percentages of targeted-OCT images (scanned on the marked site) and interpreted as correct compared to the histopathological diagnosis were higher, with percentages reaching over 97.1%; higher percentages were obtained for OSCC and OL scans (98.6%), slightly lower for OLP (97.1%) for both OCT sessions. The increase in the values of diagnoses corresponding to histopathology, based on OCT scans made on punch-targeted tissue, was statistically significant both for OPMDs ($p < 0.001$ both for OL and OLP) and for OSCC ($p = 0.001$) (Table 2).

**Table 1.** Diagnostic accuracy measures for OCT compared to histopathology findings. Pre-target indicates the OCT evaluation pre-target site registration; post-target indicates the OCT evaluation post-target site registration.

| | | | Predictive Value % (95% CI) | |
|---|---|---|---|---|
| **Observer 1** | **Sensitivity % (95% CI)** | **Specificity % (95% CI)** | **Positive** | **Negative** |
| Pre-target | | | | |
| OSCC | 82.86, (71.97–90.82) | 97.86, (93.87–99.56) | 95.08, (86.26–98.35) | 91.95, (87.21–95.03) |
| OL | 70.00, (57.87–80.38) | 85.00, (77.99–90.47) | 70.00, (60.45–78.08) | 85.00, (79.74–89.08) |
| OLP | 68.57, (56.37–79.15) | 77.86, (70.07–84.43) | 60.76, (52.21–68.70) | 83.21, (77.61–87.63) |
| Post-target | | | | |
| OSCC | 98.57, (92.30–99.96) | 100.00, (97.40–100.00) | 100.00, (94.79–100.00) | 99.29, (95.24–99.90) |
| OL | 98.57, (92.30–99.96) | 98.57, (94.93–99.83) | 97.18, (89.70–99.27) | 99.28, (95.17–99.90) |
| OLP | 97.14, (90.06–99.65) | 98.57, (94.93–99.83) | 97.14, (89.56–99.26) | 98.57, (94.62–99.63) |
| Observer 2 | | | | |
| Pre-target | | | | |
| OSCC | 82.86, (71.97–90.82) | 98.57, (94.93–99.83) | 96.67, (87.94–99.14) | 92.00, (87.29–95.06) |
| OL | 70.00, (57.87–80.38) | 84.29, (77.18–89.88) | 69.01, (59.57–77.10) | 84.89, (79.60–89.00) |
| OLP | 68.57, (56.37–79.15) | 78.57, (70.84–85.05) | 61.54, (52.88–69.52) | 83.33, (77.78–87.72) |
| Post-target | | | | |
| OSCC | 98.57, (92.30–99.96) | 100.00, (97.40–100.00) | 100.00, (94.79–100.00) | 99.29, (95.24–99.90) |
| OL | 98.57, (92.30–99.96) | 98.57, (94.93–99.83) | 97.18, (89.70–99.27) | 99.28, (95.17–99.90) |
| OLP | 97.14, (90.06–99.65) | 98.57, (94.93–99.83) | 97.14, (89.56–99.26) | 98.57, (94.62–99.63) |

**Table 2.** McNemar test for paired data conducted on OCT evaluation pre- and post-target site registration. Pre-target indicates the OCT evaluation pre-target site registration; post-target indicates the OCT evaluation post-target site registration (* 95% CI was reported as the difference percentage).

| **Observer 1** | **Pre-Target *n.* (%)** | **Post-Target *n.* (%)** | **Difference** | **95% CI, % *** | | ***p*-Value** |
|---|---|---|---|---|---|---|
| OSCC | 58 (82.9) | 69 (98.6) | 15.71% | 7.19 | 24.24 | 0.001 |
| OL | 49 (70) | 69 (98.6) | 28.57% | 17.99 | 39.15 | <0.001 |
| OLP | 48 (68.6) | 68 (97.1) | 28.57% | 17.99 | 39.15 | <0.001 |
| Observer 2 | | | | | | |
| OSCC | 57 (81.4) | 69 (98.6) | 17.14% | 8.31 | 25.97 | <0.001 |
| OL | 50 (71.4) | 69 (98.6) | 27.14% | 16.73 | 37.56 | <0.001 |
| OLP | 49 (70) | 68 (97.1) | 27.14% | 16.73 | 37.56 | <0.001 |

The Cohen's kappa value for identification of OSCC inter-observer agreement was 0.84 (95% CI = 0.76–0.92), representing very good agreement. It was equal to 0.54 (95% CI = 0.42–0.66) for OL and 0.47 (95% CI = 0.34–0.59) for OLP in pre-target, representing for both a moderate agreement. In the post-target phase, the inter-observer agreement was 0.84 (95% CI = 0.76–0.92), representing very good agreement for OSCC, 0.54 (95% CI = 0.42–0.66) for OL and 0.49 (95% CI = 0.37–0.61) for OLP, expressing for both a moderate agreement.

## 4. Discussion

The findings of this cross-sectional study suggest that the use of standardized OCT patterns, particularly defined for OSCC, OL and OLP, and standardized data acquisition procedures in the context of different morphology of oral mucosa and lesions, could enhance the accuracy of OCT in oral cancer diagnosis.

An important lack of uniformity still exists in the literature regarding the OCT in vivo preliminary interpretations and the concordance of clinical, optical, and histological exploration, especially referring to OSCC and OPMDs and OCT procedures (Table 3).

**Table 3.** Characteristics of the studies investigating in vivo/ex vivo application of OCT for preliminary assessment of OSCC and OPMDs. BM: Basement Membrane; CIS: Carcinoma in situ; EP: Squamous stratified epithelium; EP Re: Reflectivity of epithelial layer; ET: Epithelial Thickness; DG: Desquamative Gingivitis; GVHD: Graft Versus Host Disease; K-micro: Micro-invasive carcinoma; KL: Keratinized Layer; LP: Lamina Propria; LP Re: Reflectivity of lamina propria; MMP: Mucous Membrane Pemphigoid; OL: Oral Leukoplakia; OLP: Oral Lichen Planus; OSCC: Oral Squamous Cell Carcinoma; PVL: Proliferative Verrucous Leukoplakia; PV: Pemphigus Vulgaris; SEL: Stratified Epithelial Layer; SS: Stratified Squamous epithelium.

| | Author (Year) | Study Design | N. Cases | Clinical Appearance | Pathological Diagnosis | Oral Sites | OCT Patterns Parameters/Evaluation |
|---|---|---|---|---|---|---|---|
| 1 | Ridgway (2006) [41] | Case series | 41 | Not specified benign and malignant lesions | Begnin lesions, OL, CIS, OSCC | Buccal mucosa, Floor of mouth, Gingiva, Hard palate, Lip, Tongue | SS, BM/LP |
| 2 | Wilder-Smith (2009) [40] | Preliminary Study | 50 | Leukoplakia, erythro-plakia | Dysplasia (mild, moderate, severe) CIS, OSCC | Tongue, Buccal mucosa, Floor of mouth | SEL, BM, LP |
| 3 | Volgger (2012) [42] | Prospective diagnostic trial | 100 | Leukoplakia, erythro-plakia | OSCC, dysplasia, OLP | Buccal mucosa, Floor of mouth, Gingiva, Palate, Lip, Tongue (detailed only for healthy mucosa) | KL, EP, ET, BM, LP |
| 4 | Gambino (2020) [38] | Case control study | 20 | Atrophic-erosive OLP | OLP | Buccal mucosa | EP, BM, LP |
| 5 | Panzarella (2021) [43] | Observational study | 43 | DG | OLP, PV, MMP | Gingiva | SEL, BM, LP |
| 6 | Panzarella (2022) [19] | Descriptive pilot Study | 30 | Suspected OSCC | OSCC | Tongue, Gingiva, Buccal mucosa | KL, SEL, BM, LP |
| 7 | Gambino 2022 [45] | Case/control study | 50 | Non-healing Ulcerations | Traumatic lesions, OSCC | Buccal mucosa, Gingiva, Tongue | EP, BM, LP |
| 8 | Gambino (2023) [39] | Case series | 11 | White, red-white lesions, ulcers | PVL, OLP, OL, GVHD, K-MICRO | Tongue, Gingiva, Buccal mucosa | KL, EP, BM, LP |
| 9 | Gruda (2023) [44] | Case series | 15 | OLP, leukoplakia | OLP, OL, OSCC | Buccal mucosa, Tongue | EP, EP Re, LP Re, BM |

Lesions selection and histological diagnosis appear extremely heterogeneous, especially in studies where the clinical apparency is not well defined; while most studies define the lesions to be included, selecting on appearance (white, red, or white and red lesions) as clinically assimilable to OPMDs [19,38–40,42–45]. Also, the distribution of lesions within the oral cavity exhibits notable variability. All studies process OCT evaluations of the lesions by comparison with healthy mucosa, and most base this assessment on the same anatomical site [19,38–40,42–45]. In our previous investigation and recent studies of Gambino et al., OSCC lesions were compared systematically to the healthy normal mucosa of the same site, revealing the importance of site localization for OCT diagnostic accuracy [19,39,45].

In this study, the integration of in vivo OCT assessments, histologically based, with a site-targeted punch biopsy technique, coupled with the use of standardized diagnostic patterns, distinguishes this research from existing studies. Primarily, the choice to select homogeneous lesions (i.e., plaque for OL, and reticular/plaque for OLP), reflects the need to optically characterize lesions that clinically may present with sometimes overlapping and non-unique appearances. Moreover, the adoption of standardized oral site coding, based on the 2021 NIH/SEER ICD-0-3.2 topographical classification codes, offers precise location-specific OCT analysis of oral lesions and enables a comparison of results across studies, fostering scientific collaboration and data sharing. This may enhance coordination in the management of patients with suspected oral lesions and contribute to the reliability and validity of optical research findings, particularly essential for OPMDs and OSCC early diagnosis.

Furthermore, the use of uniform and validated OCT patterns for OL, OLP and OSCC discrimination guarantees the competitive development of non-invasive, rapid, reproducible, simple-to-use diagnostic algorithms that can be useful not only to oral medicine specialists.

These patterns guide both non-invasive preliminary evaluations and targeted biopsies, ensuring precise alignment between OCT-based hypotheses and histological findings. In this regard, to improve the optical evaluation of the lesions selected for our sample model, we defined a topographic correspondence system that was functional both for OCT validation and for the choice of the most appropriate biopsy site. The punch-based target site co-registration procedure enhances the diagnostic accuracy of OCT compared to histopathological reference: sensitivity and specificity for OCT scans post-target site registration were 98.57 and 100.00 for OSCC, 98.57 and 98.57 for OL, 97.14 and 98.57 for OLP, respectively, for both observers. The substantial increase in the diagnostic accuracy between pre- and post-target site registration OCT-based diagnoses corresponding to histopathology demonstrated a statistical significance: both for OPMDs ($p < 0.001$ for both OL and OLP) and for OSCC ($p = 0.001$).

The choice to perform OCT scans both before and after punch site registration contributes to the uniqueness of the study design. Moreover, the circular punch employed in this technique boasts a diameter of 6 mm, precisely matching the diameter of the scan produced by the utilized OCT probe. As a result, tissue marking with the punch enables alignment not only in terms of location but also in terms of size between the scanned target area and the histologically analyzed tissue sample.

The highest diagnostic accuracy values achieved for OSCC through post-site registration assessments were attributed to the greater OCT consistency of patterns used for this disease compared to the increased variability associated with the patterns of the OPMDs under investigation (OL, OLP). The complete absence of well-defined epithelial stratification, together with the presence of 'icicle-like' structures, suggestive of tumor progression/invasion, render the OCT patterns for OSCC more uniform and straightforward to interpret [19]. On the contrary, the report of slightly lower diagnostic accuracy for OLP, despite the morphological homogeneity of the selected lesions (i.e., hyperkeratotic/reticular) could plausibly be attributed, in our assessment, to this intrinsic heterogeneity of pathology, depending on the inflammatory portion underlying the examined layer, underscoring the importance of considering the complexity of OLP tissues when evaluating OCT results. Overall, the contribution of multiple clinical/optical/histological blinded approaches adds consistency and objectivity to this study design and more reliability to OCT-based diagnoses.

Regarding imaging depth, OCT typically provides effective visualization up to approximately 2 mm within the tissue. While this depth is generally sufficient for assessing superficial epithelial changes and all mucosal structures, it may limit the evaluation of deeper tissue layers beneath the lamina propria. For lesions or conditions involving deeper tissue changes, additional imaging techniques or diagnostic methods may be necessary. However, for the purposes of our study, the depth achieved was adequate to analyze and distinguish between various oral lesions, particularly those affecting the epithelial and superficial subepithelial layers. This study focused on these accessible layers to validate standardized OCT patterns for early diagnosis and monitoring, acknowledging that deeper tissue analysis may require complementary diagnostic approaches to fully assess lesions extending beyond this depth.

The findings of this study could have significant implications for clinical practice. The high diagnostic accuracy achieved with the site-targeted punch biopsy-based OCT technique, especially in distinguishing OSCC from OPMD, suggests that this method could be pivotal in reducing diagnostic delays and improving treatment outcomes. Moreover, the implementation of standardized OCT patterns and site-specific coding can enhance the reproducibility and consistency of diagnoses across different clinical settings, potentially leading to more widespread adoption of OCT in routine oral cancer screenings. Furthermore, the ability to accurately target biopsy sites based on OCT findings can minimize the need for multiple invasive procedures, reducing patient discomfort and the risk of sampling errors. This not only streamlines the diagnostic process but also supports more personalized treatment planning at the earliest possible stage.

As the integration of Artificial Intelligence (AI) with OCT continues to evolve, these standardization protocols could serve as a foundational framework for the development of more sophisticated, automated diagnostic algorithms, currently missing from the literature.

Kim D. H. et al. (2022) conducted a comprehensive systematic review and meta-analysis of OCT efficacy in oral oncology, highlighting the diagnostic potential of AI and automated algorithms but not noting a dearth of studies emphasizing the precise spatial overlap between OCT-scanned areas and subsequently biopsied regions for diagnostic reference [23]. This oversight introduces a notable limitation in correlating OCT findings directly with histological outcomes. Similarly, Kim J-S (2022), in their exploration of the integration of OCT and AI for discriminating oral cancerous lesions from normal mucosa, included an analysis of four relevant studies [47]. Notably, despite the confirmation of diagnoses through histological examination in all four studies, none explicitly addressed the precise spatial overlap between the biopsy-sampled areas and those identified through OCT scans [24,25,29,48].

The need for spatial concordance between OCT-scanned regions and the corresponding biopsy sites is essential to reduce the qualitative interpretative complexity of oral lesions in the early learning phase of any applied computational OCT system [47,49]. Our study could contribute to filling this gap by deliberately incorporating a site-targeted punch biopsy-based technique in new automatized OCT-supported clinical algorithms, especially designed for oral carcinogenesis diagnosis.

The limitations of this study underscore several constraints that must be considered when interpreting its findings. As a preliminary phase of multi-project research, this preliminary investigation was designed as unicentric on a relatively small sample size. Moreover, the selection of only specific anterior mucosal sites of the mouth was influenced by the limitations of the OCT probe utilized. These choices may introduce the possibility of site-specific biases and limit the broader applicability of the findings. Future studies are currently underway to validate our protocols and applications in multicenter settings, with a larger sample of patients, lesions, and mucosal sites.

## 5. Conclusions

This research study presents an innovative procedure introduced for the diagnosis of oral pre-cancer and cancer, based on OCT, adherent to a strictly standardized protocol. By providing a meticulously standardized dataset, our study lays a solid foundation for refining and advancing automated diagnostic applications, encouraging a virtuous cycle of iterative improvement in optical diagnostic precision. Thus, this work highlights the transformative potential of harmonizing standardized clinical methodologies with future AI technologies in revolutionizing early cancer detection paradigms, aiming to promote advancements in patient care and anticipate further progress in the field, leading to improved patient outcomes and overall survival rates.

**Author Contributions:** Conceptualization, V.P., F.B. and S.E.R.; data curation, V.P., F.B., G.C. and V.R.; formal analysis, V.P., F.B. and L.M.; investigation, V.P., F.B., V.D.C. and V.R.; writing—original draft, V.P., F.B., L.M., S.E.R., A.F., R.M. and G.C.; writing—review & editing, V.P., F.B. and R.M.; validation, V.P., F.B., V.R., G.C. and V.D.C.; resources, V.P., F.B., L.M., S.E.R., V.R. and V.D.C.; supervision, V.P., R.M. and G.C. All authors have read and agreed to the published version of the manuscript.

**Funding:** The authors declare that they did not receive any funding or support for this work.

**Institutional Review Board Statement:** The study was conducted in accordance with the Declaration of Helsinki and approved by the Institutional Review Board of University Hospital "Policlinico Paolo Giaccone" in Palermo (Italy), approval number 11/2016.

**Informed Consent Statement:** Informed consent was obtained from all subjects involved in the study.

**Data Availability Statement:** The datasets generated and/or analyzed during the current study are available from the corresponding author on reasonable request.

**Conflicts of Interest:** The authors declare that they have no conflicts of interest to disclose, including relevant financial interests, activities, relationships, and affiliations.

## References

1. Conway, D.I.; Purkayastha, M.; Chestnutt, I.G. The Changing Epidemiology of Oral Cancer: Definitions, Trends, and Risk Factors. *Br. Dent. J.* **2018**, *225*, 867–873. [CrossRef]
2. Su, Y.-F.; Chen, Y.-J.; Tsai, F.-T.; Li, W.-C.; Hsu, M.-L.; Wang, D.-H.; Yang, C.-C. Current Insights into Oral Cancer Diagnostics. *Diagnostics* **2021**, *11*, 1287. [CrossRef]
3. Abdul, N.S. Role of Advanced Diagnostic Aids in the Detection of Potentially Malignant Disorders and Oral Cancer at an Early Stage. *Cureus* **2023**, *15*, e34113. [CrossRef]
4. de Kleijn, B.J.; Heldens, G.T.N.; Herruer, J.M.; Sier, C.F.M.; Piazza, C.; de Bree, R.; Guntinas-Lichius, O.; Kowalski, L.P.; Vander Poorten, V.; Rodrigo, J.P.; et al. Intraoperative Imaging Techniques to Improve Surgical Resection Margins of Oropharyngeal Squamous Cell Cancer: A Comprehensive Review of Current Literature. *Cancers* **2023**, *15*, 896. [CrossRef] [PubMed]
5. Di Fede, O.; Panzarella, V.; Buttacavoli, F.; La Mantia, G.; Campisi, G. Doctoral: A Smartphone-Based Decision Support Tool for the Early Detection of Oral Potentially Malignant Disorders. *Digit. Health* **2023**, *9*, 205520762311771. [CrossRef]
6. Sung, H.; Ferlay, J.; Siegel, R.L.; Laversanne, M.; Soerjomataram, I.; Jemal, A.; Bray, F. Global Cancer Statistics 2020: GLOBOCAN Estimates of Incidence and Mortality Worldwide for 36 Cancers in 185 Countries. *CA Cancer J. Clin.* **2021**, *71*, 209–249. [CrossRef]
7. Mauceri, R.; Bazzano, M.; Coppini, M.; Tozzo, P.; Panzarella, V.; Campisi, G. Diagnostic Delay of Oral Squamous Cell Carcinoma and the Fear of Diagnosis: A Scoping Review. *Front. Psychol.* **2022**, *13*, 1009080. [CrossRef] [PubMed]
8. Wang, J.; Xu, Y.; Boppart, S.A. Review of Optical Coherence Tomography in Oncology. *J. Biomed. Opt.* **2017**, *22*, 1. [CrossRef]
9. Mauceri, R.; Coppini, M.; Vacca, D.; Bertolazzi, G.; Panzarella, V.; Di Fede, O.; Tripodo, C.; Campisi, G. Salivary Microbiota Composition in Patients with Oral Squamous Cell Carcinoma: A Systematic Review. *Cancers* **2022**, *14*, 5441. [CrossRef]
10. Lee, C.-K.; Chi, T.-T.; Wu, C.-T.; Tsai, M.-T.; Chiang, C.-P.; Yang, C.-C. Diagnosis of Oral Precancer with Optical Coherence Tomography. *Biomed. Opt. Express* **2012**, *3*, 1632. [CrossRef]
11. Hamdoon, Z.; Jerjes, W.; Al-Delayme, R.; McKenzie, G.; Jay, A.; Hopper, C. Structural Validation of Oral Mucosal Tissue Using Optical Coherence Tomography. *Head. Neck Oncol.* **2012**, *4*, 29. [CrossRef]
12. Ghosh, B.; Bhandari, A.; Mandal, M.; Paul, R.R.; Pal, M.; Mitra, P.; Chatterjee, J. Quantitative in Situ Imaging and Grading of Oral Precancer with Attenuation Corrected-Optical Coherence Tomography. *Oral. Oncol.* **2021**, *117*, 105216. [CrossRef]
13. Capocasale, G.; Panzarella, V.; Rodolico, V.; Di Fede, O.; Campisi, G. In Vivo Optical Coherence Tomography Imaging in a Case of Mucous Membrane Pemphigoid and a Negative Nikolsky's Sign. *J. Dermatol.* **2018**, *45*, 603–605. [CrossRef]
14. Ilhan, B.; Lin, K.; Guneri, P.; Wilder-Smith, P. Improving Oral Cancer Outcomes with Imaging and Artificial Intelligence. *J. Dent. Res.* **2020**, *99*, 241–248. [CrossRef] [PubMed]

15. Jerjes, W.; Upile, T.; Conn, B.; Hamdoon, Z.; Betz, C.S.; McKenzie, G.; Radhi, H.; Vourvachis, M.; El Maaytah, M.; Sandison, A.; et al. In Vitro Examination of Suspicious Oral Lesions Using Optical Coherence Tomography. *Br. J. Oral. Maxillofac. Surg.* **2010**, *48*, 18–25. [CrossRef] [PubMed]
16. Hamdoon, Z.; Jerjes, W.; McKenzie, G.; Jay, A.; Hopper, C. Optical Coherence Tomography in the Assessment of Oral Squamous Cell Carcinoma Resection Margins. *Photodiagn. Photodyn. Ther.* **2016**, *13*, 211–217. [CrossRef] [PubMed]
17. Hamdoon, Z.; Jerjes, W.; Upile, T.; McKenzie, G.; Jay, A.; Hopper, C. Optical Coherence Tomography in the Assessment of Suspicious Oral Lesions: An Immediate Ex Vivo Study. *Photodiagn. Photodyn. Ther.* **2013**, *10*, 17–27. [CrossRef]
18. Obade, A.Y.; Pandarathodiyil, A.K.; Oo, A.L.; Warnakulasuriya, S.; Ramanathan, A. Application of Optical Coherence Tomography to Study the Structural Features of Oral Mucosa in Biopsy Tissues of Oral Dysplasia and Carcinomas. *Clin. Oral. Investig.* **2021**, *25*, 5411–5419. [CrossRef]
19. Panzarella, V.; Buttacavoli, F.; Gambino, A.; Capocasale, G.; Di Fede, O.; Mauceri, R.; Rodolico, V.; Campisi, G. Site-Coded Oral Squamous Cell Carcinoma Evaluation by Optical Coherence Tomography (OCT): A Descriptive Pilot Study. *Cancers* **2022**, *14*, 5916. [CrossRef]
20. Yang, Z.; Shang, J.; Liu, C.; Zhang, J.; Liang, Y. Identification of Oral Precancerous and Cancerous Tissue by Swept Source Optical Coherence Tomography. *Lasers Surg. Med.* **2022**, *54*, 320–328. [CrossRef]
21. Yang, E.C.; Tan, M.T.; Schwarz, R.A.; Richards-Kortum, R.R.; Gillenwater, A.M.; Vigneswaran, N. Noninvasive Diagnostic Adjuncts for the Evaluation of Potentially Premalignant Oral Epithelial Lesions: Current Limitations and Future Directions. *Oral. Surg. Oral. Med. Oral. Pathol. Oral. Radiol.* **2018**, *125*, 670–681. [CrossRef]
22. Sunny, S.P.; Agarwal, S.; James, B.L.; Heidari, E.; Muralidharan, A.; Yadav, V.; Pillai, V.; Shetty, V.; Chen, Z.; Hedne, N.; et al. Intra-Operative Point-of-Procedure Delineation of Oral Cancer Margins Using Optical Coherence Tomography. *Oral. Oncol.* **2019**, *92*, 12–19. [CrossRef]
23. Kim, D.H.; Kim, S.W.; Hwang, S.H. Efficacy of Optical Coherence Tomography in the Diagnosing of Oral Cancerous Lesion: Systematic Review and Meta-analysis. *Head. Neck* **2023**, *45*, 473–481. [CrossRef]
24. Yuan, W.; Cheng, L.; Yang, J.; Yin, B.; Fan, X.; Yang, J.; Li, S.; Zhong, J.; Huang, X. Noninvasive Oral Cancer Screening Based on Local Residual Adaptation Network Using Optical Coherence Tomography. *Med. Biol. Eng. Comput.* **2022**, *60*, 1363–1375. [CrossRef]
25. Yang, Z.; Shang, J.; Liu, C.; Zhang, J.; Liang, Y. Identification of Oral Cancer in OCT Images Based on an Optical Attenuation Model. *Lasers Med. Sci.* **2020**, *35*, 1999–2007. [CrossRef] [PubMed]
26. Xu, Y.; Deng, X.; Sun, Y.; Wang, X.; Xiao, Y.; Li, Y.; Chen, Q.; Jiang, L. Optical Imaging in the Diagnosis of OPMDs Malignant Transformation. *J. Dent. Res.* **2022**, *101*, 749–758. [CrossRef]
27. Ramezani, K.; Tofangchiha, M. Oral Cancer Screening by Artificial Intelligence-Oriented Interpretation of Optical Coherence Tomography Images. *Radiol. Res. Pract.* **2022**, *2022*, 1614838. [CrossRef]
28. Jerjes, W.; Hamdoon, Z.; Yousif, A.A.; Al-Rawi, N.H.; Hopper, C. Epithelial Tissue Thickness Improves Optical Coherence Tomography's Ability in Detecting Oral Cancer. *Photodiagn. Photodyn. Ther.* **2019**, *28*, 69–74. [CrossRef]
29. Heidari, A.E.; Suresh, A.; Kuriakose, M.A.; Chen, Z.; Wilder-Smith, P.; Sunny, S.P.; James, B.L.; Lam, T.M.; Tran, A.V.; Yu, J.; et al. Optical Coherence Tomography as an Oral Cancer Screening Adjunct in a Low Resource Settings. *IEEE J. Sel. Top. Quantum Electron.* **2019**, *25*, 1–8. [CrossRef]
30. Tsai, M.-T.; Lee, C.-K.; Lee, H.-C.; Chen, H.-M.; Chiang, C.-P.; Wang, Y.-M.; Yang, C.-C. Differentiating Oral Lesions in Different Carcinogenesis Stages with Optical Coherence Tomography. *J. Biomed. Opt.* **2009**, *14*, 044028. [CrossRef]
31. Yang, C.C.; Tsai, M.-T.; Lee, H.-C.; Lee, C.-K.; Yu, C.-H.; Chen, H.-M.; Chiang, C.-P.; Chang, C.-C.; Wang, Y.-M.; Yang, C.C. Effective Indicators for Diagnosis of Oral Cancer Using Optical Coherence Tomography. *Opt. Express* **2008**, *16*, 15847. [CrossRef] [PubMed]
32. Agha, R.; Abdall-Razak, A.; Crossley, E.; Dowlut, N.; Iosifidis, C.; Mathew, G.; Beamishaj; Bashashati, M.; Millham, F.H.; Orgill, D.P.; et al. STROCSS 2019 Guideline: Strengthening the Reporting of Cohort Studies in Surgery. *Int. J. Surg.* **2019**, *72*, 156–165. [CrossRef] [PubMed]
33. Warnakulasuriya, S.; Kujan, O.; Aguirre-Urizar, J.M.; Bagan, J.V.; González-Moles, M.Á.; Kerr, A.R.; Lodi, G.; Mello, F.W.; Monteiro, L.; Ogden, G.R.; et al. Oral Potentially Malignant Disorders: A Consensus Report from an International Seminar on Nomenclature and Classification, Convened by the WHO Collaborating Centre for Oral Cancer. *Oral. Dis.* **2021**, *27*, 1862–1880. [CrossRef]
34. Muller, S.; Tilakaratne, W.M. Update from the 5th Edition of the World Health Organization Classification of Head and Neck Tumors: Tumours of the Oral Cavity and Mobile Tongue. *Head. Neck Pathol.* **2022**, *16*, 54–62. [CrossRef] [PubMed]
35. Essat, M.; Cooper, K.; Bessey, A.; Clowes, M.; Chilcott, J.B.; Hunter, K.D. Diagnostic Accuracy of Conventional Oral Examination for Detecting Oral Cavity Cancer and Potentially Malignant Disorders in Patients with Clinically Evident Oral Lesions: Systematic Review and Meta-analysis. *Head. Neck* **2022**, *44*, 998–1013. [CrossRef]
36. Fritz, A.; Percy, C.; Jack, A.; Shanmugaratnam, K.; Sobin, L.; Parkin, M.; Whelan, S. *ICD-O International Classification of Diseases for Oncology*; First Revision; World Health Organization: Geneva, Switzerland, 2013.
37. National Cancer Institute. Surveillance, Epidemiology, and E.R.P.-(NIH/SEER). Head and Neck Equivalent Terms and Definitions C000-C148, C300-C339, C410, C411, C442, C479 Excludes Lymphoma and Leukemia M9590–M9992 and Kaposi Sarcoma M9140. 2021; pp. 1–50. Available online: https://seer.cancer.gov/tools/solidtumor/Head_Neck_STM.pdf (accessed on 15 August 2024).

38. Gambino, A.; Cabras, M.; Cafaro, A.; Broccoletti, R.; Carossa, S.; Hopper, C.; Chiusa, L.; El Haddad, G.; Porter, S.R.; Arduino, P.G. In-Vivo Usefulness of Optical Coherence Tomography in Atrophic-Erosive Oral Lichen Planus: Comparison between Histopathological and Ultrastructural Findings. *J. Photochem. Photobiol. B* **2020**, *211*, 112009. [CrossRef]
39. Gambino, A.; Martina, E.; Panzarella, V.; Ruggiero, T.; El Haddad, G.; Broccoletti, R.; Arduino, P.G. Potential Use of Optical Coherence Tomography in Oral Potentially Malignant Disorders: In-Vivo Case Series Study. *BMC Oral. Health* **2023**, *23*, 540. [CrossRef]
40. Wilder-Smith, P.; Lee, K.; Guo, S.; Zhang, J.; Osann, K.; Chen, Z.; Messadi, D. In Vivo Diagnosis of Oral Dysplasia and Malignancy Using Optical Coherence Tomography: Preliminary Studies in 50 Patients. *Lasers Surg. Med.* **2009**, *41*, 353–357. [CrossRef] [PubMed]
41. Ridgway, J.M.; Armstrong, W.B.; Guo, S.; Mahmood, U.; Su, J.; Jackson, R.P.; Shibuya, T.; Crumley, R.L.; Gu, M.; Chen, Z.; et al. In Vivo Optical Coherence Tomography of the Human Oral Cavity and Oropharynx. *Arch. Otolaryngol. Head. Neck Surg.* **2006**, *132*, 1074. [CrossRef]
42. Volgger, V.; Stepp, H.; Ihrler, S.; Kraft, M.; Leunig, A.; Patel, P.M.; Susarla, M.; Jackson, K.; Betz, C.S. Evaluation of Optical Coherence Tomography to Discriminate Lesions of the Upper Aerodigestive Tract. *Head. Neck* **2013**, *35*, 1558–1566. [CrossRef]
43. Panzarella, V.; Bartolone, A.; Coniglio, R.; Rodolico, V.; Maniscalco, L.; Capocasale, G.; Iurato Carbone, M.; Campisi, G. Diagnostic Concordance between Optical Coherence Tomography and Histological Investigations for Immune-Mediated Desquamative Gingivitis: Observational Study. *Int. J. Environ. Res. Public Health* **2021**, *18*, 9095. [CrossRef]
44. Gruda, Y.; Albrecht, M.; Buckova, M.; Haim, D.; Lauer, G.; Koch, E.; Joehrens, K.; Schnabel, C.; Golde, J.; Li, J.; et al. Characteristics of Clinically Classified Oral Lichen Planus in Optical Coherence Tomography: A Descriptive Case-Series Study. *Diagnostics* **2023**, *13*, 2642. [CrossRef]
45. Gambino, A.; Cafaro, A.; Broccoletti, R.; Turotti, L.; Karimi, D.; El Haddad, G.; Hopper, C.; Porter, S.R.; Chiusa, L.; Arduino, P.G. In Vivo Evaluation of Traumatic and Malignant Oral Ulcers with Optical Coherence Tomography: A Comparison between Histopathological and Ultrastructural Findings. *Photodiagn. Photodyn. Ther.* **2022**, *39*, 103019. [CrossRef]
46. Mercaldo, N.D.; Lau, K.F.; Zhou, X.H. Confidence intervals for predictive values with an emphasis to case-control studies. *Stat. Med.* **2007**, *26*, 2170–2183. [CrossRef] [PubMed]
47. Kim, J.-S.; Kim, B.G.; Hwang, S.H. Efficacy of Artificial Intelligence-Assisted Discrimination of Oral Cancerous Lesions from Normal Mucosa Based on the Oral Mucosal Image: A Systematic Review and Meta-Analysis. *Cancers* **2022**, *14*, 3499. [CrossRef]
48. James, B.L.; Sunny, S.P.; Heidari, A.E.; Ramanjinappa, R.D.; Lam, T.; Tran, A.V.; Kankanala, S.; Sil, S.; Tiwari, V.; Patrick, S.; et al. Validation of a Point-of-Care Optical Coherence Tomography Device with Machine Learning Algorithm for Detection of Oral Potentially Malignant and Malignant Lesions. *Cancers* **2021**, *13*, 3583. [CrossRef]
49. Yang, Z.; Pan, H.; Shang, J.; Zhang, J.; Liang, Y. Deep-Learning-Based Automated Identification and Visualization of Oral Cancer in Optical Coherence Tomography Images. *Biomedicines* **2023**, *11*, 802. [CrossRef]

diagnostics

MDPI

*Article*

# Influencing Factors Regarding the Severity of Peri-Implantitis and Peri-Implant Mucositis

**Csilla Benedek [1], Bernadette Kerekes-Máthé [2,*], Liana Bereșescu [3], Imola Zsuzsa Buka [1], Zsuzsanna Bardocz-Veres [4], Ildikó Geréb [5], Krisztina Ildikó Mártha [6] and Kinga Mária Jánosi [7]**

1 Department of Periodontology and Oral Diagnosis, "George Emil Palade" University of Medicine, Pharmacy, Science and Technology of Târgu Mureș, 540142 Târgu Mureș, Romania; imola.buka@umfst.ro (I.Z.B.)
2 Department of Tooth and Dental Arch Morphology, "George Emil Palade" University of Medicine, Pharmacy, Science and Technology of Târgu Mureș, 540142 Târgu Mureș, Romania
3 Department of Preventive and Community Dentistry, "George Emil Palade" University of Medicine, Pharmacy, Science and Technology of Târgu Mureș, 540142 Târgu Mureș, Romania
4 Department of Prosthodontics and Oral Rehabilitation, "George Emil Palade" University of Medicine, Pharmacy, Science and Technology of Târgu Mureș, 540142 Târgu Mureș, Romania; zsuzsanna.bardocz-veres@umfst.ro
5 Windisch Dental-Wident, 1053 Budapest, Hungary; gerebildiko23@gmail.com
6 Department of Orthodontics, "George Emil Palade" University of Medicine, Pharmacy, Science and Technology of Târgu Mureș, 540142 Târgu Mureș, Romania; krisztina.martha@umfst.ro
7 Department of Fixed Prosthodontics, "George Emil Palade" University of Medicine, Pharmacy, Science and Technology of Târgu Mureș, 540142 Târgu Mureș, Romania
* Correspondence: bernadette.kerekes-mathe@umfst.ro; Tel.: +40-746-239180

**Abstract:** The scientific literature is increasingly focused on peri-implant mucositis and peri-implantitis, which are biological outcomes of dental implant treatment. Background/Objectives: The present study aimed to evaluate the two most critical complications of dental implantation, peri-implant mucositis and peri-implantitis, through the prism of different influencing factors. Methods: We followed 40 patients, with a total number of 92 dental implants, divided into three age groups: under 35 years, between 35 and 55 years, and older than 55 years. Patients were also divided into groups according to the time since implant placement: 1–3 years, 4–7 years, and more than 7 years. The patients were examined, and periodontal pocket depth, peri-implant pocket depth, Löe–Silness gingival index, mucosal thickness, and keratinized mucosal width were recorded; bone resorption was measured on radiographs using a 2D image analysis method; and a questionnaire was also conducted. Results: Bone resorption was highest in the 35–55 age group (3.09 $\pm$ 0.04 mm) and for implants placed 4–7 years ago (3.39 $\pm$ 0.12 mm). Females had a mean bone resorption of 3.4 $\pm$ 0.15 mm and males of 2.45 $\pm$ 0.07 mm. Statistically, there was a significant difference only in the Löe–Silness index: the 35–55 age group had the highest values ($p = 0.04$). Conclusions: There were no statistically significant differences between the time since implant placement and the degree of bone resorption, nor between sexes. Peri-implant inflammation may occur at any age, regardless of the lifetime of the implants.

**Keywords:** peri-implantitis; peri-implant mucositis; bone resorption

## 1. Introduction

Dental implants have many advantages over the classic and traditional fixed partial dentures: a much higher success rate, as shown by the majority of the studies conducted in this field (over 97% success rate for ten years), better preservation of bone in the edentulous areas, a lower risk of caries formation, a reduction in adjacent natural teeth sensitivity, and less endodontic damage to neighboring teeth [1–3].

### 1.1. The Success Rate of the Implantation

The implant can be successful if it is stable during the examination and if the tissues surrounding it are inflammation-free [4].

The success rate depends, among other things, on primary stability, which means that the implant is firmly seated in the socket. Factors influencing primary stability include bone density, the size and character of the bone–implant interface, the implant's shape, and the surgical technique [5–7].

The stability and overall health of the hard and soft tissues around implants, among other factors influencing the implant–prosthetic complex, are critical to the outcome of implant therapy [8–10]. The integrity of the hard and soft tissues surrounding a dental implant can be compromised by peri-implant diseases such as peri-implant mucositis and peri-implantitis, which are inflammatory lesions that develop due to plaque accumulation in the surrounding tissues [9].

### 1.2. Peri-Implant Mucositis

The 2017 World Workshop on the Classification of Periodontal and Peri-Implant Diseases and Conditions describes peri-implant mucositis as "a disease that involves inflammation of the soft tissues surrounding a dental implant without additional bone loss after the initial bone remodeling that may occur during healing after the surgical placement of the implant" [9,11–13].

Peri-implant mucosal inflammation and a lack of progressive marginal peri-implant bone loss are the primary diagnostic criteria for peri-implant mucositis [14,15]. Peri-implant mucositis is a reversible, treatable condition. It is thought to be a precursor to peri-implantitis. Once clinical signs of peri-implant mucositis are found during an exam, an X-ray that shows no bone loss confirms the diagnosis [14,16].

### 1.3. Peri-Implantitis

Peri-implantitis is a plaque-associated pathologic modification of the tissues surrounding the implant, characterized by inflammatory cells in the peri-implant mucosa and progressive bone loss around dental implants [9,12]. It is believed to be the primary factor in implant failure after osseointegration [9,17].

Sites of peri-implantitis show signs of mucosal inflammation surrounding the implant and/or gingival recession, accompanied by increased probing depths around implants due to radiologically detected bone loss. Suppuration of the peri-implant pockets indicates the active nature of the pocket [11]. In the absence of peri-implant probing depth values from a previous examination or in the absence of previous radiographs, which are the most important indicators, a positive diagnosis of peri-implantitis can be established based on the following: positive bleeding index on probing; 6 mm or more peri-implant probing depth values; and 3 mm or more marginal bone level apical to the most coronal area of the endosseous component of the implant [11,14].

The shape of bone resorption in peri-implantitis is circular around the implant. The development of bone loss is rapid, does not follow a linear pattern, and occurs during the first three years of use [14,18–21]. In this order, peri-implantitis causes accelerated and severe bone loss and subsequent implant failure and loss [22].

### 1.4. Risk Factors for Developing Peri-Implant Inflammations

Several risk factors, such as smoking, poor oral hygiene, prior periodontal disease, and lack of professional and personal maintenance, have been associated with an increased likelihood of developing peri-implantitis [9,23]. Notably, these elements are also recognized as a risk factor for developing periodontitis [9,24]. The relationship between peri-implantitis and periodontitis has been studied over time, and a strong link has been observed: both conditions are the result of bacterial inflammation [22,25].

Individuals who do not practice good dental hygiene have an odds ratio of 14.3, which increases their likelihood of developing peri-implantitis [9,24,26]. Inconsistent or nonexistent complementary supportive and maintenance therapy has also been shown to increase the risk of tooth loss and relapse of periodontal disease [27].

Smoking has direct and indirect effects on the periodontium by inhibiting cytokine production, altering humoral immune system function, impairing neutrophil activities, stimulating capillary vasoconstriction and fibrosis, and increasing the prevalence of periodontal pathogens in periodontal pockets [9,24]. These modifications may increase the subject's risk of developing peri-implantitis in addition to making them more susceptible to periodontitis.

Local predisposing factors play a significant role in the prevalence of peri-implant conditions. Prosthetic parameters, including implant location, the type and pattern of prosthetic connection emergence, and residual cement in the tissues surrounding implants, have been shown to influence these peri-implant conditions [28].

The main objective of the present study was to evaluate the two most critical complications of dental implantation, peri-implant mucositis and peri-implantitis, through the prism of various influencing factors.

## 2. Materials and Methods

Forty patients were selected from cases treated at a dental clinic in Mures County between November 2022 and February 2024. Power calculations with G*Power version 3.1.9.6. software (Franz Faul, Universität Kiel, Kiel, Germany) determined the sample size calculation with 80% power, alpha = 0.05.

The following inclusion criteria were used:

- At least one dental implant placed.
- Absence of systemic diseases in the background, especially those that directly affect the success and survival rate of dental implants, such as osteoporosis, diabetes, neurological disorders, HIV, hypothyroidism, and cardiovascular diseases.
- Absence of oral cavity changes, such as autoimmune mucocutaneous diseases, necrotizing periodontal diseases, scurvy, and extensive necrosis in agranulocytosis.
- Absence of medication: Only patients who were not taking any medication were included in this study. The most important drugs that could affect the survival rate of dental implants are bisphosphonates, non-steroidal anti-inflammatory drugs (NSAIDs), glucocorticoids, proton pump inhibitors (PPIs), and serotonin reuptake inhibitors (SSRIs).
- Non-smoking patients.
- Good or acceptable patient oral hygiene protocol, performed at least twice daily. Oral hygiene habits were considered by designing a questionnaire.

An evaluative digital panoramic radiograph was taken during periodic checkups.

Exclusion criteria:

- No inserted dental implant;
- Presence of systemic diseases;
- Presence of oral cavity changes;
- Long-term daily medication of the patient;
- Smoking patients;
- Poor oral hygiene;
- Absence of evaluable digital panoramic X-rays.

Our study was approved by the Scientific Research Ethics Committee of the "George Emil Palade" University of Medicine, Pharmacy, Science and Technology of Targu Mures (1895/19 October 2022).

The gender distribution of the investigated cases: 21 women and 19 men. Cases were divided into three groups according to age: those under 35 years (group A), those between 35 and 55 years (group B), and those over 55 years (group C). The cases were also divided into three groups according to the time since implant placement: implants 1–3 years old (group 1), implants 4–7 years old (group 2), and implants older than 7 years (group 3).

In all cases, clinical and radiological examinations were performed (Figure 1a,b)

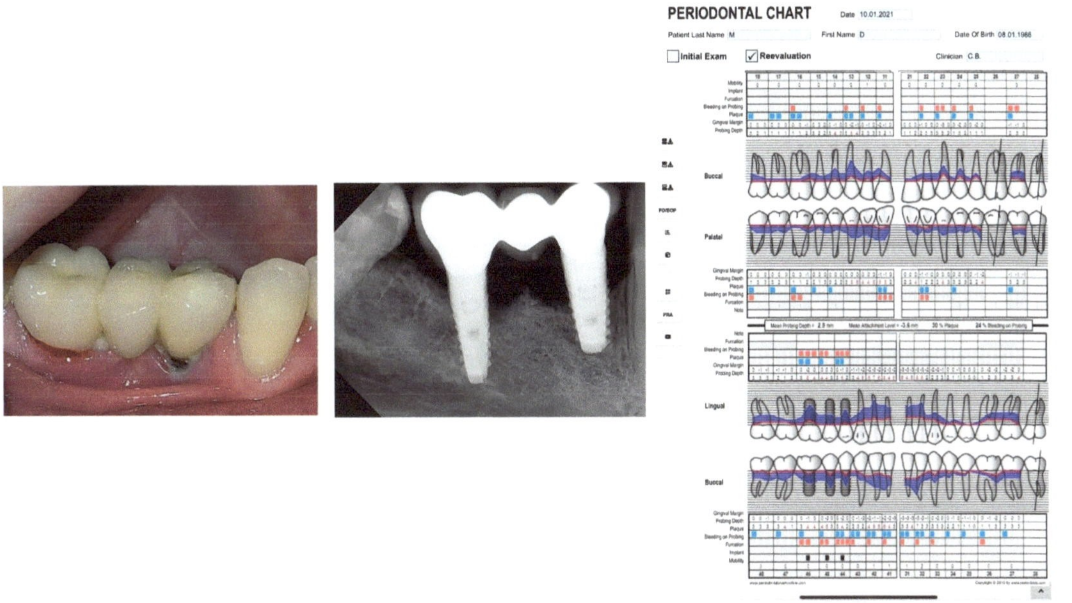


(a) (b) (c)

**Figure 1.** The peri-implantitis of a 36-year-old female at 5 years from implant placement: (**a**) intraoral aspect, (**b**) radiological aspect, (**c**) periodontal chart of the patient.

During the clinical examination, the following parameters were determined: periodontal pocket depth of the natural teeth present in the oral cavity to evaluate the periodontal status of the patients, peri-implant pocket depth, Löe–Silness gingival index, peri-implant mucosal thickness, and peri-implant keratinized mucosal width. The same periodontology specialist evaluated all the above parameters. Intraoral photographs of the implant site were taken, and a ten-question questionnaire was completed. The questionnaire was used to collect data on the patient's experience with the implant, and the instruments and methods used to clean the areas around the implants.

The periodontal status of the existing natural teeth was assessed by determining the depth of the periodontal pocket at 6 points around each tooth: mesio-buccal, buccal, disto-buccal, mesio-oral, oral, and disto-oral points, using the William probe (Hu-Friedy Italy Srl, Milano, Italy), which contains gradations from 1 to 10 mm, omitting the 4 and 6 mm gradations for better operator orientation (Figure 1c).

Similarly, the peri-implant pocket depth was evaluated in the same 6 points using a plastic periodontal probe (Hu-Friedy Italy Srl, Milano, Italy) with gradations from 1 to 15 mm (Figure 1a).

Using the Löe–Silness gingival index, we evaluated the condition of the gingiva, i.e., the presence and degree of peri-implant mucositis, as follows:

0—No visible inflammation.

1—Slight discoloration, without gingival bleeding.

2—Obvious inflammation, gingival bleeding appears a few seconds after probing.

3—Visible gingivitis and spontaneous gingival bleeding [29].

Regarding the thickness of the peri-implant mucosa, it is essential to know that two final phenotypes can be distinguished. One extreme is thin, wavy mucosa; the other is thick mucosa with a flat bone margin. To evaluate the peri-implant mucosal thickness, a plastic periodontal probe was inserted under the gingival margin: a value of 0 was taken for thin mucosa if the probe penetrated the gingiva; a value of 1 was registered for thick mucosa if the probe did not penetrate the gingiva [29].

The width of the peri-implant mucosa was determined in mm by placing the periodontal probe centrally between the muco-gingival junction and the most coronal point where the attached mucosa emerges [29].

The panoramic radiographs were then evaluated and measured. Measurements were performed using the two-dimensional image analysis method with the Image-Pro Insight 9.3 program (Media Cybernetics, Rockville, MD, USA). After calibrating the images, measuring points were taken on the mesial and distal sides of the implants, at the junction of the bone surface and the mucosa. Then, the amount of bone resorption was measured in millimeters (Figure 2).

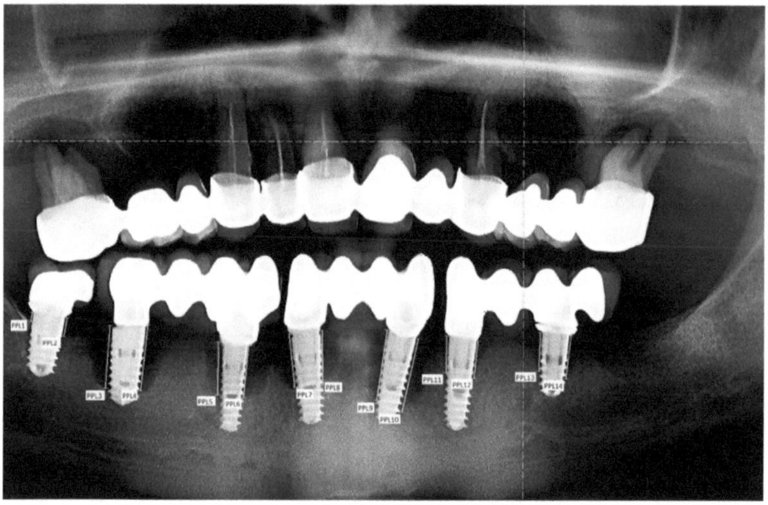

**Figure 2.** Lower arch: measurement points on the mesial and distal surfaces of the implants—61-year-old male patient; implant placement: 11 years ago.

Data were collected using Excel 2019, statistical analysis was performed using GraphPad Prism 9.5.1 (GraphPad Software, Boston, MA, USA), outliers were filtered using the Grubbs test, data distribution was examined using the Kolmogorov–Smirnov test, and groups were compared using ANOVA and t-tests. The significance level was set at 0.05.

## 3. Results

Overall, 15% of the cases examined were in the under-35 age group, 52.5% were in the 35–55 age group, and 32.5% were in the over-55 age group. Females and males were almost equally represented in all age groups.

The degree of bone resorption was first examined by age group. In the under-35 age group, the amount of bone resorption was 3.08 ± 0.03 mm; in the 35–55 age group, it was 3.09 ± 0.04 mm; and in those over 55 years, it was 2.05 ± 0.09 mm. Statistically, there was no significant difference in the degree of bone resorption between the age groups ($p$ = 0.62). A similar result was obtained according to the time elapsed since implant placement. In implants placed 1–3 years ago, the degree of bone resorption was 2.82 ± 0.04 mm; in implants placed 4–7 years ago, it was 3.39 ± 0.12 mm, while in implants older than 7 years it was 2.08 ± 0.05 mm. Statistically, there were no significant differences between the groups ($p$ = 0.57). More bone resorption can be observed in the first years, which does not necessarily worsen in the future.

No statistically significant differences were found between genders ($p = 0.71$), although a slightly higher degree of bone resorption was observed in females (3.4 mm ± 0.15) than in males (2.45 ± 0.07 mm ).

The periodontal status of the patients was evaluated by measuring the periodontal pocket depths around the natural teeth present in the oral cavity (Tables 1 and 2) (Figure 3a,b). The periodontal pocket depth around implants showed significantly greater values ($p = 0.0006$) than natural teeth.

**Table 1.** Mean values of the measured parameters by age groups, with *p* values showing statistically significant differences. (PPD = periodontal pocket depth; PD = probing depth; SD = standard deviation).

| Age Group | PPD around Natural Teeth (Mean ± SD) | PD around Implants (Mean ± SD) | *p* Value | Peri-Implant Mucosa Width (Mean ± SD) |
|---|---|---|---|---|
| Under 35 years | 4.14 ± 1.16 | 4.75 ± 1.32 | 0.188 | 3.43 ± 1.82 |
| 35–55 years | 4.24 ± 0.83 | 5.08 ± 0.95 | 0.002 | 2.54 ± 1.32 |
| Over 55 years | 4.09 ± 0.91 | 5.12 ± 1.30 | 0.014 | 2.07 ± 2.10 |

**Table 2.** Mean values of the measured parameters grouped by the time elapsed since implant placement, with *p* values showing statistically significant differences. (PPD = periodontal pocket depth; PD = probing depth; SD = standard deviation).

| Insertion of the Implant (s) | PPD around Natural Teeth (Mean ± SD) | PD around Implants (Mean ± SD) | *p* Value | Peri-Implant Mucosa Width (Mean ± SD) |
|---|---|---|---|---|
| 1–3 years ago | 4.14 ± 0.88 | 4.86 ± 1.08 | 0.04 | 3.29 ± 1.52 |
| 4–7 years ago | 4.09 ± 0.91 | 5.12 ± 1.30 | 0.014 | 2.07 ± 2.10 |
| more than 7 years ago | 4.27 ± 0.95 | 5.13 ± 1.03 | 0.016 | 2.29 ± 1.32 |

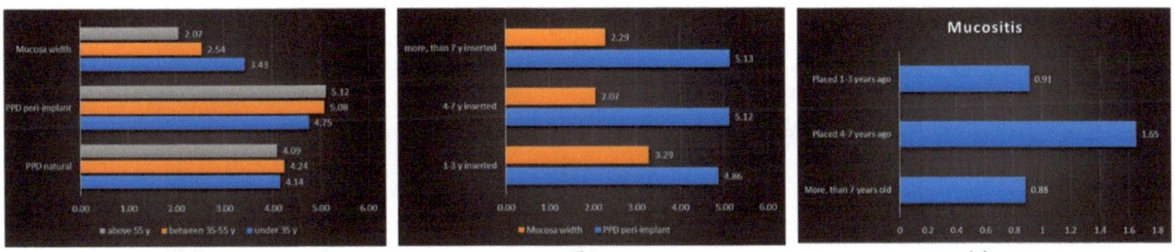


(a) (b) (c)

**Figure 3.** The changes following peri-implant parameters: (**a**) periodontal pocket depth changes reported for age groups; (**b**) the width of the keratinized mucosa compared with the peri-implant periodontal pocket depth according to the time elapsed since the implant placement; (**c**) average values of Löe–Silness gingival index as a function of the time elapsed since implant placement.

From a statistical point of view, the peri-implant periodontal pocket depth did not show a significant difference between age groups ($p = 0.78$), or in the time elapsed since implant placement ($p = 0.75$).

The comparison of the PPD (periodontal pocket depth) values of the natural teeth with the peri-implant probing depth values is shown in Tables 1 and 2. These values were compared within the different age groups. In the group under 35 years of age, there is no significant difference between the probing depth values around the implant and the PPD around the natural teeth of the same person.

For the 35–55 and over-55 years age groups, the peri-implant probing depths were significantly higher than the PPD values of the natural teeth of the same person in each group concerning the time elapsed since implant placement. The mean values of PPD and peri-implant probing depth and the corresponding *p* values are shown in Tables 1 and 2.

The highest values for the Löe–Silness gingival index were found for the 35–55 age group and implants placed 4–7 years ago (Figure 3c), indicating status between level 1 and 2 inflammations. The values for the 35–55 age group show a significant difference compared to those of the other age groups ($p = 0.04$). However, no statistically significant differences were found between the other groups ($p > 0.05$). We found no differences between the genders in the degree of inflammation ($p = 0.45$).

Both mucosal thickness and keratinized mucosal width ($p < 0.0001$) showed significant differences compared with peri-implant periodontal pocket depth (Figures 1a and 3a). There was a tendency for an inverse relationship between the thickness and width of the keratinized mucosa and the peri-implant periodontal pocket depth, with the mucosal parameters increasing as the peri-implant periodontal pocket depth decreased.

There were no significant differences in mucosal thickness between age groups ($p = 0.06$) or time since implant placement ($p = 0.106$) (Figure 1a).

The width of the keratinized mucosa was not affected by age ($p = 0.24$) or time since implant placement ($p = 0.15$). The mean values of mucosal thickness around implants according to age groups and time since implant placement are highlighted in Tables 1 and 2.

Based on the questionnaires, the most frequent subjective symptoms experienced by people with implants were collected: the most frequent was the squeezing of food next to the implant (22.5% of the respondents reported it), followed by bleeding gums (20%), the visible perception of receding gums (in 17.5%), and, to a lesser extent, halitosis and the visibility of the metal border along the gingival margin as perceived discomforts. All patients reported receiving information on how to clean the area around the implant after the treatment. In addition, they learned about this topic from friends and the Internet. In addition to the toothbrush, most of the patients used mouthwash (77.5%), dental floss (35%), and interdental brushes (32.5%) as additional methods; some of them used water-flossers (25%), and the fewest used a single-bristle toothbrush (10%) and super floss (10%) as additional oral hygiene products.

## 4. Discussion

Dental implantation is a modern method of tooth replacement. Its technology is constantly developing, but this treatment method can still have many complications. The dentist, the patient, or the implant system itself may cause unintended consequences. Complications can be intraoperative (e.g., nerve injury, sinus opening—especially with sinus lift) or postoperative (e.g., implant exposure, inflammation, bone resorption) [30].

The present study evaluated the peri-implant complications related to age, gender, time elapsed since implant placement, periodontal health, mucosal thickness and width, subjective symptoms, and the oral hygiene habits of the patients. According to our findings, the age and gender of the patients do not influence bone loss around implants, but it can occur slightly more in females and 4–7 years after implant placement. Other studies from the literature support our findings related to the gender of the patients [31] but highlight a high correlation between bone loss and the patient's age [32].

According to the "Consensus Report of the Sixth European Workshop in Periodontology," the incidence of peri-implantitis is 28–56%, while that of peri-implant mucositis is around 80%. Risk factors include periodontitis, smoking, poor oral hygiene, and diabetes [13,33,34]. The patients included in this study were non-smokers, had good or acceptable oral hygiene, and had no systemic diseases.

The biological causes of complications include bacterial invasion of the peri-implant tissues, leading to inflammatory changes in the soft tissues and rapid bone destruction. In addition, personal factors, tissue deficiencies, systemic factors (osteoporosis, smoking, mental illness, diabetes mellitus, alcohol consumption), and biomechanical and overload factors may also lead to the development of complications [33,35]. Our study only included patients who did not have any pre-existing systemic disorders, which could have potentially affected the outcomes of our research. We were interested in studying the implant's behavior and survival rate in intraoral conditions without being influenced by systemic diseases. This topic could be the subject of another study.

According to Ferreira's study, the incidence of peri-implantitis and peri-implant mucositis is influenced by smoking and the thickness of the keratinized mucosa. A keratinized mucosa thickness of less than 2 mm significantly increases the incidence of inflammation around the implants [36]. In this research, the smoking factor was eliminated due to the protocol of the dental clinic: the surgeon refuses to place implants in smoking patients. The average width of keratinized mucosa around dental implants placed 1–3 years ago was more than 3 mm, associated with a peri-implant pocket depth of less than 5 mm, and around implants older than 4 years the average width of keratinized mucosa was less than 2.3 mm, associated with a peri-implant pocket depth of more than 5 mm. Our study was consistent with Ferreira's findings: the lower the keratinized mucosal thickness around implants, the higher the incidence of peri-implant inflammation. Peri-implant mucositis precedes the development of peri-implantitis, so mucositis occurs in a much higher percentage than peri-implantitis itself. This is also supported by data from the literature [32,37,38]. An important clinical feature of prosthodontic consideration is the restoration's fixation type: there can be screw-retained or cemented prosthetic works. All prosthetic works in the present research were cemented following the dental clinic's protocol, resulting in a more esthetic appearance. Both methods have their advantages and disadvantages. Cemented restorations without an early and periodical screening can lead to early bone loss around implants with subgingivally placed restorations because of the undetectable excess cement [39]. Properly selecting the cement and the adequate, individualized treatment protocol can significantly decrease the risk of peri-implant bone loss [40]. Screw-retained bridges have a better long-term prognosis compared to cemented ones because of the missing excess cement on the cervical third; they are more feasible, and they can be removed for any future adjustment or repair, which would not be possible in the case of classic cemented restorations. However, the latter is more esthetic as the access hole is absent on the occlusal area. It allows for some angulation of the underlying implants [41–44].

Hard and soft tissue changes around the implant are multifactorial. They may be caused by trauma, periodontitis, anatomical conditions, thin mucosa, lack of keratinized mucosa, incorrect implant placement, tooth migration, and systemic diseases [45]. Another study demonstrated that the risk of developing peri-implantitis increases with smoking and the presence of the TNF$\alpha$-308 GA/AA genotype [46]. Patients with background periodontal disease have a higher risk of developing peri-implantitis or peri-implant mucositis [47]. During this study, significantly greater PPD was observed around implants compared to natural teeth, which was related to the age of the examined patients and the time elapsed since implant placement. Only the under-35 age group and those with implants placed 1–3 years ago showed similar values. Periodically monitoring periodontal health can minimize the risk of peri-implant complications. This study's results agree with other findings in the literature [48,49]. In patients with periodontal disease, bone loss and periodontal pocket depth around implants were greater than around natural teeth, without significant differences related to age or gender.

The leading cause of inflammation around the implants is bacterial colonization at the head and body of the implant. Therefore, perfect epithelial attachment is one of the fundamental factors for the long-term survival of the implants. Developing this epithelial attachment at the mucosal level also depends on the establishment of perfect cleaning of the implant head [25]. Each patient in this study who underwent implant placement in our dental clinic signed an informed consent form and committed to using the complementary oral hygiene methods previously presented by the surgeon. Another study is planned to evaluate the effects of using different adjunctive oral hygiene methods around dental implants.

Long-term experience in the dental implant literature indicates that a positive papillary bleeding index, a probing depth greater than 4 mm, and a slight bone loss in most cases reflect dental implants that are still functioning well, considering that healing after dental implant placement is the result of a foreign body reaction, with the formation of scar tissue. Therefore, measuring the probing depth and determining the papilla bleeding index in evaluating periodontal status around implants may lead to overdiagnosis and possibly overtreatment of suspected biofilm-mediated peri-implantitis conditions. The authors of the study state that treatment should be initiated only when clinical symptoms (discomfort, pain, swelling, discoloration, and the presence of pus) and significant bone loss over time, as confirmed by radiographs, are present. The goal of treatment should be to eradicate the infection, which may include implant removal [50].

As the loss rate of placed implants has increased, specific follow-up protocols have been established for daily practice. In the case of peri-implant mucositis, the diagnostics protocol includes a visual inspection that shows signs of inflammation around the implants (red color of the peri-implant mucosa, swollen soft tissues), significant bleeding (line or tear-shaped), the presence of pus on probing, deeper probing depths that exceed the standard, non-pathological range, and the absence of additional bone loss after initial bone remodeling [12,50]. In the case of peri-implantitis, the diagnostic protocol includes visible soft tissue inflammatory processes around the implants, a positive papilla bleeding index, pus on probing, deeper pocket depth compared to values measured at superstructure placement, and progressive bone loss after one year compared to previous radiographic bone level assessment. Without initial radiographs and previous probing depth values, radiographic evidence of 3 mm or higher bone loss and 6 mm or greater probing depth with significant bleeding suggests peri-implantitis. Assessment of the annual rate of bone loss might be helpful in daily clinical practice [11,14,50].

In epidemiologic studies, the same criteria should be used to determine the health of peri-implant tissues and detect peri-implant mucositis as in daily practice. The problem with epidemiologic studies is that radiographic and clinical information on suprastructure placement may not be available. Under these circumstances, the diagnosis of peri-implantitis requires 3 mm or more from the implant platform to the bone contact and a positive bleeding index [12,50,51].

Although the findings of the current study are consistent with those mentioned earlier, it is crucial to acknowledge the limitations. The small sample size is an important constraint. Further studies with larger cohorts and standardized evaluation protocols are needed. This will provide a more comprehensive understanding of peri-implant disease. Moreover, additional research is needed to evaluate the influence of various factors such as different types of tobacco, implant-supported prostheses, adjunctive oral hygiene methods, and systemic diseases on dental implants' longevity and survival rate.

## 5. Conclusions

In the cases examined in this study, there were no statistically significant differences between the time since implant placement and the degree of bone resorption: a large amount of bone resorption can be detected from the first years, similar to implants placed ten years ago. The degree of bone resorption, peri-implant periodontal pocket depth, and mucosal thickness and width did not differ significantly between genders and age groups. Within each group, the peri-implant probing depth was significantly greater than the periodontal pocket depth values of the natural teeth of the same individual concerning the time elapsed since implant placement. Periodontitis is a significant risk factor for the development of peri-implant inflammation, and patients with periodontitis had more significant bone loss and periodontal pocket depth around implants. In the population we studied, peri-implant mucositis was less common in the under-35 age group than in the 35–55 age group. Peri-implant inflammation can occur at any age, regardless of the lifetime of the implant.

**Author Contributions:** Conceptualization, C.B. and B.K.-M.; methodology, L.B.; software, B.K.-M.; validation, Z.B.-V.; formal analysis, I.Z.B. and B.K.-M.; investigation, I.G. and I.Z.B.; resources, I.G. and C.B.; data curation, L.B. and Z.B.-V. writing—original draft preparation, C.B.; writing—review and editing, B.K.-M. and K.M.J.; visualization, K.I.M.; supervision, K.M.J. and K.I.M. All authors have read and agreed to the published version of the manuscript.

**Funding:** This research received no external funding.

**Institutional Review Board Statement:** The study was conducted in accordance with the Declaration of Helsinki on experimentation involving human subjects, as revised in 2013, and approved by the Ethical Committee of University of Medicine, Pharmacy, Science and Technology "G. E. Palade" of Târgu Mureș, Romania (protocol code: 1895; date of approval: 19 October 2022).

**Informed Consent Statement:** Each patient in this study who underwent implant placement in our dental clinic signed an informed consent form. Written informed consent has been obtained from the patients to publish this paper.

**Data Availability Statement:** The datasets analyzed during this study are available from the first author on request.

**Conflicts of Interest:** The authors declare no conflicts of interest.

## References

1. Block, M.S. Dental implants: The last 100 years. *J. Oral Maxillofac. Surgery* **2018**, *76*, 11–26. [CrossRef] [PubMed]
2. Buser, D.; Sennerby, L.; De Bruyn, H. Modern implant dentistry based on osseointegration: 50 years of progress, current trends and open questions. *Periodontol. 2000* **2017**, *73*, 7–21. [CrossRef] [PubMed]
3. Nervins, M. Implant dentistry: A continuing evolution. *Int. J. Periodontics Restor. Dent.* **2014**, *34*, 7. [CrossRef] [PubMed]
4. Vajdovich, I.; Orosz, M. Realization of tissue care concept by the use of Denti bone level implants. Three years of clinical experience in applying Denti BL implants. *Fogorvosi Szle.* **2012**, *105*, 155–156.
5. Karthik, K.; Sivaraj, S. Evaluation of implant success: A review of past and present concepts. *J. Pharm. Bioallied Sci.* **2013**, *5*, 117–119. [CrossRef] [PubMed]
6. Makary, C.; Menhall, A. Primary stability optimization by using fixtures with different thread depth according to bone density: A clinical prospective study on early loaded implants. *Materials* **2019**, *12*, 2398. [CrossRef]
7. Cicciu, M. Bioengineering methods of analysis and medical devices: Current trends and state of the art. *Materials* **2020**, *13*, 797. [CrossRef] [PubMed]
8. Raghavendra, S.J.; Dhinakarsamy, V. Osseoinegration. *J. Pharm. Bioallied Sci.* **2015**, *7*, 226–229. [CrossRef]
9. Iacono, V.J.; Bassir, S.H.; Wang, H.H.; Myneni, S.R. Peri-implantitis: Effects of periodontitis and its risk factors—A narrative review. *FOMM* **2023**, *5*, 27. [CrossRef]
10. Papaspyridakos, P.; Chen, C.J.; Singh, M.; Weber, H.P.; Gallucci, G. Success criteria in implants dentistry: A systematic review. *J. Dent. Res.* **2012**, *91*, 242–248. [CrossRef]
11. Berglundh, T.; Armitage, G.; Araujo, M.G.; Avila-Ortiz, G.; Blanco, J.; Camargo, P.M.; Chen, S.; Cochran, D.; Derks, J.; Figuero, E.; et al. Peri-implant diseases and conditions: Consensus report of workgroup 4 of the 2017 World Workshop on the Classification of periodontal and peri-implant diseases and conditions. *J. Periodontol.* **2018**, *89*, 313–318. [CrossRef] [PubMed]
12. Renvert, S.; Persson, G.R.; Pirih, F.Q.; Camargo, P.M. Peri-implant health, peri-implant mucositis, and peri-implantitis: Case definitions and diagnostic considerations. *J. Clin. Periodontol.* **2018**, *45*, 278–285. [CrossRef] [PubMed]
13. Lindhe, J.; Meyle, J. Group D of European Workshop on Periodontology. Peri-implant diseases: Consensus report of the Sixth European Workshop on Periodontology. *J. Clin. Periodontol.* **2008**, *35*, 282–285. [CrossRef] [PubMed]
14. Heitz-Mayfield, L. Peri-implant mucositis and peri-implantitis: Key features and differences. *Br. Dent. J.* **2024**, *236*, 791–794. [CrossRef] [PubMed]
15. Heitz-Mayfield, L.; Salvi, G.E. Peri-implant mucositis. *J. Periodontol.* **2018**, *89*, 257–266. [CrossRef] [PubMed]
16. Salvi, G.E.; Aglietta, M.; Eick, S.; Sculean, A.; Lang, N.P.; Ramseier, C.A. Reversibility of experimental peri-implant mucositis compared with experimental gingivitis in humans. *Clin. Oral Implant. Res.* **2012**, *23*, 182–190. [CrossRef] [PubMed]
17. Hammerle, C.H.; Chen, S.T.; Wilson, T.G. Consensus statements and recommended clinical procedures regarding the placement of implants in extraction sockets. *Int. J. Oral Maxillofac. Implant.* **2004**, *19*, 26–28.
18. Derks, J.; Schaller, D.; Hakansson, J.; Wennström, J.L.; Tomasi, C.; Berglundh, T. Peri-implantitis—Onset and pattern of progression. *J. Clin. Periodontol.* **2016**, *43*, 383–388. [CrossRef] [PubMed]
19. Kowalski, J.; Lapinska, B.; Nissan, J.; Lukomska-Szymanska, M. Factors influencing marginal bone loss around dental implants: A narrative review. *Coatings* **2021**, *11*, 865. [CrossRef]
20. Galindo-Moreno, P.; Catena, A.; Pérez-Sayáns, M.; Fernández-Barbero, J.E.; O'Valle, F.; Padial-Molina, M. Early marginal bone loss around dental implants to define success in implant dentistry: A retrospective study. *Clin. Implant. Dent. Relat. Res.* **2022**, *24*, 630–642. [CrossRef] [PubMed]

21. Saravi, B.E.; Putz, M.; Patzelt, S.; Alkalak, A.; Uelkuemen, S.; Boeker, M. Marginal bone loss around oral implants supporting fixed versus removable prostheses: A systematic review. *Int. J. Implant. Dent.* **2020**, *6*, 20. [CrossRef] [PubMed]
22. Robitaille, N.; Reed, D.N.; Walters, J.D.; Kumar, P. Periodontal and peri-implant diseases: Identical or fraternal infections? *Mol. Oral Microbiol.* **2016**, *31*, 285–301. [CrossRef] [PubMed]
23. Schwarz, F.; Derks, J.; Monje, A.; Wang, H. Peri-implantitis. *J. Clin. Periodontol.* **2018**, *45*, 246–266. [CrossRef] [PubMed]
24. Genco, R.J.; Borgnakke, W.S. Risk factors for periodontal disease. *Periodontol. 2000* **2013**, *62*, 59–94. [CrossRef] [PubMed]
25. Zheng, H.; Xu, L.; Wang, Z.; Li, L.; Zhang, J.; Zhang, Q.; Chen, T.; Lin, J.; Chen, F. Subgingival microbiome in patients with healthy and ailing dental implants. *Sci. Rep.* **2015**, *16*, 10948. [CrossRef] [PubMed]
26. Ferreira, S.D.; Silva, G.L.; Cortelli, J.R.; Costa, J.E.; Costa, F.O. Prevalence and risk variables for peri-implant disease in Brazilian subjects. *J. Clin. Periodontol.* **2006**, *33*, 929–935. [CrossRef] [PubMed]
27. Lee, C.T.; Huang, H.Y.; Sun, T.C.; Karimbux, N. Impact of patient compliance on tooth loss during supportive periodontal therapy: A systematic review and meta-analysis. *J. Dent. Res.* **2015**, *94*, 777–786. [CrossRef] [PubMed]
28. Rokaya, D.; Srimaneepong, V.; Wisitrasameewon, W.; Humagain, M.; Thunyakitpisal, P. Peri-implantitis update: Risk indicators, diagnosis, and treatment. *Eur. J. Dent.* **2020**, *14*, 672–682. [CrossRef]
29. Gera, I. *Periodontology*, 1st ed.; Semmelweis Kiadó: Budapest, Hungary, 2009; pp. 30, 421.
30. Causes and Treatment of the Failure of Dental Implant Restorations. Available online: https://www.semmelweis.hu/szajsebeszet (accessed on 29 June 2018).
31. Dreyer, H.; Grischke, J.; Tiede, C.; Eberhard, J.; Schweitzer, A.; Toikkanen, S.E.; Glöckner, S.; Krause, G.; Stiesch, M. Epidemiology and risk factors of peri-implantitis: A systematic review. *J. Periodontal Res.* **2018**, *53*, 657–681. [CrossRef] [PubMed]
32. Devi, S.; Duraisamy, R. Crestal Bone Loss in Implants Postloading and Its Association with Age, Gender, and Implant Site: A Retrospective Study. *J. Long-Term Eff. Med. Implant.* **2020**, *30*, 205–211. [CrossRef] [PubMed]
33. Vajdovich, I. *Dental Implantology*, 1st ed.; Semmelweis: Budapest, Hungary, 2017; pp. 40–52, 245–259.
34. Ogata, Y.; Nakayama, Y.; Tatsumi, J.; Kubota, T.; Sato, S.; Nishida, T.; Takeuchi, Y.; Onitsuka, T.; Sakagami, R.; Nozaki, T.; et al. Prevalence and risk factors for peri-implant diseases in Japanese adult dental patients. *J. Oral Sci.* **2017**, *59*, 1–11. [CrossRef] [PubMed]
35. Dental Implants—Esthetic Complications. Available online: https://www.dental.hu/fogaszati-implantatumok-esztetikai-komplikaciok (accessed on 6 February 2024).
36. Ferreira, C.F.; Buttendorf, A.R.; de Souza, J.G.; Dalago, H.; Guenther, S.F.; A Bianchini, M. Prevalence of peri-implant diseases: Analyses of associated factors. *Eur. J. Prosthodont. Restor. Dent.* **2015**, *23*, 199–206. [PubMed]
37. Mahardawi, B.; Jiaranuchart, S.; Damrongsirirat, N.; Arunjaroensuk, S.; Mattheos, N.; Somboonsavatdee, A.; Pimkhaokham, A. The lack of keratinized mucosa as a risk factor for peri-implantitis: A systematic review and meta-analysis. *Sci. Rep.* **2023**, *13*, 3778. [CrossRef] [PubMed] [PubMed Central]
38. Afrashtehfar, K.I.; Oh, K.C.; Jurado, C.A.; Lee, H. Lack of keratinized mucosa increases peri-implantitis risk. *Evid.-Based Dent.* **2023**, *24*, 118–120. [CrossRef] [PubMed]
39. Staubli, N.; Walter, C.; Schmidt, J.C.; Weiger, R.; Zitzmann, N.U. Excess cement and the risk of peri-implant disease—A systematic review. *Clin. Oral Implant. Res.* **2017**, *28*, 1278–1290. [CrossRef] [PubMed]
40. Kotsakis, G.; Zhang, L.; Gaillard, P.; Raedel, M.; Walter, M.; Konstantinidis, I. Investigation of the Association Between Cement-Retention and Prevalent Peri-Implant Diseases: A Cross-Sectional Study. *J. Periodontol.* **2015**, *87*, 1–14. [CrossRef] [PubMed]
41. Rosenstiel, S.F.; Land, M.F.; Fujimoto, J. *Contemporary Fixed Prosthodontics*, 5th ed.; Elsevier Inc.: St. Louis, MO, USA, 2016; pp. 334, 358–361.
42. Chio, A.; Hatai, Y. Restoration of two implants using custom abutments and transverse screw-retained zirconia crowns. *Am. J. Esthet. Dent.* **2012**, *2*, 264–280.
43. Wittneben, J.G.; Joda, T.; Weber, H.P.; Bragger, U. Screw retained vs. cement retained implant-supported fixed dental prosthesis. *Periodontol. 2000* **2017**, *73*, 141–151. [CrossRef] [PubMed]
44. Jánosi, K.M.; Cerghizan, D.; Berneanu, F.D.; Kovács, A.; Szász, A.; Mureșan, I.; Hănțoiu, L.G.; Albu, A.I. Full-mouth rehabilitation of a patient with gummy smile—Multidisciplinary approach: Case Report. *Medicina* **2023**, *59*, 197. [CrossRef]
45. Hammerle, C.H.; Tarnow, D. The etiology of hard- and soft-tissue deficiencies at dental implants: A narrative review. *J. Periodontol.* **2018**, *89*, 291–303. [CrossRef] [PubMed]
46. Petkovic-Curcin, A.; Zeljic, K.; Cikota-Aleksic, B.; Dakovic, D.; Tatic, Z.; Magic, Z. Association of cytokine gene polymorphism with peri-implantitis risk. *Int. J. Oral Maxillofac. Implant.* **2017**, *32*, 241–248. [CrossRef] [PubMed]
47. Altay, M.A.; Tozoğlu, S.; Yıldırımyan, N.; Özarslan, M. Is history of periodontitis a risk factor for peri-implant disease? A pilot study. *Int. J. Oral Maxillofac. Implant.* **2018**, *33*, 152–160. [CrossRef] [PubMed]
48. Lv, P.-X.; Zhong, J.-S.; Ouyang, X.-Y.; Iao, S.; Liu, J.; Xie, Y. Investigation of peri-implant diseases prevalence and related risk indicators in patients with treated severe periodontitis over 4 years after restoration. *J. Dent. Sci.* **2024**, *19*, 894–899. [CrossRef] [PubMed]
49. Astolfi, V.; Ríos-Carrasco, B.; Gil-Mur, F.J.; Ríos-Santos, J.V.; Bullón, B.; Herrero-Climent, M.; Bullón, P. Incidence of Peri-Implantitis and Relationship with Different Conditions: A Retrospective Study. *Int. J. Environ. Res. Public Health* **2022**, *19*, 4147. [CrossRef] [PubMed] [PubMed Central]

50. Coli, P.; Christiaens, V.; Sennerby, L.; de Bruyn, H. Reliability of periodontal diagnostic tools for monitoring peri-implant health and disease. *Periodontol. 2000* **2017**, *73*, 203–217. [CrossRef] [PubMed]
51. Araujo, M.G.; Lindhe, J. Peri-implant health. *J. Clin. Periodontol.* **2018**, *45*, 230–236. [CrossRef] [PubMed]

diagnostics

MDPI

*Review*

# Prognosis, Controversies and Assessment of Bone Erosion or Invasion of Oral Squamous Cell Carcinoma

**Ahmed Ata Alfurhud**

Oral and Maxillofacial Surgery and Diagnostic Sciences Department, College of Dentistry, Jouf University, King Khalid Road, Sakaka 72388, Saudi Arabia; aalfarhood@ju.edu.sa or dr.aalfurhud@jodent.org; Tel.: +966-501738443

**Abstract: Objectives**: To discuss the prognostic outcomes, controversies and assessment of bone erosion or invasion of oral squamous cell carcinoma (OSCC). **Methods:** A structured literature review was conducted to critically analyse relevant evidence. The Web of Science database was searched using specific keywords aligned with the review question. After identifying initial studies, their references were also reviewed to include any additional relevant publications, ensuring a comprehensive evaluation of the available evidence. **Results:** The search identified 11 relevant studies, including 5 from the initial search and 6 from reference review. The significance of bone involvement is unclear in OSCC, with varying definitions of cortical bone erosion and medullary bone infiltration contributing to conflicting results regarding the prognostic significance of bone involvement. The majority of evidence stems from retrospective cohort studies without clear study criteria and a lack of power to draw valid conclusions. **Conclusions:** There are currently a lack of high-quality studies assessing bone invasion in OSCC. While there appears to be some evidence that medullary bone infiltration is prognostic, further well-designed studies are warranted.

**Keywords:** cortical bone; medullary carcinomas; oral squamous cell carcinoma; outcome; prognosis

## 1. Introduction

Oral squamous cell carcinoma (OSCC) is the most common malignant tumour arising in the oral cavity [1]. It is usually preceded by dysplastic changes in the stratified squamous epithelium lining the mouth [2]. OSCC has a wide range of clinical presentations, which makes the diagnosis difficult in some cases, particularly in the early stages [3]. Tumours may also arise in close proximity to the maxillary and mandibular bone.

According to the Tumour Node Metastasis (TNM) staging classification, OSCC that invades the cancellous bone (medullary bone infiltration) is upgraded to T stage T4a (regardless of size), whereas cortical bone erosion limited to the cortical plate does not result in a T stage upgrade to T4a. If no bone involvement has occurred or there is only superficial cortical bone erosion, the T stage is based on the size and depth of the tumour or invasion into adjacent structures [4].

In the present paper, the term 'Bone Involvement' refers specifically to two distinct patterns: (1) cortical bone erosion and (2) medullary bone infiltration. However, distinguishing between these two patterns of bone involvement can be challenging in certain cases, with significant implications for both treatment and prognosis.

There are a number of published studies describing the significance of bone involvement, but unfortunately, the majority of them do not sufficiently distinguish between the two patterns of bone involvement [5], which is important to achieve optimal surgical margins, to determine which patients may require adjunctive therapy and to correctly stage patients [6,7].

Medullary bone infiltration involves complete perforation of the cortical bone and extension into the medullary cavity, and establishing this can be challenging, particularly in the erosive pattern [8], as the bone of the maxilla and the mandible have naturally occurring perforations. In edentulous patients, there is atrophy of the maxillary and mandibular bones due to physiological remodelling which happens after tooth extraction [9]. This can also be problematic because it may be difficult to differentiate between patients with bone involvement and those with bone loss due to periodontal disease and bone resorption following tooth extraction [10]. The overall aim of this study was to review and discuss the prognostic outcomes, controversies and assessment of bone erosion or invasion of OSCC.

## 2. Materials and Methods

This study employed a narrative review design to analyse the existing literature, aiming to identify knowledge gaps and provide a comprehensive overview of the prognostic implications, controversies, and assessment of bone erosion or invasion in OSCC. A systematic search was conducted in the Web of Science and PubMed databases using the keywords: "cortical bone", "medullary carcinomas", "oral squamous cell carcinoma", "outcome", and "prognosis", combined with the Boolean operator "AND" to ensure comprehensive retrieval of relevant studies. The references of the identified studies were also manually reviewed to identify any additional relevant research that met the specified selection criteria.

The inclusion and exclusion criteria for references were carefully designed to ensure the selection of relevant studies while aligning with the research objectives. The timeframe for inclusion focused on research articles published between 1990 and 2020, as the research and writing process began after this date. Specifically, studies that addressed the role of bone erosion or invasion as an independent prognostic factor and its association with survival rates and poor clinical outcomes were included. The analysis was further refined to focus on studies providing evidence linking cortical or medullary bone invasion by OSCC to adverse prognostic outcomes. No restrictions were applied to study design, allowing for the inclusion of all studies that discussed the significance of bone erosion and invasion, regardless of methodology. However, commentaries and empirical articles were excluded to maintain consistency in the type of evidence analysed, and unpublished studies were excluded to ensure the reliability of peer-reviewed and publicly accessible work. Although no language restrictions were applied during the search, all identified articles were published in English, and no relevant articles in other languages were found.

## 3. Results

The initial database search identified five relevant articles. An additional six studies meeting the inclusion criteria were identified through a review of the references, resulting in a total of 11 studies included in the analysis. A summary of the selected studies is provided in Table 1.

**Table 1.** A summary of studies included in this review.

| Reference (Type of Study) | Location of Tumour | No. of Patients | Average Age (Years) | Bone Invasion Assessment |
|---|---|---|---|---|
| [5] (Retrospective cohort study) | Oral tongue, FOM, Alveolus RMT, Buccal, Hard palate, Other. | 498 | 63.5 | The authors clearly defined and assessed the patterns of bone involvement, categorizing it into three distinct types: (1) No Bone Involvement (Absent): Absence of any bone involvement. (2) Cortical Bone Invasion: Involvement limited to the cortical layer of the bone. (3) Medullary Bone Invasion: Extension into the cancellous (spongy) bone. |
| [11] (Retrospective cohort study) | Alveolar ridge, Buccal, FOM, Gingiva, Hard Palate, Oral tongue, RMT | 254 | --------- | Patient Cohorts Based on Tumour Size and Bone Invasion: Patients were classified into three groups according to primary tumour size and bone invasion status: (1) ≤4 cm Without Bone Invasion: Tumours ≤ 4 cm in size with no evidence of bone involvement (AJCC T1/T2). (2) ≤4 cm With Bone Invasion Only: Tumours ≤ 4 cm in size where bone invasion was the sole factor contributing to an AJCC T4 classification. (3) >4 cm or Additional T4 Factors: Tumours > 4 cm in size or those with other features (e.g., skin invasion or deep muscle invasion) qualifying for an AJCC T4 classification, regardless of bone invasion pattern. |
| [12] (Retrospective cohort study) | FOM, Gingiva, RMT, Tongue, Buccal mucosa, others | 106 | 57.7 | In this study, bone involvement was evaluated preoperatively using clinical examination, panoramic radiographs and/or computed tomography scans. Postoperatively, bone involvement was confirmed based on the extent of bone resection. However, the researchers did not differentiate between the two patterns of bone involvement: cortical erosion or medullary bone infiltration histopathology, and no specific histopathological criteria for assessment were provided. |

**Table 1.** *Cont.*

| Reference (Type of Study) | Location of Tumour | No. of Patients | Average Age (Years) | Bone Invasion Assessment |
|---|---|---|---|---|
| [13] (Retrospective cohort study) | Base of tongue, Soft palate, RMT, Buccal mucosa, Lateral tongue, Anterior and Lateral FOM, others. | 82 | Men: 59<br>Women: 63 | The authors assessed bone involvement through clinical and radiographic examinations, with postoperative confirmation based on pathological reports. However, they did not specify whether the bone involvement pattern was cortical or medullary, nor did they provide clear criteria for pathologists to distinguish between these patterns. Data on two indicators of bone involvement were analysed: clinical examination findings, such as tumour fixation to the bone, and radiological evidence of bone involvement. |
| [14] (Retrospective cohort study) | FOM, RMT Alveolus, Tongue, Buccal or Cheek | 100 | 63 | The medullary infiltrative pattern, the tumour penetrates the cancellous bone spaces as small islands or projections, without an intervening layer of connective tissue and with minimal osteoclast activity. In contrast, the cortical erosive pattern features tumour invasion along a broad front, where a connective tissue layer and active osteoclasts separate the tumour from the bone. |
| [6] (Retrospective cohort study) | ----------- | 111 | 63 | While the patterns of bone involvement were evaluated, the authors did not specify distinct features for "cortical bone erosion" and "medullary bone infiltration." According to the authors, the cortical bone erosion was considered to occur when the tumour was clinically observed to be "adherent to" or "superficially involving" the bone. In contrast, the medullary bone infiltration was identified when the tumour extended deeply into the medullary cavity or when the mandible was atrophy. |
| [7] (Retrospective cohort study) | Buccal mucosa, RMT, Lower gingiva, Lip | 43 | 49.4 | The pattern of bone involvement was assessed using the same criteria as described in [14]. |
| [15] (Retrospective cohort study) | Tongue, FOM Alveolar crest, Buccal region | 982 | 60.3 | The bone involvement was assessed using the methodology described in [6]. Although the evaluation categorized bone as either invaded or not invaded, the authors did not establish clear histopathological criteria to differentiate between cortical bone erosion and medullary bone infiltration. |

**Table 1.** *Cont.*

| Reference (Type of Study) | Location of Tumour | No. of Patients | Average Age (Years) | Bone Invasion Assessment |
|---|---|---|---|---|
| [16] (Retrospective cohort study) | Lower gingiva | 142 | 62.7 | The assessment of bone involvement was based on a thorough perioperative evaluation, clinical and imaging examinations, intraoperative frozen section analysis, tumour proximity to or fixation on the underlying bone, and the depth of bony invasion. Histopathological analysis confirmed the presence of bone involvement, which the authors categorized into cortical and medullary types. However, they did not provide a clear definition or criteria for distinguishing between these two patterns of bone involvement. |
| [17] (Retrospective cohort study) | FOM, Lower alveolus, RMT | 96 | 62.6 | The extent of bone involvement was categorized as either macroscopic (visible destruction of bone by the tumour observed during gross examination of the specimen) or microscopic (detected only under a microscope). The level of bone involvement was classified into two categories: cortical only (limited to the outer bone layer) and medullary (involving malignant cell infiltration into the cancellous bone of the medullary cavity). |
| [18] (Retrospective cohort study) | Buccal Mucosa FOM, Lower Gum, RMT, Tongue | 326 | 64 | The bone involvement was recorded as cortical and medullary. However, no clear criteria were mentioned, except in medullary bone infiltration when the cancer cells reach into medullary spaces. |

Abbreviations: FOM, floor of mouth; RMT, Retromolar trigone; AJCC, American Joint Committee on Cancer.

## 4. Review of Literature on Bone Invasion

The controversies surrounding patterns of bone invasion—specifically, cortical bone erosion and medullary bone infiltration—have been discussed to determine whether bone erosion or infiltration by OSCCs is an independent prognostic factor [19]; however, the studies have shown conflicting results [5]. For instance, it has been argued the survival rate difference between two surgical procedures (marginal and segmental mandibulectomy) give no significant difference in the survival rates between these two procedures, even for cortical bone erosion or medullary bone infiltration [6]. In contrast, a strong relationship between the patterns of bone involvement and poor outcomes has also been reported in the literature, showing a correlation with the extent of bone invasion [5,11–14]. However, research from other authors does not support this position [6,7,20].

Ebrahimi et al. [5] conducted a retrospective cohort study by dividing the patients based on: 1. absent (without bone involvement); 2. cortical bone erosion (limited to cortical plate); and 3. medullary bone infiltration (extension into cancellous bone), and reported that patients with medullary bone infiltration had significantly lower 5-year overall survival (29% vs. 65%) and disease-specific survival (DSS) (36% vs. 77%) compared to those without bone involvement ($p < 0.001$). In contrast, patients with cortical bone erosion alone showed no significant difference in survival compared to those without bone involvement. Distant metastases were more common in patients with medullary bone infiltration (9.8%) compared to cortical bone erosion (4.9%) and no bone involvement (3.8%). Univariate analysis showed a 330% higher risk of distant metastases in patients with medullary bone infiltration versus those without bone involvement. Therefore, medullary bone infiltration was an independent indicator of reduced overall and DSS and had a worse prognosis compared with the others.

Fried et al. [11] investigated the impact of bone involvement in small OSCCs using histopathological criteria to evaluate the depth and severity of invasion. Patients were divided into three cohorts (details in Table 1). Cohorts 1 and 2 demonstrated similar clinical outcomes regardless of bone involvement, whereas cohort 3 exhibited worse overall survival, DSS, distant metastasis and regional control. The study concluded that small tumours with cortical bone erosion may have outcomes comparable to T1 and T2 tumours, but medullary bone infiltration is a significant prognostic factor associated with poorer control and survival rates. Medullary bone infiltration was identified as the strongest predictor of poor outcomes.

Another retrospective study was conducted to assess bone involvement. The results showed a 5-year observed survival rate of 60.35%. Local recurrence (LR) was significantly lower in early-stage tumours ($p = 0.02$). Patients undergoing bone resections greater than 4 cm had lower survival rates compared to those with resections of less than 4 cm ($p = 0.01$). Advanced-stage tumours ($p = 0.006$) and involvement of surgical margins ($p = 0.0001$) or bone ($p = 0.003$) were also significantly associated with reduced survival [12].

Jones et al. [13] found that patients without bone involvement had a 5-year survival rate of 53%, while those with suspected bone involvement had a significantly lower rate of 25% ($p < 0.02$). Bone involvement is a strong indicator of poor prognosis in oral cavity cancers. The findings of Shaw et al. [14] highlight the critical role of bone involvement in predicting recurrence and DSS. The 5-year DSS was 68%, and the crude survival rate was 50%. Notably, the pattern of bone involvement proved to be a significant prognostic factor. Tumours with cortical bone erosion were associated with a relatively favourable prognosis, while medullary bone infiltration indicated more aggressive tumour behaviour and worse outcomes.

However, contrary to previous findings, various theories in the literature suggest differing perspectives on bone involvement. Patel et al. [6] demonstrated that the presence of medullary bone infiltration and the extent of bone invasion did not significantly affect the 5-year local control rate. Similarly, no differences in local control or survival rates were observed between cases with cortical bone erosion versus medullary bone infiltration. However, LR was found to be associated with soft tissue margin involvement in the context of bone involvement. The study concluded that soft tissue margin involvement, when coupled with bone involvement, is the most critical indicator of poor prognosis.

This view is supported by Chen et al. [7], who analysed local control rates in two groups. Among patients with bone involvement, the local control rate was 85.7%, compared to 77.8% in patients without bone involvement. Although the bone involvement was categorized as "None", "Cortex" and "Medullary" (the latter represented by only one patient), no statistically significant difference was observed between the groups.

Mücke et al. [15] reported findings consistent with those of Patel et al. [6] and Chen et al. [7], showing that bone involvement was not an independent predictor of survival. The mean survival for patients with bone involvement was 71.6 $\pm$ 46.2 months, compared to 72.9 $\pm$ 48.1 months for those without bone involvement. They concluded that overall survival was primarily influenced by factors such as the extent of mandibulectomy, age, tumour stage, N stage, recurrence and tumour grade, while bone involvement had little impact on prognosis. Thus, although bone involvement does not directly affect survival, the extent of bone involvement in mandibular tumours remains crucial for surgical planning and prognosis. The study of Mücke et al. [15] highlights that while bone involvement is not significantly correlated with survival in OSCC patients, achieving tumour-free margins through surgery tailored to the tumour's extent is essential for better outcomes.

Three studies have presented conflicting results regarding the impact of bone involvement in OSCCs. Du et al. [16] reported a significantly higher risk of recurrence in OSCCs with bone involvement, although DSS rates were similar regardless of bone involvement. Fives et al. [17] found that medullary bone infiltration significantly worsened local control and overall survival in tumours $\leq$ 4 cm. In contrast, Petrovic et al. [18] concluded that bone involvement did not adversely affect prognosis, as local recurrence-free survival and DSS were comparable between OSCCs with and without bone involvement.

## 5. Discussion

The study by Ebrahimi et al. [5] underscores the critical prognostic role of bone involvement in patient outcomes. Medullary bone infiltration, as identified in their cohort, was associated with markedly reduced overall and DSS, highlighting its aggressive clinical nature. Moreover, the significantly increased risk of distant metastases, with a 330% higher likelihood compared to patients without bone involvement, further establishes medullary infiltration as a key indicator of poor prognosis. These findings suggest that medullary bone infiltration not only serves as an independent prognostic factor but also emphasizes the need for more aggressive therapeutic strategies for affected patients. In contrast, the finding that survival rates were similar between patients with cortical bone erosion and those without bone involvement suggests that cortical erosion has a less significant impact on prognosis compared to medullary bone infiltration. This highlights that different types of bone involvement affect patient outcomes to varying degrees. These distinctions provide valuable insight into tailoring treatment strategies and improving risk stratification for patients with varying degrees of bone involvement.

Based on the findings of Ebrahimi et al. [5], it is recommended that the T staging system be revised to enable better stratification for DSS. In their study, an alternative T staging system was proposed to more accurately reflect the prognostic differences associated with varying degrees of bone involvement. This system initially classifies tumours based on size as T1, T2, and T3, with the recommendation that tumours should be upstaged by one category (e.g., from T2 to T3) in the presence of medullary bone infiltration. This recommendation is based on evidence showing a significant increase in mortality associated with medullary bone infiltration, regardless of the tumour's size. Importantly, when bone involvement was only categorized as "present" or "absent", it was not identified as a significant independent predictor of overall survival or DSS. In contrast, medullary bone infiltration was shown to be a critical criterion for tumour staging.

The current American Joint Committee on Cancer (AJCC) T staging system does not adequately stratify DSS outcomes, as there is considerable overlap between T3 and T4 tumours. However, the alternative T staging system proposed by Ebrahimi et al. [5] provides better stratification of patient prognoses. This highlights the need to establish standardised criteria that differentiate patterns of bone involvement, ensuring that not all tumours with bone involvement are automatically classified as T4.

The findings of Fried et al. [11] align closely with those reported by Ebrahimi et al. [5], further emphasising the critical prognostic implications of medullary bone infiltration OSCC. Both studies highlight that while cortical bone erosion may not significantly affect survival outcomes, medullary involvement is strongly associated with poorer prognosis, including reduced survival rates and increased distant metastasis. Fried et al. [11] emphasised that small tumours (<4 cm) with bone involvement, currently classified as T4 under the AJCC staging system, exhibit outcomes comparable to small tumours without bone involvement. These findings reinforce the need to differentiate between cortical bone erosion and medullary bone infiltration within the staging framework. Furthermore, Fried et al. [11] validated a modified T staging system using their dataset, which offered improved stratification of patient outcomes compared to the existing AJCC system. Their study supports the consideration of modifications to the AJCC staging system to better reflect the prognostic differences between types of bone involvement, thus enhancing the accuracy of staging and treatment planning.

Muñoz Guerra et al. [12] investigated bone involvement in OCSCC using preoperative clinical exams, panoramic radiographs, and/or CT scans, with confirmation based on the extent of postoperative bone resection. However, their study lacked differentiation between cortical bone erosion and medullary bone infiltration and did not specify histopathological criteria for evaluating bone involvement. Compared to the more rigorous methodologies employed by Ebrahimi et al. [5] and Fried et al. [11], particularly in histopathological assessment, the approach used by Muñoz Guerra et al. [12]. was less reliable. This discrepancy in assessment methods raises the possibility that bone involvement may have been underestimated in the study by Muñoz Guerra et al. [12]. The findings highlight the importance of employing standardised criteria to define cortical bone erosion and medullary bone infiltration in future studies. Such standardization would not only improve the accuracy of bone involvement assessments but also enhance the comparability of findings across studies. Additionally, it would contribute to the establishment of more consistent prognostic and staging frameworks for OCSCC, ultimately aiding in the management and treatment of this disease.

Intra and inter-rater reliability is a known issue in pathology where scoring of dysplasia and grading of tumours can give varying results. For example, in numerous fields of pathology, particularly breast and prostate grading, different experienced pathologists favour different features when grading, leading to poor reproducibility [21,22]. It is not unreasonable to assume that similar issues exist when pathologists assess tumour for bone involvement, although no studies examining this issue were identified.

The methodology used in the study by Jones et al. [13] relied mainly on clinical and radiographic examinations to assess bone involvement, without providing a detailed description of the bone involvement patterns (e.g., erosion versus true infiltration). Instead, bone involvement was simply classified as either invaded or non-invaded. While the authors considered clinical examination a safe and reliable method for detecting bone involvement, this approach has limitations. Radiological and clinical assessments may fail to identify smaller or subtler areas of bone involvement that could be detected through microscopic examination. Histopathological analysis, as a more sensitive and precise method, allows for a clearer identification of invasion patterns and could detect smaller areas of invasion that radiological and clinical investigations could miss. This highlights the need for incorporating microscopic evidence into assessment protocols to improve diagnostic accuracy and ensure comprehensive evaluation of invasion patterns. Accordingly, it is suggested that the pattern of invasion was not classified as cortical bone erosion or medullary bone infiltration because the authors focused more on the clinical and radiographic examination without considering that histopathological examination can be better utilized to differentiate between the two patterns.

Some studies have been unable to demonstrate the prognostic significance of bone involvement, as discussed earlier. However, in the study by Patel et al. [6], the authors did not provide clear definitions or criteria for distinguishing between cortical bone erosion and medullary bone infiltration. Additionally, they acknowledged the absence of histological data regarding medullary bone infiltration. In some cases, the determination of bone involvement may rely on discussions between pathologists and radiologists, particularly in cases where the diagnosis is unclear or difficult to assess.

The pattern of bone involvement was assessed using the same criteria in two studies [7,14], yet their results were conflicting. According to Chen et al. [7], histological evidence of bone involvement did not significantly affect local tumour control or overall survival. However, the sample size in this study was relatively small compared to other studies, and the presence of medullary bone infiltration in only a single patient was insufficient to reliably determine its prognostic impact. To draw valid conclusions or demonstrate meaningful differences between cohorts, studies should have adequate statistical power. Without this, the findings may not be reliable due to the study being underpowered. Furthermore, if the criteria used by Ebrahimi et al. [5] and Fried et al. [11] were applied to the cohort in Chen et al. [7], where bone involvement was almost absent, the findings would likely align with those of Ebrahimi et al. [5] and Fried et al. [11]. This is because the presence of medullary bone infiltration is a critical factor in determining the prognostic significance of bone invasion.

The study by Mücke et al. [15] concluded that bone involvement should not be considered an independent predictor of survival. However, their assessment of bone involvement was based solely on whether the bone was invaded or not, without considering the specific pattern of bone involvement. Additionally, bone involvement was evaluated using a combination of clinical examination, CT and MRI, but histopathological examination was not included. As a result, true bone involvement may not have been accurately assessed, which could explain why the study did not find a significant impact of bone involvement on survival.

A systematic review with meta-analysis conducted by Li et al. [19] provided significant insights into the differences between cortical bone erosion and bone infiltration in OSCC. The study concluded that medullary bone infiltration is distinct from cortical bone erosion, with medullary bone infiltration associated with a higher rate of distant metastasis. This increased metastatic potential is attributed to the tumour's ability to access the circulation through the blood vessels in the cancellous bone. The review included 18 studies with a total of 3756 participants. Among these, 7 studies were classified as having an unclear risk of bias, while the remainder were deemed to have a high risk of bias. The meta-analysis revealed a significant relationship between medullary bone infiltration and overall survival ($p = 0.04$). Notably, medullary bone infiltration was found to significantly decrease overall survival ($p = 0.0001$), while cortical bone erosion showed no significant effect ($p = 0.66$). When focusing on DSS, mandibular medullary bone infiltration involvement was identified as a predictor of poor DSS ($p < 0.0001$), whereas cortical bone erosion did not impact DSS ($p = 0.66$). These findings underscore the importance of differentiating between the two types of bone involvement in prognostic assessments for OSCC.

In the paper by Jimi et al. [23], the authors describe the "the erosive pattern of bone invasion as is marked by a broad pushing front, a sharp interface between tumour and bone, osteoclastic bone resorption and fibrosis along the tumour front and an absence of bone islands within the tumour mass". However, this definition is problematic. Bone involvement can also present with a "pushing front" and "sharp interface" when a cohesive tumour pushes through the cortical bone into the medullary bone. As such, labelling this as an "erosion pattern" is misleading, as it may suggest that bone involvement is only associated with a discohesive invasive front. This could lead other studies to incorrectly conclude that bone involvement can only occur in such a manner, when in fact it may occur with different patterns of invasion.

In reviewing the literature, the included studies showed conflicting results, which may be due to differences in either the cohort or the methodology of assessment. One major factor is the variation in cohort characteristics, such as the distribution of tumour sites. For instance, in the studies by Ebrahimi et al. [5] and Fried et al. [11], tongue cancer was reported in 204 and 90 patients, respectively, whereas in the cohort of Patel et al. [6], only 9 cases of tongue cancer were included. Furthermore, the number of cases with involved margins was much higher in the studies by Ebrahimi et al. [5] and Fried et al. [11], with 79 and 63 cases, respectively, compared to just 16 cases in Patel et al. [6]. In contrast, the study by Chen et al. [7] did not include any cases involving the tongue or floor of mouth. These differences emphasize the importance of ensuring that patients' clinicopathological and demographic characteristics are comparable in order to draw reliable conclusions and minimize confounding factors, both within individual studies and when comparing studies. In addition to differences in patient characteristics, the cohort size was much smaller in some studies compared to others. This difference in cohort size could be a contributing factor to the conflicting results observed across these studies.

For future research, developing an objective set of criteria to differentiate between cortical bone erosion and medullary bone infiltration is essential for advancing future research and improving clinical diagnostics. Key areas of focus include analysing osteoclastic activity through immunohistochemical markers to assess the density and presence of osteoclasts in affected regions. Evaluating bone-lining cell integrity using markers can help distinguish reactive processes associated with erosion from infiltrative processes indicative of invasion. Additionally, studying the peritumoural fibro-osseous response may reveal that erosion often involves minimal desmoplasia, while medullary bone infiltration is typically associated with a pronounced desmoplastic reaction. The tumour-bone interface may also be examined, with erosion showing smooth borders and non-infiltrative morphology, while medullary bone infiltration presents irregular, spiculated borders and infiltrative tumour clusters. Advanced imaging techniques, such as micro-CT or confocal microscopy, can further enhance understanding by providing three-dimensional visualization of the bone-soft tissue interface. Future efforts should aim to validate these criteria through large-scale studies, ensure consistency in definitions and incorporate quantitative tools for more precise differentiation.

## 6. Conclusions

This review aimed to evaluate the significance of bone involvement in OSCCs and its influence on survival rates, specifically in relation to two distinct patterns of bone involvement. Additionally, it sought to examine whether consistent definitions exist for cortical bone erosion and medullary bone infiltration. The findings highlight that it is currently not possible to confirm whether bone involvement is a definitive prognostic indicator due to conflicting results and inconsistencies in the definitions of these patterns. The lack of consensus among researchers and pathologists on histological criteria for assessing bone involvement and differentiating between the patterns undermines the reliability of the existing evidence. This ambiguity limits the ability to draw actionable conclusions and implement effective clinical protocols. Despite the previous systematic review conducted in 2017 [19], there remains a critical gap in high-quality evidence to support standardised recommendations.

The practical impact of this review lies in its ability to highlight the challenges in diagnosing and prognosing OSCC patients, while underscoring the need to address current gaps in standardized definitions and assessment criteria. By addressing the lack of standardized definitions for cortical bone erosion and medullary bone infiltration, clinicians can achieve more consistent and accurate assessments of bone involvement, leading to better staging and treatment planning. Clarifying the prognostic significance of these patterns through high-quality studies could enable personalised treatment approaches and more reliable outcome predictions. Additionally, standardised criteria would enhance collaboration among multidisciplinary teams and form the basis for evidence-based clinical guidelines, ultimately ensuring more effective and uniform care for OSCC patients.

To address this, future research must prioritize the development and adoption of standardised definitions and assessment criteria for bone involvement. Such standardization will enable the design of robust, high-quality studies that can clarify whether and how prognosis is impacted by the two patterns of bone involvement.

**Funding:** This research received no external funding.

**Conflicts of Interest:** The author declares no conflicts of interest.

## Abbreviations

| | |
|---|---|
| OSCC | Oral Squamous Cell Carcinoma |
| TNM | Tumour Node Metastasis |
| DSS | Disease-Specific Survival |
| LR | Local Recurrence |
| FOM | Floor of mouth |
| RMT | Retromolar trigone |
| AJCC | American Joint Committee on Cancer |

## References

1. Montero, P.H.; Patel, S.G. Cancer of the oral cavity. *Surg. Oncol. Clin. N. Am.* **2015**, *24*, 491–508. [CrossRef] [PubMed]
2. Tilakaratne, W.M.; Jayasooriya, P.R.; Jayasuriya, N.S.; de Silva, R.K. Oral epithelial dysplasia: Causes, quantification, prognosis, and management challenges. *Periodontology 2000* **2019**, *80*, 126–147. [CrossRef]

3. Singh, T.; Schenberg, M. Delayed diagnosis of oral squamous cell carcinoma following dental treatment. *Ann. R. Coll. Surg. Engl.* **2013**, *95*, 369–373. [CrossRef]
4. Brierley, J.D.; Gospodarowicz, M.K.; Wittekind, C. (Eds.) *TNM Classification of Malignant Tumours*, 8th ed.; John Wiley & Sons: Chichester, UK, 2017; ISBN 978-1-119-26357-9.
5. Ebrahimi, A.; Murali, R.; Gao, K.; Elliott, M.S.; Clark, J.R. The prognostic and staging implications of bone invasion in oral squamous cell carcinoma. *Cancer* **2011**, *117*, 4460–4467. [CrossRef] [PubMed]
6. Patel, R.S.; Dirven, R.; Clark, J.R.; Swinson, B.D.; Gao, K.; O'Brien, C.J. The prognostic impact of extent of bone invasion and extent of bone resection in oral carcinoma. *Laryngoscope* **2008**, *118*, 780–785. [CrossRef]
7. Chen, Y.L.; Kuo, S.W.; Fang, K.H.; Hao, S.P. Prognostic impact of marginal mandibulectomy in the presence of superficial bone invasion and the nononcologic outcome. *Head Neck* **2011**, *33*, 708–713. [CrossRef] [PubMed]
8. Bullock, M.J. Current challenges in the staging of oral cancer. *Head Neck Pathol.* **2019**, *13*, 440–448. [CrossRef]
9. Pagni, G.; Pellegrini, G.; Giannobile, W.V.; Rasperini, G. Postextraction alveolar ridge preservation: Biological basis and treatments. *Int. J. Dent.* **2012**, 151030. [CrossRef] [PubMed]
10. Woolgar, J.A.; Triantafyllou, A. Pitfalls and procedures in the histopathological diagnosis of oral and oropharyngeal squamous cell carcinoma and a review of the role of pathology in prognosis. *Oral Oncol.* **2009**, *45*, 361–385. [CrossRef]
11. Fried, D.; Mullins, B.; Weissler, M.; Shores, C.; Zanation, A.; Hackman, T.; Shockley, W.; Hayes, N.; Chera, B.S. Prognostic significance of bone invasion for oral cavity squamous cell carcinoma considered T1/T2 by American Joint Committee on Cancer size criteria. *Head Neck* **2014**, *36*, 776–781. [CrossRef]
12. Muñoz Guerra, M.F.; Naval Gías, L.; Campo, F.R.; Pérez, J.S. Marginal and segmental mandibulectomy in patients with oral cancer: A statistical analysis of 106 cases. *J. Oral Maxillofac. Surg.* **2003**, *61*, 1289–1296. [CrossRef] [PubMed]
13. Jones, A.S.; England, J.; Hamilton, J.; Helliwell, T.R.; Field, J.; Gerlinger, I.; Karkanevatos, T. Mandibular invasion in patients with oral and oropharyngeal squamous carcinoma. *Clin. Otolaryngol. Allied Sci.* **1997**, *22*, 239–245. [CrossRef]
14. Shaw, R.J.; Brown, J.S.; Woolgar, J.A.; Lowe, D.; Rogers, S.N.; Vaughan, E.D. The influence of the pattern of mandibular invasion on recurrence and survival in oral squamous cell carcinoma. *Head Neck* **2004**, *26*, 861–869. [CrossRef] [PubMed]
15. Mücke, T.; Hölzle, F.; Wagenpfeil, S.; Wolff, K.D.; Kesting, M. The role of tumour invasion into the mandible of oral squamous cell carcinoma. *J. Cancer Res. Clin. Oncol.* **2011**, *137*, 165–171. [CrossRef] [PubMed]
16. Du, W.; Fang, Q.; Wu, Y.; Wu, J.; Zhang, X. Oncologic outcome of marginal mandibulectomy in squamous cell carcinoma of the lower gingiva. *BMC Cancer* **2019**, *19*, 775. [CrossRef] [PubMed]
17. Fives, C.; Nae, A.; Roche, P.; O'Leary, G.; Fitzgerald, B.; Feeley, L.; Sheahan, P. Impact of mandibular invasion on prognosis in oral squamous cell carcinoma four centimeters or less in size. *Laryngoscope* **2017**, *127*, 849–854. [CrossRef] [PubMed]
18. Petrovic, I.; Montero, P.H.; Migliacci, J.C.; Palmer, F.L.; Ganly, I.; Patel, S.G.; Shah, J.P. Influence of bone invasion on outcomes after marginal mandibulectomy in squamous cell carcinoma of the oral cavity. *J. Cranio-Maxillofac. Surg.* **2017**, *45*, 252–257. [CrossRef] [PubMed]
19. Li, C.; Lin, J.; Men, Y.; Yang, W.; Mi, F.; Li, L. Does medullary versus cortical invasion of the mandible affect prognosis in patients with oral squamous cell carcinoma? *J. Oral Maxillofac. Surg.* **2017**, *75*, 403–415. [CrossRef] [PubMed]
20. Ash, C.S.; Nason, R.W.; Abdoh, A.A.; Cohen, M.A. Prognostic implications of mandibular invasion in oral cancer. *Head Neck* **2000**, *22*, 794–798. [CrossRef]
21. Dalton, L.W.; Page, D.L.; Dupont, W.D. Histologic grading of breast carcinoma: A reproducibility study. *Cancer* **1994**, *73*, 2765–2770. [CrossRef]
22. Allsbrook, W.C.; Mangold, K.A.; Johnson, M.H.; Lane, R.B.; Lane, C.G.; Amin, M.B.; Bostwick, D.G.; Humphrey, P.A.; Jones, E.C.; Reuter, V.E.; et al. Interobserver reproducibility of Gleason grading of prostatic carcinoma: Urologic pathologists. *Hum. Pathol.* **2001**, *32*, 74–80. [CrossRef] [PubMed]
23. Jimi, E.; Furuta, H.; Matsuo, K.; Tominaga, K.; Takahashi, T.; Nakanishi, O. The cellular and molecular mechanisms of bone invasion by oral squamous cell carcinoma. *Oral Dis.* **2011**, *17*, 462–468. [CrossRef] [PubMed]

diagnostics

MDPI

Review

# Clinical and Morphological Aspects of Aggressive Salivary Gland Mixed Tumors: A Narrative Review

**Alexandra Corina Faur [1], Alina Maria Șișu [1,*], Laura Andreea Ghenciu [2], Roxana Iacob [1,3], Emil Robert Stoicescu [4], Ovidiu Alin Hațegan [5] and Mărioara Cornianu [6]**

1 Department of Anatomy and Embryology, "Victor Babeș" University of Medicine and Pharmacy Timișoara, Eftimie Murgu Square, No. 2, 300041 Timișoara, Romania; faur.alexandra@umft.ro (A.C.F.); roxana.iacob@umft.ro (R.I.)

2 Department of Functional Sciences, "Victor Babeș" University of Medicine and Pharmacy Timișoara, Eftimie Murgu Square, No. 2, 300041 Timișoara, Romania; bolintineanu.laura@umft.ro

3 Doctoral School, "Victor Babes" University of Medicine and Pharmacy Timisoara, Eftimie Murgu Square No. 2, 300041 Timisoara, Romania

4 Department of Radiology and Medical Imaging, "Victor Babeș" University of Medicine and Pharmacy Timisoara, Eftimie Murgu Square No. 2, 300041 Timisoara, Romania; stoicescu.emil@umft.ro

5 Discipline of Anatomy and Embryology, Medicine Faculty, "Vasile Goldis" Western University of Arad, Revolution Boulevard 94, 310025 Arad, Romania; hategan.ovidiu@uvvg.ro

6 Department of Microscopic-Morphology-Morphopathology, ANATPATMOL Research Center, "Victor Babeș" University of Medicine and Pharmacy Timișoara, Eftimie Murgu Square, No. 2, 300041 Timișoara, Romania; cornianu.marioara@umft.ro

* Correspondence: alinasisu@umft.ro

**Abstract:** Salivary gland tumors are a rare and heterogeneous group of neoplasms of the head and neck region. The mixed category of these tumors include the following entities: pleomorphic adenoma (PA), carcinoma ex pleomorphic adenoma (CEPA), salivary carcinosarcoma (CS), and metastasizing PA (MPA). The most common benign tumor of the salivary glands is PA. Metastasis and malignant degeneration have been reported in cases of PA of a salivary gland origin. Judging by their behavior, MPA, CEPA, and CS can be considered aggressive tumors. Invasive CEPA has been identified in the parotid gland more frequently. MPA and CS cases reported in the current literature are rare. In this paper, we present, narratively, the clinico-morphological features of this group of mixed tumors.

**Keywords:** carcinoma ex pleomorphic adenoma; salivary carcinosarcoma; metastasizing pleomorphic adenoma; mixed tumors of the salivary glands; minor salivary glands; salivary tumors

## 1. Introduction

Salivary gland tumors are a heterogeneous group of neoplasms accounting for 5% of malignant lesions in the head and neck region [1]. The entities usually included in the category of salivary gland mixed tumors are pleomorphic adenomas (PAs), carcinoma ex pleomorphic adenoma (CEPA), carcinosarcoma (CS), and metastasizing PA (MPA). PA is the most common benign tumor of the salivary glands, with an incidence rate of up to 70%. Approximately 6.2% of PAs can undergo malignant transformation. CEPA is a generic term that defines malignant epithelial tumors developed from a pre-existing PA. For a CEPA diagnosis, both carcinomatous areas and benign PA must be observed in the histopathological section or there must be a previously diagnosed PA at the respective location. CS, or a true malignant mixed tumor, is a biphasic tumor with both epithelial/myoepithelial and mesenchymal malignant elements, arising de novo or from a preexisting PA. MPA is a rare occurrence, histologically similar to PA, but produces secondary tumors in distant sites [2–5].

CEPA represents 3.6% of salivary tumors (varying between 0.9 and 14% depending on the study) and 12% of malignant salivary tumors (varying between 2.8 and 42.4%), with an incidence rate of 0.17 tumors per 1 million inhabitants [6–9]. CEPA has a slight female predilection and typically develops in patients aged 60–80 years, with a median age of 60 years, making CEPA patients on average 12 years older than those with PA [10,11]. A study focusing on CEPA in major salivary glands reports a higher frequency among male patients in their 5th decade of life, while another study indicates that invasive CEPA is more common in males over 60 years old [12,13]. CEPA is more frequently found in the parotid gland but can also be observed in the submandibular gland and, in less than 7% of cases, in the minor salivary glands of the palate, nasopharynx, oral mucosa, maxilla, nasal cavity, lower lip, and less often in the upper lip [6,10,11,14–16]. More unusual locations include the lacrimal glands or the accessory parotid gland [17,18]. Few studies have identified malignant salivary gland tumors in the sublingual gland, with even fewer cases of CEPA in this location [19,20]. Some authors report that aggressive variants of CEPA are more frequently located in the parotid gland (81.7%), with 18% of cases in the submandibular gland, 0.3% in the sublingual gland, and some cases affecting minor salivary glands, such as the palatine glands [13,14,21,22].

CS is a malignant salivary tumor composed of both carcinomatous and sarcomatous elements. CS, described by Kirklin in 1951, and termed true mixed malignant tumor (carcinosarcoma) by King OH Jr. in 1976 [3,23], represents less than 1% of malignant mixed tumors (0.04–1%), with only about 100 cases reported in the current literature [3,7,23–25]. Most patients have a history of PA or present with histopathological aspects of PAs. In rare cases (0.2%), CS arises de novo [26]. CS is more common in patients in their 6th to 7th decades of life, with a slight male preponderance and an average presentation age of 58 years (ranging from 14–87 years). About two-thirds of the tumors develop in the parotid gland, approximately 19% in the submandibular gland, and 14% in the palate. Some studies report more frequent CS occurrence in the larynx and less often in the nasopharynx, tongue, oral floor, gingivae, or major salivary glands [3,7,27].

MPA is a benign tumor that inexplicably metastasizes regionally or distantly [28]. These rare tumors, with only a few cases described, develop in the parotid gland (over 75%), the submandibular gland (13%), and the palate (9%). Some studies hypothesize that MPA and CEPA represent different stages of PA malignancy [6,29,30]. CEPA with metastatic deposits in the kidney, lung, and bone composed exclusively of MPA has been described [6]. Knight J and Rathasingham K reviewed 81 cases of MPA in the salivary glands over 72 years (1942–2014) and found that these tumors most commonly metastasize to bone, lung, and neck lymph nodes. The mean age at diagnosis is 49.5 years, with 74.1% of cases in the parotid gland, 14.8% in the submandibular gland, 6.2% in the palate, 2.5% in the nasal septum, and 1% in the tongue. The reported male-to-female ratio is 34:46, with 80.4% of patients alive at a 1-year follow-up. In their study, MPAs were identified in bone (36.6%), lung (33.8%), cervical lymph nodes (20.1%), renal (8.6%), cutaneous (8.6%), liver (4.9%), and brain (3.7%). Thirty-three of these cases had multiple sites of metastases. Isolated cases of MPA have been described in the sinus, retroperitoneal space, abdominal wall, pharynx, mediastinum, and breast [4]. This is the largest series of MPAs described in a review paper identified in the current literature. Additional studies report individual cases of MPA mainly localized to lymph nodes, with fewer cases in the lung, bone, and kidney. The distribution of MPA cases is illustrated in Figure 1 [4,30–36].

In this narrative review, we discuss the morphological and clinical aspects that characterize the mixed tumors of the salivary glands that may aid in the understanding of their diagnosis and the evolutionary course.

*Materials and Methods*

We have chosen to prepare the review in the narrative form because of the rarity of the salivary gland neoplastic lesions reported in the literature (mostly case report articles). We consulted the PRISMA criteria and adapted the method for our study [37]. We had a purpose of identifying the articles with the subject of mixed salivary gland tumors. English-language literature covering the diagnosis of salivary gland tumors was searched by accessing the PubMed electronic database and other sources (Google scholar, Scopus).

The scientific publications were hand-searched in the internet data using the following key words: "carcinoma ex pleomorphic adenoma", "salivary carcinosarcoma", "metastasising pleomorphic adenoma", "mixed tumors of the salivary glands", "minor salivary glands," and "salivary tumors". We identified and overviewed a database comprising 205 research papers addressing salivary gland neoplasms, comprising both individual studies and reviews. Abstracts, duplicates, irrelevant topics, publications in other languages than English, and articles not in the field of interest or with repetitive information were excluded from the study. The final number of obtained articles was 80. We categorized these remaining articles into four datasets. One dataset comprised studies investigating salivary glands tumors with an emphasis on the subject of mixed salivary neoplasms. The remaining three datasets each focused on a specific type of the mixed salivary gland tumor (CEAP, CS, and MPA). The algorithm used for this research paper selection is explained in Figure 2.

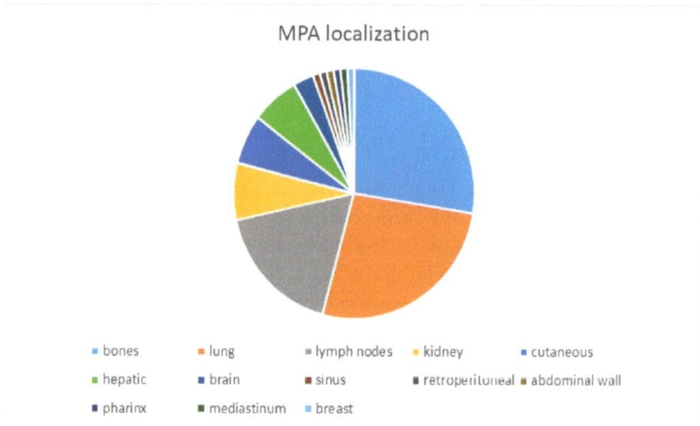


**Figure 1.** Distribution of MPA localization; from literature-data-counted cases, the MPAs identified were 28% in bone (30 cases), 29% in the lung (29 cases), 17% in lymph nodes (19 cases), 7% in the kidney (8 cases), 6% cutaneous and hepatic (each with 7 cases cited), and 3% in the brain (3 cases identified), and the rest represents 1% being isolated cases [4,30–36].

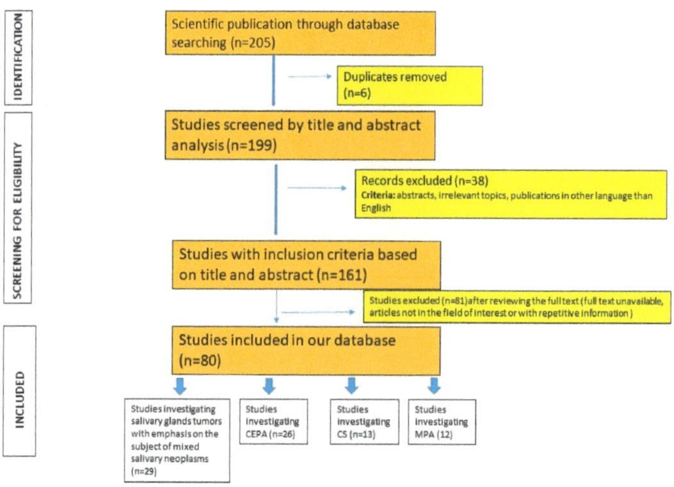


**Figure 2.** Algorithm used for article selection; n = number of studies; CEPA = carcinoma ex pleomorphic adenoma, CS = carcinosarcoma, MPA = metastasizing PA.

## 2. Clinico-Morphological Aspects of CEPA

### 2.1. Clinical Aspects

Clinical data considered, suggestive of the possibility of malignancy of a PA, are as follows: the submandibular location of the tumor, a longer period of time for development, older patient age (average 61 years), and tumors larger than 4 cm [2]. In cases of CEPA, two main clinical aspects are present: either the patients report the presence of a slow growing tumor mass, which is rapidly increasing in size, or the malignant evolution of a PA is noted in a patient that has underwent several surgeries [10]. However, most CEPAs, although invasive, are asymptomatic [7].

The typical history of a patient with CEPA is represented by the presence of a tumor mass for a period longer than 3 years (10–15 years), which begins to increase rapidly in a few months (on average 3–6 months). There are patients with tumors increasing in a shorter period [6,7]. Tumors arising in the minor salivary glands represent 9–23% of all salivary neoplasms. The incidence of minor salivary gland CEPA cases is difficult to determine due to their rarity [21,38–42]. In 30% of cases (especially those located in the major salivary glands), patients complain of pain and facial nerve paralysis, enlarged lymph nodes, dysphagia, toothache, skin ulcerations, and masses of tumors fixed to the skin. The periods for which the symptoms lead the patient to seek medical advice vary from one month to 52 years. In cases with a sinonasal location, a symptomatology (of variable duration in time from 1 to 60 months) represented by symptoms of obstruction-difficulties in breathing and chronic sinusitis, but also epistaxis, headache, tooth dislocations, or otitis media, was described [6–9]. A patient with CEPA of the minor salivary glands with lung metastasis presented with a painful ulcerative lesion of the wall of the oropharynx [21].

### 2.2. Gross Aspects

On average, CEPA is twice as large as its benign counterpart, ranging from 1.5 to 25 cm in diameter. Most of these tumors are poorly circumscribed and infiltrative, though if PA is the dominant component, they may be well circumscribed, encapsulated, or fibrotic [7,43]. Extensive sampling of the PA surgical specimen is crucial to evaluate possible CEPA, and multiple serial sections are sometimes required to identify the malignant area. Grossly, PAs in the major salivary glands are generally well circumscribed and encapsulated, while non-encapsulated tumors are more frequently identified in the minor salivary glands. The degree of encapsulation in PAs varies, with some areas lacking a capsule and showing tumor extension into adjacent tissue. However, if these areas are continuous with the PA, they should not be considered as tumor invasion. Tumor extension from the capsule is seen in recurrent or slow-growing PAs. In invasive CEPA, the carcinomatous area is often more extensive than the benign tumor. The cross-sectional surface of CEPA may exhibit any of the macroscopic features found in PAs and in the corresponding types of carcinomatous components. More commonly, bluish-grey, transparent, or whitish-yellow tumor masses with areas of calcification are described. In some cases, where the malignant component is dominant, areas of hemorrhage and necrosis are present [2,9,13].

### 2.3. Microscopic Aspects

Any type of carcinoma can be identified as the carcinomatous component of CEPA. Most commonly, the carcinomatous component is represented by adenocarcinoma not otherwise specified (42.4%) and salivary duct carcinoma (32.8%). Less frequent types include mucoepidermoid carcinoma (MEC), adenoid cystic carcinoma (ACC), undifferentiated carcinoma (UC), myoepithelial and epithelial–myoepithelial carcinoma (EMC), and polymorphous adenocarcinoma [7,13,43–45]. The MEC component must be graded into low-, intermediate-, and high-grade tumors, as identifying high-grade transformation areas in CEPA is crucial for predicting patient outcomes [28,46]. Figures 3 and 4 illustrate examples of CEPA with salivary duct carcinoma (SDC), adenocarcinoma not otherwise specified (ADK NOS), and MEC as malignant components.

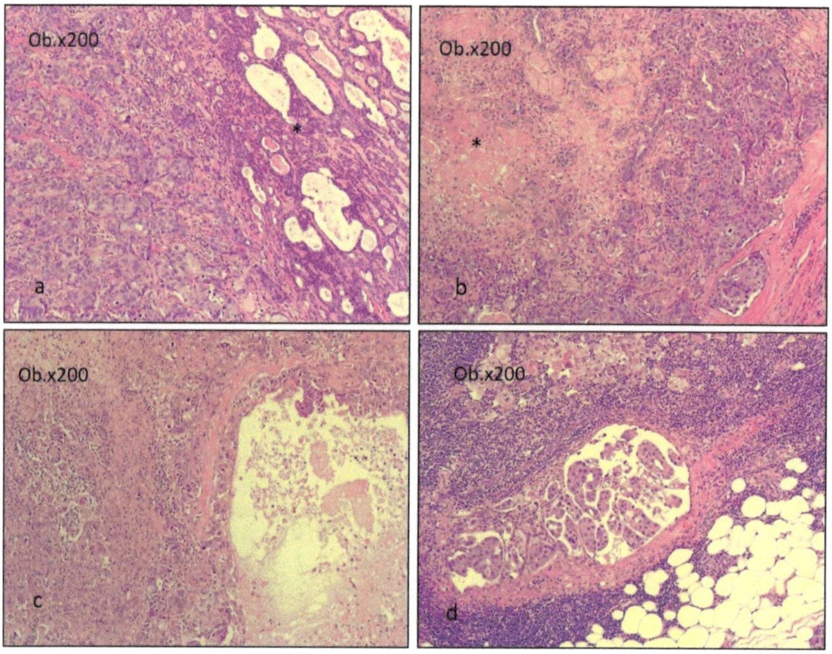


**Figure 3.** SDC as the malignant component of CEAP. The benign PA is presented in images (**a**,**b**) and is marked with *. Image (**c**) is only the SDC component, and (**d**) illustrates the metastasis in the lymph node of the SDC malignant component of CEAP. The images were obtained using a Leica DM750 microscope with a digital camera, 200× magnification (Ob. = objective).

Rare occurrences of CEPA are reported in the literature, such as small-cell carcinomas developed on parotid PA or ACC developed in sinonasal PA [10,47]. Iino et al. identified a case of CEPA with a clear cell squamous cell carcinoma (SCCcc) as the carcinomatous component. Histochemical staining, including the absence of Alcian Blue-positive mucinous cells, ruled out mucoepidermoid carcinoma, making SCCcc a diagnosis of exclusion [48]. Karpowicz et al. described a CEPA with melanoma as the malignant component [24,49]. Reports of acinic cell carcinomas as the malignant component in CEPA are few [50,51].

In CEPA, the proportion of benign versus malignant components varies. Some authors categorize CEPA, based on the malignant component's appearance, into cases with only an epithelial component and those with a myoepithelial component. Cases with exclusively myoepithelial components are rare and tend to have a higher recurrence rate [9,12]. The carcinomatous component can occupy 50% to 100% of the tumor [9,43]. The PA areas in CEPA can be challenging to detect, sometimes represented by few epithelial elements or a chondromyxoid stroma. Occasionally, only hyalinized nodules from the remaining pleomorphic adenoma are observed [7]. If the malignant component grows to occupy the entire tumor, detecting PA relies on clinicopathologic data.

In PA, malignancy criteria include pleomorphic and hyperchromatic nuclei, intense mitotic activity, atypical mitoses, necrosis, stromal hyalinization (especially if calcified), capsule invasion, perineural and perivascular invasion, and hemorrhage [9]. Immunohistochemistry can aid in diagnosis [44,45], with intense and diffuse androgen receptor, p53, and HER-2/neu immunoreactivity reported in CEPA [2]. GFAP expression is more common in PA [52,53]. A high Ki67 index (>5%), increased EGFR expression, and loss of Bcl-2 immunopositivity support a diagnosis of malignancy [54–56]. Genetic alterations are also present, with PLAG1 and HMGA2 gene fusions/amplification described in both

CEPA and PA. TP53 mutations are noticed in 60% of CEPA cases, along with additional mutations, like c-MYC, RAS, P21, and PIK3R1 [56–58].

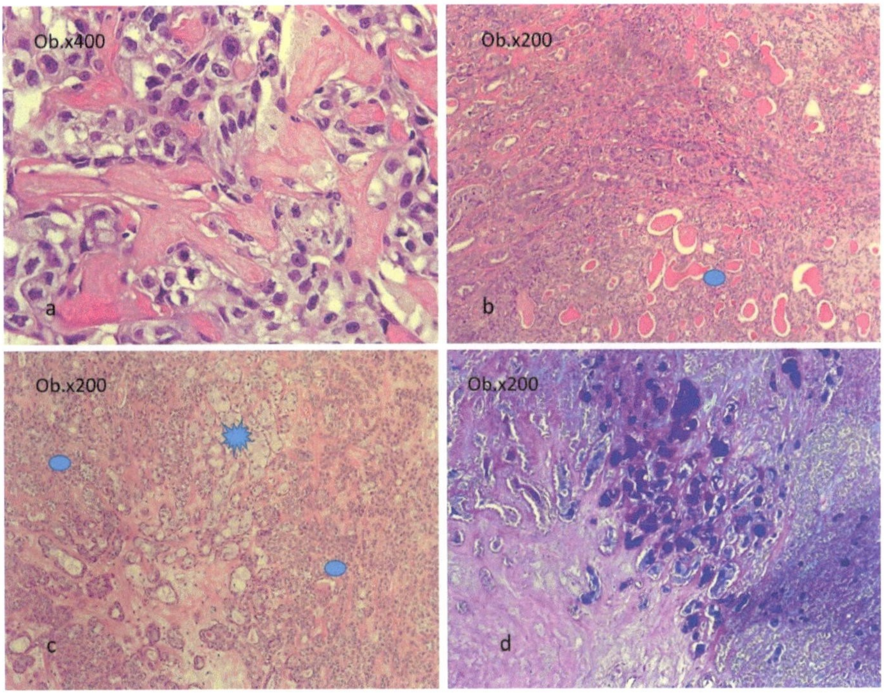


**Figure 4.** CEPA. (**a**). Benign component of PA with myoepithelial cells. (**b**). ADK NOS as the malignant component with PA marked with a blue oval shape. In images (**c**,**d**), MEC is the malignant component marked with a blue star and PA is marked with oval shapes. In image (**d**), the Alcian Blue histochemical stain highlights the MEC component. The images were obtained using a Leica DM750 microscope with a digital camera, 200× and 400× magnification (Ob. = objective).

### 2.4. Patterns of Invasion in CEPA

The destructive and infiltrative growth pattern is an important diagnostic criterion [53]. When analyzing a CEPA case, particular attention should be given to the degree of tumor invasion. The term "non-invasive carcinoma developed in a PA" was introduced by LiVolsi and Perzin in 1977 when they described 47 CEPA cases, of which six showed no invasion and did not relapse or metastasize [2,13,59].

Non-invasive carcinomas that develop in PA are classified as in situ or intracapsular. Histologically, these types are characterized by the abrupt transition from typical PA to an area with malignant cytological changes but limited to the pre-existing adenoma. Non-invasive carcinomas can show PA matrix invasion without extracapsular invasion, and these aspects are not considered clinically invasive if the capsule is not penetrated. Microscopically, a clear contrast can be noted between areas of PA replaced by larger cells with pleomorphic and hyperchromatic nuclei and increased mitotic activity and the benign cells of PA. Intense mitotic activity and tumor aspects in the carcinomatous component can be highlighted using markers, such as Ki-67, Her-2/neu, p53, and the androgen receptor, but results must be interpreted with caution as 5–10% of PA may also express these markers [2,7].

The meaning of the term "minimal capsular invasion" has changed over time. Originally reported in 1984 by Tortoledo et al., their study evaluated 40 cases of CEPA, where the majority had tumors with malignant areas showing invasion less than 8 mm from the capsule. The follow-up reported favorable outcomes, with none of these patients dying due to disease progression. However, sixteen patients with invasion exceeding 8 mm died of the disease. The frequency of tumor recurrences was related to the extent of invasion and the status of the resection margins [13,60].

Minimally invasive CEPA is defined as carcinoma with invasion not exceeding more than 1.5 mm of the tumor capsule, though distinguishing between benign tumor pseudopods and true invasion can sometimes be difficult. Mushroom-type invasion into and through the tumor capsule—similar to that described for thyroid carcinomas—is considered indicative of malignancy. For a CEPA diagnosis, histopathologic features of atypical cells always accompany invasion. Atypical changes within these tumors vary from focal to diffuse, with multifocal carcinomatous areas frequently developing and replacing many benign elements. Although some tumors may demonstrate minimal atypia, criteria, such as nuclear hyperchromia and pleomorphism, are common, necrosis is often present, and mitoses are easily observed [2,7].

The cut-off value for CEPA to be considered invasive is still debated, ranging from 1.5 to 100 mm [9,13,28,43,61–63]. Early studies reported lesser values for invasion. Brandwein et al. studied 12 patients with non-invasive and minimally invasive CEPA ($\leq$1.5 mm), finding that 8 of these patients did not experience recurrences or metastases 2.5 years after diagnosis [13,61]. Lewis and Olsen reported that for 66 CEPA cases studied, patients with extracapsular invasion of less than 5 mm did not experience tumor recurrences or metastases, but survival rates decreased drastically for those with invasion of at least 15 mm. They concluded that patients with tumors with extracapsular invasion of less than 5 mm had favorable outcomes and responded well to surgical treatment [43]. Based on these studies, CEPAs were classified as non-invasive (in situ, intracapsular), minimally invasive ($\leq$1.5 mm), and invasive (>1.5 mm) [2,7,43]. However, some studies showed that the area of extracapsular extension might be 4–6 mm and even up to 100 mm [9,28].

Silvana Di Palma's study proposed classifying CEPA into two categories: early CEPA and widely invasive CEPA. Early CEPA is further subclassified into non-invasive, in situ, intratubular, intraductal tumors, and invasive variants represented by intracapsular invasive type, minimally invasive tumors (less than 1.5 mm), and those with invasion not exceeding 6 mm. This proposal is based on recent studies analyzing CEPA with invasion exceeding 1.5 mm, which reported a significant proportion of cases where invasion did not exceed 6 mm and the patients did not show disease progression [13]. The prognostic implications of this classification need further investigation.

### 2.5. The Evolutionary Course of CEPA

Depending on the histopathologic type and the level of invasion, the 5-year survival rate for patients with CEPA can vary widely, from over 90% to just over 20%. Patients with non-invasive or minimally invasive CEPA generally have a prognosis similar to PA, with metastases being rarely reported. In contrast, invasive CEPA is considered extremely aggressive, with 23–50% of patients developing one or more recurrences. Tumor recurrences and metastases are indicators of a poor prognosis, with metastases observed in 30–70% of cases, commonly found in the lungs, bone, and kidney. In these cases, the 5-year survival rate is approximately 50%. CEPA typically metastasizes as carcinoma, although there are reports of metastases with histological features of PA [6,7,64–68].

Non-invasive CEPA metastases are reported in fewer than 2% of cases; thus, non-invasive and minimally invasive CEPA generally have an excellent prognosis, whereas invasive CEPA has a poor prognosis [7]. Non-invasive carcinomas with negative resection margins do not require adjuvant treatments after surgical excision. Minimally invasive carcinomas are treated based on the resection margin status and the presence of perineural invasion—if either is observed, additional surgery and/or radiotherapy is required [2].

Invasive CEPA often includes highly malignant components, such as SDC, ADK NOS, or UC [46]. The 5-year survival rate for CEPA can vary between 30% and 96% depending on the histological type of the malignant component. Specifically, 5-year survival rates are 62% for SDC, 50% for myoepithelial carcinoma, and 30% for UCa as malignant components of CEPA [68,69]. In a series of CEPAs with sinonasal localization and a malignant component of adenoid cystic carcinoma, the overall survival rate was 7.7 years, with a 5-year survival rate of 50% and a 10-year survival rate of 29% [47].

## 3. Clinico-Morphological Aspects in CS

CS cases represent 0.04–0.16% of all malignant salivary gland tumors with distant metastasis occurring in 54% of patients. The CS metastasis is usually described in the lung, but liver, bone, abdominal cavity, and brain metastases are being reported. Patients are in their sixth and seventh decade of life, and mostly there is no gender predilection reported [69,70]. Clinically, patients typically present with a rapidly growing tumoral mass that may be accompanied by pain and facial nerve palsy. Tumors can be well or poorly circumscribed [2,7,25].

### 3.1. Gross and Microscopic Aspects

Salivary carcinosarcomas are biphasic tumors, composed mostly of carcinomatous and sarcomatous elements in variable proportions (Figure 5).

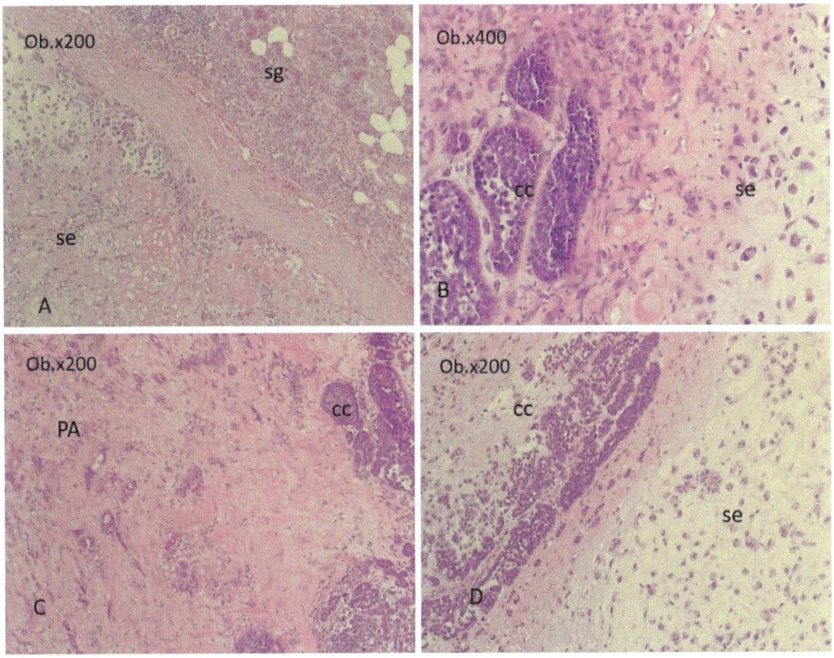


**Figure 5.** CS with PA, sarcomatous elements (se) of chondrosarcoma, and basal cell adenocarcinoma (BC ADK) as the carcinomatous element (cc). (**A**). CS-condrosarcoma (se) and adjacent salivary gland (sg). (**B**). CS with BC ADK (cc) and condrosarcoma (se) areas. (**C**). CS with PA and BC ADK (cc) areas. (**D**). CS with BC ADK (cc) and condrosarcoma (se) areas (lower magnification). Abbreviations: sg = salivary gland, se = sarcomatous element, cc = carcinomatous element, PA = pleomorphic adenoma. The images were obtained using a Leica DM750 microscope with a digital camera, 200× magnification (Ob. = objective).

Chondrosarcoma and osteosarcoma are the most common sarcomatous elements of CS. Fibrosarcoma, myxosarcoma, leiomyosarcoma, liposarcoma, rhabdomyosarcoma, and even malignant fibrous histiocytoma are less frequently observed as components of CS. The carcinomatous components of CS are mainly represented by a differentiated/moderately differentiated SDC, UC, adenocarcinomas, or squamous cell carcinoma. Small cell carcinoma, EMC, myoepithelial carcinoma, or ACC were reported in isolated cases as CS components. Invasion and local destruction are characteristics of this neoplasm [3,7,25,26,71–74].

In one third of the cases, the benign PA area can also be noted. Petersson F and Loh KS described a rare case of CS developed on a PA for which the carcinomatous component was represented by large cells of neuroendocrine carcinoma and a sarcomatous one based on a spindle cell sarcoma with myofibroblastic differentiation [24]. Geraldes Filho et al. described a case of salivary CS with features represented by undifferentiated carcinoma and the mesenchymal component with chondrosarcoma, high-grade undifferentiated sarcoma, and malignant giant cell tumor aspects [73].

### 3.2. The Evolutionary Course of CS

Salivary CSs are aggressive tumors with an average survival rate of 29.3 months, with most patients (60%) dying within 30 months of initial diagnosis. Median survival rates of 3.6 years have also been reported, but the 5-year survival rate is 0%. CS presents local recurrences and metastases. However, due to their rarity, the long-term prognosis is difficult to predict [3,7,68–74].

There is still no standardized treatment for salivary CS, but the most recent data indicate that the therapy of these tumors is represented by wide surgical excision supplemented by radiotherapy and in selected cases by chemotherapy [74]. Future research should focus on pathogenetically oriented therapies for rarely diagnosed or insufficiently studied diseases [69,70,75–77].

Due to their rarity and the heterogeneous morphological aspects, the diagnosis of CS is challenging. The differential diagnosis of salivary CS must include the sarcomatoid variant of a SDC and synovial sarcoma. In SDC, the epithelial component is similar to breast carcinoma, and the sarcomatoid component is immunopositive (but not always) for cytokeratins. Synovial sarcoma resembles a salivary CS both morphologically and in the immunohistochemical profile, but in synovial sarcoma, compact bundles can be identified intersecting spindle cells and glandular structures, while the cells that make up CS are more pleomorphic and poorly differentiated [26,78]. Collision, hybrid, and dedifferentiated tumors must also be excluded. Also, it is not clear if the carcinomatous and sarcomatous elements occur through the collision of two tumors or if these two components are of a clonal origin. The study of genomic profiles of the epithelial and mesenchymal components of the CSs showed an overall homology of 75% between their profiles, which was considered indicative of a monoclonal origin [79]. However there are hypotheses suggesting that CSs are multiclonal and derived from two or more types of stem cells [70]. Further studies are needed to investigate the phenotypes of the components of CS.

## 4. Clinico-Morphological Aspects of MPA

MPA is described in the literature data mostly in female patients, in their third and sixth decades of life. The primary PA is in the parotid gland (79% of cases), submandibular gland (13%), and palate (9%) [34]. MPA is histologically and molecularly identical with the primary PA. Both the PA and its metastasis consist of a mixture of benign epithelial, myoepithelial, and mesenchymal components. The tumors are well circumscribed (both primary and secondary) [29,80]. Most studies show that the histology of the PA is not important for the metastatic ability of this type of tumor. In some cases, pleomorphic cells with mitotic activity were identified. However, these features are not considered sufficient proof for the PA to be classified as a malignant tumor. There are authors who believe that the presence of mitotic activity and the absence of the capsule are aspects indicative of the metastatic potential of PA [81]. Some studies have shown that in MPAs, the stromal or myoepithelial components form the bulk of the tumor mass, and the cells have a high rate of mitoses [6]. A case with local recurrence of PA and simultaneous MPA in 58/59 ipsilateral cervical lymph nodes was reported [33]. Cervical lymph node MPA and infiltration of the sternocleidomastoid muscle were identified by Catarzi et al. [35]. There are reports of patients that died of disease [29]

*The Evolutionary Course of MPA*

With a benign histological appearance but malignant behavior, MPA represents a rare aspect of salivary neoplasms. The malignant behavior of these tumors is often associated with multiple local recurrences of PA following surgical interventions or incomplete excision of the primary tumor. Surgical manipulation is believed to lead to the intravascular implantation of tumor cells. Additionally, radiation-induced malignant transformation or metastasis due to investigative maneuvers, such as fine-needle aspiration, are risk factors for developing MPA after the primary tumor has been excised [6,31].

A long interval (1.5–55 years) between the development of the primary tumor and its metastases has been reported [31]. Half of these tumors metastasize to bone, and 30% metastasize to the lungs and neck lymph nodes. Less frequently, MPAs are identified in other parts of the body [4,7,32,69]. In the current literature data, there have been MPAs with localization, such as intra-abdominal (in the liver, kidneys, retroperitoneal), skull, central nervous system, pharynx, in the paranasal sinuses, external auditory canal, larynx, and even in the skin (of the gluteal region). Some authors reported that the metastasis developed on average 15–16 years after the initial PA diagnosis. A case with PA of the minor salivary glands of the palate vault untreated for 40 years developed an MPA in the cervical lymph nodes [82]. There are other studies that have identified situations where PAs have metastasized 51–55 years after the primary diagnosis [4,32,81–84].

The prevention and treatment options for MPA remain subjects of ongoing debate. Complete tumor resection with adequate margins can prevent local recurrence and distant metastasis. For the minor salivary gland, the reported recurrence rate of PA is low (with this, the incidence of MPA from this location also decreases) [85]. Therapeutic agents targeting progesterone receptor molecular signals are considered potential candidates for treating recurrent PA [31,81]. The treatment of choice for MPA is the surgical excision of the metastasis with wide tissue margins. In some cases, postoperative radiotherapy and chemotherapy were used as adjunctive treatments with variable results [82].

Ongoing documentation and long-term follow-up are mandatory so a survival rate for MPA can be assessed. According to the literature data, about 40% of MPA patients die with disease [82].

## 5. Conclusions

CEAP, MPA, and CS represent mixed salivary gland tumors with aggressive behavior. Different tumors can develop in a CEPA, so treatments must take into account the histological type of carcinoma developed in the PA. The pathologist must look at these CEPAs not as a unique type of tumor but as a group of distinct tumors, for which the gross and microscopic appearance must be adequately evaluated. The pathologist's report for CEPA cases must include, in addition to the type of tumor, the presence and degree of invasion, as these are important aspects for prognosis and therapy. CEPA with malignant components represented by UC, SDC, and ACC or with high-grade transformation areas usually receive a more complex treatment. The subtype of CEPA with extensive extracapsular invasion is aggressive and has an increased risk of recurrence and metastasis. In practice, the extent of invasion in the cases of CEPA and the identification of the benign component may be challenging. Even though PAs are common tumors of the salivary glands, their metastatic potential has to be acknowledged. Understanding the tumorigenesis of MPAs may help in the prevention of the malignant behavior of the PA. In cases with CS, recognizing the biphasic morphology is of paramount importance in the differential diagnosis. The mesenchymal PA component of the CEAP has to be differentiated from the malignant component of CS. CSs are aggressive tumors that have a poor prognosis.

**Author Contributions:** Conceptualization, A.C.F. and A.M.Ş.; methodology, L.A.G.; investigation, A.C.F.; resources, R.I.; writing—original draft preparation, E.R.S., O.A.H. and M.C.; writing—review and editing, A.C.F. and M.C.; visualization, L.A.G.; supervision, A.C.F. All authors have read and agreed to the published version of the manuscript.

**Funding:** This research received no external funding.

**Institutional Review Board Statement:** Not applicable.

**Informed Consent Statement:** Not applicable.

**Data Availability Statement:** No new data created.

**Acknowledgments:** We would like to acknowledge VICTOR BABES UNIVERISTY OF MEDICINE AND PHARMACY TIMISOARA for its support in covering the costs of publication for this research paper.

**Conflicts of Interest:** The authors declare no conflicts of interest.

## References

1. Locati, L.D.; Ferrarotto, R.; Licitra, L.; Benazzo, M.; Preda, L.; Farina, D.; Gatta, G.; Lombardi, D.; Nicolai, P.; Vander Poorten, V.; et al. Current management and future challenges in salivary glands cancer. *Front. Oncol.* **2023**, *13*, 1264287. [CrossRef] [PubMed] [PubMed Central]
2. McHugh, J.B.; Visscher, D.W.; Barnes, E.L. Update on selected salivary gland neoplasms. *Arch. Pathol. Lab. Med.* **2009**, *133*, 1763–1774. [CrossRef] [PubMed]
3. Jain, S.; Abdelwahed, M.; Chavarria, D.H.; Pereira, L.; Stone, G.; Johnson, A.; Li, J.Y. Carcinosarcoma of the parotid gland: A case report and review of the literature. *J. Med. Case Rep.* **2024**, *18*, 24. [CrossRef] [PubMed] [PubMed Central]
4. Knight, J.; Ratnasingham, K. Metastasising pleomorphic adenoma: Systematic review. *Int. J. Surg.* **2015**, *19*, 137–145. [CrossRef] [PubMed]
5. Alsanie, I.; Rajab, S.; Cottom, H.; Adegun, O.; Agarwal, R.; Jay, A.; Graham, L.; James, J.; Barrett, A.W.; van Heerden, W.; et al. Distribution and Frequency of Salivary Gland Tumours: An International Multicenter Study. *Head Neck Pathol.* **2022**, *16*, 1043–1054. [CrossRef] [PubMed] [PubMed Central]
6. Matsushima, M.; Ohara, R.; Ishida, M.; Kanao, K.; Shimokava, R.; Nakajima, Y. Carcinoma ex pleomorphic adenoma of the submandibular gland with renal metastases composed exclusively of metastasizing pleomorphic adenoma. *Int. Cancer Conf. J.* **2012**, *1*, 116–120. [CrossRef]
7. Gnepp, D.R.; Brandwein-Gensler, M.S.; El-Naggar, A.K.; Nagao, T. Carcinoma ex pleomorphic adenoma. In *Pathology & Genetics of Head and Neck Tumours*; Barnes, L., Eveson, J.W., Reichart, P., Sindranski, D., Eds.; World Health Organization Classification of Tumours; IARC Press: Lyon, France, 2005; Volume 5, pp. 242–243.
8. Yamada, S.; Nabeshima, A.; Tabata, T.; Guo, X.; Tasaki, T.; Wang, K.Y.; Shimajiri, S.; Sasaguri, Y. Invasive salivary duct carcinoma ex pleomorphic adenoma of the parotid gland: A teaching case giving rise to the genuine diagnostic difficulty on an inadequate cytology specimen. *Diagn. Pathol.* **2012**, *7*, 61. [CrossRef] [PubMed] [PubMed Central]
9. Antony, J.; Gopalan, V.; Smith, R.A.; Lam, A.K. Carcinoma ex pleomorphic adenoma: A comprehensive review of clinical, pathological and molecular data. *Head Neck Pathol.* **2012**, *6*, 1–9. [CrossRef] [PubMed] [PubMed Central]
10. Cimino-Mathews, A.; Lin, B.M.; Chang, S.S.; Boahene, K.D.; Bishop, J.A. Carcinoma ex pleomorphic adenoma of the nasal cavity. *Head Neck Pathol.* **2011**, *5*, 405–409. [CrossRef] [PubMed] [PubMed Central]
11. Nakamura, S.; Inui, M.; Matsumura, Y.; Takeoka, T.; Okumura, K.; Tagawa, T. A case of carcinoma ex pleomorphic adenoma in the buccal mucosa: Review of the literature. *J. Maxillofac. Oral Surg.* **2013**, *12*, 224–227. [CrossRef] [PubMed] [PubMed Central]
12. Zhao, J.; Wang, J.; Yu, C.; Guo, L.; Wang, K.; Liang, Z.; Lou, J. Prognostic factors affecting the clinical outcome of carcinoma ex pleomorphic adenoma in the major salivary gland. *World J. Surg. Oncol.* **2013**, *11*, 180. [CrossRef] [PubMed] [PubMed Central]
13. Di Palma, S. Carcinoma ex pleomorphic adenoma, with particular emphasis on early lesions. *Head Neck Pathol.* **2013**, *7* (Suppl. S1), S68–S76. [CrossRef] [PubMed] [PubMed Central]
14. Furukawa, M.; Suzuki, H.; Matsuura, K.; Takahashi, E.; Suzuki, H.; Tezuka, F. Carcinoma ex pleomorphic adenoma of the palatal minor salivary gland with extension into the nasopharynx. *Auris Nasus Larynx* **2001**, *28*, 279–281. [CrossRef] [PubMed]
15. Mitate, E.; Kawano, S.; Kiyoshima, T.; Kawazu, T.; Chikui, T.; Goto, Y.; Matsubara, R.; Nakamura, S. Carcinoma ex pleomorphic adenoma of the upper lip: A case of an unusual malignant component of squamous cell carcinoma. *World J. Surg. Oncol.* **2013**, *11*, 234. [CrossRef] [PubMed] [PubMed Central]
16. Reichart, P.A.; Kalz, S.; Rabel, A.; Bornstein, M.M. Carcinoma ex pleomorphic adenoma in a minor salivary gland: Report of a case. *Oral Maxillofac. Surg.* **2010**, *14*, 59–62. [CrossRef] [PubMed]
17. Kini, Y.K.; Halli, R.; Mishra, S.; Kalburge, J.V. Comprehensive management of a rare carcinoma ex pleomorphic adenoma of the lacrimal gland with a modified lateral orbitotomy access osteotomy. A case report. *Oral Maxillofac. Surg.* **2012**, *16*, 123–126. [CrossRef] [PubMed]

18. Tamiolakis, D.; Chimona, T.S.; Georgiou, G.; Proimos, E.; Nikolaidou, S.; Perogamvrakis, G.; Papadakis, C.E. Accessory parotid gland carcinoma ex pleomorphic adenoma. Case study diagnosed by fine needle aspiration. *Stomatologija* **2009**, *11*, 37–40. [PubMed]
19. Yu, T.; Gao, Q.H.; Wang, X.Y.; Wen, Y.M.; Li, L.J. Malignant sublingual gland tumors: A retrospective clinicopathologic study of 28 cases. *Oncology* **2007**, *72*, 39–44. [CrossRef] [PubMed]
20. Kroul, R.; Dubey, A.; Binhamed, A.; Butler, J.; Cooke, A.; Abdoh, A.; Nason, R. Prognostic factors depicting overall survival in lesser major (submandibular, sublingual) and minor salivary gland tumors. *Turk. J. Cancer* **2008**, *38*, 159–166.
21. Akan, H.; Yildiz, L.; Unal, R. Carcinoma ex pleomorphic adenoma of the minor salivary gland with pulmonary metastasis. *Diagn. Interv. Radiol.* **2008**, *14*, 3–5. [PubMed]
22. Beckhardt, R.N.; Weber, R.S.; Zane, R.; Garden, A.S.; Wolf, P.; Carrillo, R.; Luna, M.A. Minor salivary gland tumors of the palate: Clinical and pathologic correlates of outcome. *Laryngoscope* **1995**, *105*, 1155–1160. [CrossRef] [PubMed]
23. Feng, D.; Fidele, N.B.; Agustin, M.M.; Jian, G.; Bourleyi, S.I.; Augustin, L.; Olivier, N.K. Carcinosarcoma of parotid gland (malignant mixed tumor). *Ann. Maxillofac. Surg.* **2015**, *5*, 240–243. [CrossRef] [PubMed] [PubMed Central]
24. Petersson, F.; Loh, K.S. Carcinosarcoma ex non-recurrent pleomorphic adenoma composed of TTF-1 positive large cell neuroendocrine carcinoma and myofibrosarcoma: Apropos a rare Case. *Head Neck Pathol.* **2013**, *7*, 163–170. [CrossRef] [PubMed] [PubMed Central]
25. Andreadis, D.; Poulopoulos, A.; Epivatianos, A.; Nomikos, A.; Christidis, K.; Barbatis, C. Carcinosarcoma of the parotid gland: Immunohistochemical analysis with emphasis in cell cycle mitotic activity and cell adhesion molecules expression. *Oral Oncol.* **2006**, *42*, 140–143. [CrossRef]
26. Kim, H.S.; Cho, H.J.; Chung, Y.T.; Park, S.A.; Cho, H.J.; Kim, J.M. Carcinosarcoma (true malignant mixed tumor) of the parotid gland –a report of a case with small cell carcinoma as the carcinomatous component. *J. Pathol. Transl. Med.* **2008**, *42*, 175–180.
27. Lim, A.L.; Zahirrudin, Z.; Pua, K.C. A rare case of nasopharyngeal carcinosarcoma. *Med. J. Malays.* **2012**, *67*, 428–429. [PubMed]
28. Seethala, R.R.; Stenman, G. Update from the 4th Edition of the World Health Organization Classification of Head and Neck Tumours: Tumors of the Salivary Gland. *Head Neck Pathol.* **2017**, *11*, 55–67. [CrossRef]
29. Rodríguez-Fernández, J.; Mateos-Micas, M.; Martínez-Tello, F.J.; Berjón, J.; Montalvo, J.J.; Forteza-González, G.; Galan-Hernández, R. Metastatic benign pleomorphic adenoma. Report of a case and review of the literature. *Med. Oral Patol. Oral Cir. Bucal.* **2008**, *13*, E193–E196. [PubMed]
30. Marioni, G.; Marino, F.; Stramare, R.; Marchese-Ragona, R.; Staffieri, A. Benign metastasizing pleomorphic adenoma of the parotid gland: A clinicopathological puzzle. *Head Neck* **2003**, *25*, 1071–1076. [CrossRef]
31. Fonseca, D.; Arya, S.S.; Kodandapani, S.; Chandini, A.; Kurapati, S.; Rao, C.; Gadepalli, T.; Ali, Z. Metastasising Pleomorphic Adenoma: A Rare Entity. *Indian J. Otolaryngol. Head. Neck Surg.* **2022**, *74* (Suppl. S3), 6321–6323. [CrossRef] [PubMed] [PubMed Central]
32. Koyama, M.; Terauchi, T.; Koizumi, M.; Tanaka, H.; Sato, Y. Metastasizing pleomorphic adenoma in the multiple organs: A case report on FDG-PET/CT imaging. *Medicine* **2018**, *97*, e11077. [CrossRef] [PubMed]
33. Santaliz-Ruiz, L.E.; Morales, G.; Santini, H.; Arroyo, A. Metastasizing pleomorphic adenoma: A fascinating enigma. *Case Rep. Med.* **2012**, 148103. [CrossRef] [PubMed]
34. Soltedo, J.; Aranaga, N. Metastasizing pleomorphic adenoma of the parotid gland. *Ecancermedicalscience* **2017**, *11*, 758.
35. Catarzi, L.; Catarzi, L.; Gabriele, G.; Gabriele, G.; Pulli, B.; Pulli, B.; Cascino, F.; Cascino, F.; Gennaro, P.; Gennaro, P. Metastasizing Pleomorphic Adenoma of Parotid Gland: A Case Report and Literature Review. *Indian J. Otolaryngol. Head. Neck Surg.* **2024**, *76*, 1123–1125. [CrossRef]
36. Nakai, A.; Suzuki, K.; Furuse, H.; Tsuda, T.; Masaki, Y.; Shinno, H.; Ito, Y.; Miyazawa, H.; Taniguchi, H. Multiple Metastasizing Pleomorphic Adenomas of the Lung. *Intern. Med.* **2017**, *56*, 691–694. [CrossRef] [PubMed] [PubMed Central]
37. Parums, D.V. Editorial: Review Articles, Systematic Reviews, Meta-Analysis, and the Updated Preferred Reporting Items for Systematic Reviews and Meta-Analyses (PRISMA) 2020 Guidelines. *Med. Sci. Monit.* **2021**, *27*, e934475. [CrossRef] [PubMed] [PubMed Central]
38. Aluffi Valletti, P.; Campagnoli, M.; Dell'Era, V.; Garzaro, M.; Boffano, P.; Neirotti, F.; Mazzer, A.M.; Brucoli, M. Oral and oropharyngeal malignant minor salivary gland tumors: A retrospective study. *J. Stomatol. Oral. Maxillofac. Surg.* **2024**, *125*, 101893. [CrossRef] [PubMed]
39. Varghese, B.T.; Sebastian, P.; Abraham, E.K.; Mathews, A. Pleomorphic adenoma of minor salivary gland in the parapharyngeal space. *World J. Surg. Oncol.* **2003**, *1*, 2. [CrossRef] [PubMed] [PubMed Central]
40. Sarmento, D.J.; Morais, M.L.; Costa, A.L.; Silveira, É.J. Minor intraoral salivary gland tumors: A clinical-pathological study. *Einstein* **2016**, *14*, 508–512. [CrossRef] [PubMed] [PubMed Central]
41. Hiyama, T.; Kuno, H.; Sekiya, K.; Oda, S.; Kobayashi, T. Imaging of Malignant Minor Salivary Gland Tumors of the Head and Neck. *Radiographics* **2021**, *41*, 175–191. [CrossRef] [PubMed]
42. Tondi-Resta, I.; Hobday, S.B.; Gubbiotti, M.A.; Jalaly, J.B.; Rassekh, C.H.; Montone, K.T.; Baloch, Z.W. Carcinoma Ex Pleomorphic Adenomas: An Institutional Experience and Literature Review. *Am. J. Clin. Pathol.* **2023**, *159*, 502–515. [CrossRef] [PubMed]
43. Lewis, J.E.; Olsen, K.D.; Sebo, T.J. Carcinoma ex pleomorphic adenoma: Pathologic analysis of 73 cases. *Hum. Pathol.* **2001**, *32*, 596–604. [CrossRef] [PubMed]

44. Quereshi, A.; Barakzai, A.; Ui, N.; Gulzar, R.; Ahmad, Z.; Hasan, S. Spectrum of maignacy in mixed tumors nof salivary gland: A morphological and immunohistochemical review of 23 cases. *Ind. J. Pathol. Microbiol.* **2009**, *52*, 150–154. [CrossRef] [PubMed]
45. Klijanienko, J.; El Naggar, A.K.; Servois, V.; Rodriguez, J.; Validire, P.; Viehl, P. Mucoepidermoid carcinoma ex pleomorphic adenoma: Nonspecific preoperative cytologic findings in six cases. *Cancer* **1998**, *84*, 231–234. [CrossRef]
46. Nishida, H.; Kusaba, T.; Kawamura, K.; Oyama, Y.; Daa, T. Histopathological Aspects of the Prognostic Factors for Salivary Gland Cancers. *Cancers* **2023**, *15*, 1236. [CrossRef] [PubMed] [PubMed Central]
47. Toluie, S.; Thompson, L.D.R. Sinonasal tract adenoid cystic carcinoma ex-pleomorphic adenoma: A clinicopathologic and immunophenotypic study of 9 cases combined with a comprehensive review of the literature. *Head Neck Pathol.* **2012**, *6*, 409–421. [CrossRef]
48. Iino, M.; Yamada, H.; Ishikawa, H.; Suzuki, M.; Shomura, E.; Ide, F.; Saito, I.; Mori, Y. Carcinoma ex pleomorphic adenoma of the submandibular gland: Report of a case with unusual malignant component of clear squamous cell carcinoma. *Oral Surg. Oral Med. Oral Pathol Oral Radiol. Endod.* **2008**, *106*, e30–e34. [CrossRef]
49. Karpowicz, M.K.; Shalmon, B.; Molberg, K.H.; El-Naggar, A.K. Melanoma in a carcinoma ex pleomorphic adenoma of the parotid gland: A case report and putative histogenesis. *Hum. Pathol* **2011**, *42*, 1355–1358. [CrossRef]
50. Krishna, P.S.; Sivapathasudharam, B. Acinic cell adenocarcinoma-a case report. *J. Oral Maxillofac. Pathol.* **2003**, *7*, 15–18. [CrossRef]
51. Tawfik, O.; Namiq, A. Tumors of the salivary glands. In *Cancer Grading Manual*; Damjanov, I., Fang, F., Eds.; Springer: New York, NY, USA, 2007; pp. 13–18.
52. Curran, A.E.; Allen, C.M.; Beck, F.M.; Damm, D.D.; Murrah, V.A. Distinctive pattern of glial fibrillary acidic protein immunoreactive useful in distinguishing fragmented pleomorphic adenoma, canalicular adenoma and polymorphous low grade adenocarcinoma of minor salivary glands. *Head Neck Pathol.* **2007**, *1*, 27–32. [CrossRef]
53. Santos, G.C.; Carvalho, K.C.; Falzoni, R.; Simoes, A.C.; Rocha, R.M.; Lopes, A.; Vassallo, J.; Reis, L.F.; Soares, F.A.; da Cunha, I.W. Glial fibrillary acidic protein in tumor types with cartilaginous differentiation. *Mod. Pathol.* **2009**, *22*, 1321–1327. [CrossRef] [PubMed]
54. Nagao, T.; Sato, E.; Inoue, R.; Oshiro, H.; H Takahashi, R.; Nagai, T.; Yoshida, M.; Suzuki, F.; Obikane, H.; Yamashina, M.; et al. Immunohistochemical analysis of salivary gland tumors: Application for surgical pathology practice. *Acta Histochem. Cytochem.* **2012**, *45*, 269–282. [CrossRef] [PubMed] [PubMed Central]
55. Bussari, S.; Ganvir, S.M.; Sarode, M.; Jeergal, P.A.; Deshmukh, A.; Srivastava, H. Immunohistochemical Detection of Proliferative Marker Ki-67 in Benign and Malignant Salivary Gland Tumors. *J. Contemp. Dent. Pract.* **2018**, *19*, 375–383. [CrossRef] [PubMed]
56. Faur, A.C.; Buzaş, R.; Lăzărescu, A.E.; Ghenciu, L.A. Current Developments in Diagnosis of Salivary Gland Tumors: From Structure to Artificial Intelligence. *Life* **2024**, *14*, 727. [CrossRef]
57. Żurek, M.; Fus, Ł.; Niemczyk, K.; Rzepakowska, A. Salivary gland pathologies: Evolution in classification and association with unique genetic alterations. *Eur. Arch. Oto-Rhino-Laryngol.* **2023**, *280*, 4739–4750. [CrossRef]
58. Valstar, M.H.; Mast, H.; Ten Hove, I.; Moonen, L.R.; Balm, A.J.; Smeele, L.E.; Koljenović, S.; Dinjens, W.N.; van Velthuysen, M.F. Malignant transformation of salivary gland pleomorphic adenoma: Proof of principle. *J. Pathol. Clin. Res.* **2021**, *7*, 432–437. [CrossRef] [PubMed] [PubMed Central]
59. LiVolsi, V.A.; Perzin, K.H. Malignant mixed tumors arising in salivary glands. I. Carcinomas arising in benign mixed tumors: A clinicopathologic study. *Cancer* **1977**, *39*, 2209–2230. [CrossRef] [PubMed]
60. Tortoledo, M.E.; Luna, M.A.; Batsakis, J.G. Carcinomas ex pleomophic adenoma and malignant mixed tumors: Histomorphologic indexes. *Arch. Otolaryngol* **1984**, *110*, 172–176. [CrossRef]
61. Brandwein, M.; Huvos, A.G.; Dardick, I.; Thomas, M.J.; Theise, N.D. Noninvasive and minimally invasive carcinoma ex mixed tumor: A clinicopathologic and ploidy study of 12 patients with major salivary tumors of lo (or no?) malignant potential. *Oral Surg. Oral Med. Oral Pathol. Oral Radiol. Endod.* **1996**, *81*, 655–664. [CrossRef]
62. Speight, P.M.; Barett, A.W. Prognostic factors in malignant tumours of the salivary glands. *Br. J. Oral Maxillofac. Surg.* **2009**, *47*, 587–593. [CrossRef]
63. Speight, P.M.; Barett, A.W. Salivary gland tumors: Diagnostic challenges and an update on the latest WHO classification. *Diagn. Histopathol.* **2020**, *26*, 147–158. [CrossRef]
64. Seethala, R.R.; Altemani, A.; Ferris, R.L.; Fonseca, I.; Gnepp, D.R.; Ha, P.; Nagao, T.; Skalova, A.; Stenman, G.; Thompson, L.D.R. Data Set for the Reporting of Carcinomas of the Major Salivary Glands: Explanations and Recommendations of the Guidelines from the International Collaboration on Cancer Reporting. *Arch. Pathol. Lab. Med.* **2019**, *143*, 578–586. [CrossRef] [PubMed]
65. Ettl, T.; Schartz-Furlan, S.; Gosau, M.; Reichert, T. Salivary gland carcinomas. *Oral Maxillofac. Surg.* **2012**, *16*, 267–283. [CrossRef]
66. Felix, A.; Rosa, J.C.; Nunes, J.F.; Fonseca, I.; Cidado, A.; Soares, J. Hyalinizing clear cell carcinoma of salivary glands: A study of extracellular matrix. *Oral Oncol.* **2002**, *38*, 364–368. [CrossRef]
67. Sheedy, S.P.; Welker, K.M.; DeLone, D.R.; Gilbertson, J.R. CNS metstasis of carcinoma ex pleomorphic adenoma of the parotid gland. *Am. J. Neuroradiol.* **2006**, *27*, 1483–1485.
68. Peel, R.L.; Seethala, R.R. Pathology of salivary glands. In *Salivary Glands Disorders*; Myers, E., Ferris, R., Eds.; Springer: Berlin/Heidelberg, Germany, 2007; Chapter 3; pp. 33–104.
69. Keh, S.M.; Tait, A.; Ahsan, F. Primary carcinosarcoma of the parotid gland. *Clin. Pract.* **2011**, *1*, e117. [CrossRef] [PubMed] [PubMed Central]

70. Woo, C.G.; Son, S.M. Carcinosarcoma of the parotid gland with abdominal metastasis: A case report and review of literature. *World J. Surg. Oncol.* **2018**, *16*, 103. [CrossRef] [PubMed] [PubMed Central]
71. Gnepp, D.R. Malignant mixed tumors of the salivary glands: A review. *Pathol. Annu.* **1993**, *28*, 279–328.
72. Kwon, M.Y.; Gu, M. True Malignant mixed tumor (carcinosarcoma) of the parotid gland with unusual Mesenchymal component. A case report and review of the literature. *Arch. Pathol. Lab. Med.* **2001**, *125*, 812–815. [CrossRef]
73. Geraldes Filho, J.C.; Carvalho, L.G.M.; Pinheiro, N.F., Jr.; de Freitas, L.A.R.; Fontes Athanazio, P.R.; Abensur Athanazio, D. Carcinosarcoma of the parotid gland featuring foci of malignant giant cell tumor. *J. Bras. Pathol. Med. Lab.* **2012**, *48*, 129–134. [CrossRef]
74. Jang, S.E.; Jun, Y.J.; Han, H.; Jang, K.S.; Paik, S.S. Parotid gland carcinosarcoma with osteosarcoma as sarcomatous component: A case report with fine needle aspiration cytologic findings. *Korean J. Pathol.* **2011**, *45*, 412–416. [CrossRef]
75. Ghenciu, L.A.; Hațegan, O.A.; Bolintineanu, S.L.; Dănilă, A.-I.; Faur, A.C.; Prodan-Bărbulescu, C.; Stoicescu, E.R.; Iacob, R.; Șișu, A.M. Immune-Mediated Ocular Surface Disease in Diabetes Mellitus—Clinical Perspectives and Treatment: A Narrative Review. *Biomedicines* **2024**, *12*, 1303. [CrossRef] [PubMed]
76. Septimiu-Radu, S.; Gadela, T.; Gabriela, D.; Oancea, C.; Rosca, O.; Lazureanu, V.E.; Fericean, R.M.; Bratosin, F.; Dumitrescu, A.; Stoicescu, E.R.; et al. A Systematic Review of Lung Autopsy Findings in Elderly Patients after SARS-CoV-2 Infection. *J. Clin. Med.* **2023**, *12*, 2070. [CrossRef]
77. Georgescu, D.; Ancusa, O.E.; Azoulay, D.; Lascu, A.; Ionita, I.; Calamar-Popovici, D.; Ionita, M.; Rosca, C.I.; Brează, G.M.; Reisz, D.; et al. Portal Vein Thrombosis in Patients with Liver Cirrhosis: What Went Wrong? *Int. J. Gen. Med.* **2023**, *16*, 3889–3906. [CrossRef] [PubMed] [PubMed Central]
78. Colizza, A.; Di Stadio, A.; Ralli, M.; De Luca, P.; Cavaliere, C.; Gilardi, A.; Zoccali, F.; Riminucci, M.; Greco, A.; Corsi, A.; et al. Systematic Review of Parotid Gland Sarcomas: Multi-Variate Analysis of Clinicopathologic Findings, Therapeutic Approaches and Oncological Outcomes That Affect Survival Rate. *Cancers* **2022**, *14*, 4862. [CrossRef] [PubMed] [PubMed Central]
79. Vékony, H.; Leemans, C.R.; Ylstra, B.; Meijer, G.A.; van der Waal, I.; Bloemena, E. Salivary gland carcinosarcoma: Oligonucleotide array CGH reveals similar genomic profiles in epithelial and mesenchymal components. *Oral Oncol.* **2009**, *45*, 259–265. [CrossRef] [PubMed]
80. Matsumiya-Matsumoto, Y.; Morita, Y.; Uzawa, N. Pleomorphic Adenoma of the Salivary Glands and Epithelial-Mesenchymal Transition. *J. Clin. Med.* **2022**, *11*, 4210. [CrossRef] [PubMed] [PubMed Central]
81. Manucha, V.; Ioffe, O.B. Metastasizing pleomorphic adenoma of the salivary gland. *Arch. Pathol. Lab. Med.* **2008**, *132*, 1445–1447. [CrossRef]
82. Watson, M.; McAllister, P.; Conn, B.; MacNeill, M.; Handley, T.P.B. Metastasising Pleomorphic Salivary Adenoma: A Rare Case Report of a Massive Untreated Minor Salivary Gland Pleomorphic Adenoma with Concurrent Ipsilateral Cervical Node Metastases. *Head. Neck Pathol.* **2019**, *13*, 500–506. [CrossRef] [PubMed] [PubMed Central]
83. Nouraei, S.A.R.; Ferguson, M.S.; Clarke, P.M.; Sandison, A.; Sadhu, G.S.; Michaels, L.; Rhys-Evans, P. Metastasizing pleomorphic salivary adenoma. *Arch. Otolaryngol. Head. Neck Surg.* **2006**, *137*, 788–793. [CrossRef]
84. Manelli, G.; Rucci, L.; Gallo, O. Unusual metastases from a pleomorphic adenoma of the parotid gland: A case and literature review. *Int. J. Otolaryngol. Head Neck Surg.* **2013**, *2*, 232–235. [CrossRef]
85. Khan, M.N.; Raza, S.S.; Hussain Zaidi, S.A.; Haq, I.U.; Hussain, A.K.; Nadeem, M.D.; Farid, K. Pleomorphic Adenoma of Minor Salivary Glands. *J. Ayub Med. Coll. Abbottabad* **2016**, *28*, 620–622. [PubMed]

diagnostics

MDPI

*Case Report*

# One-Year Follow-Up of Non-Healing Socket in Hodgkin's Lymphoma Patient: Case Report and Literature Review on Management Strategies

**Ahmed Ata Alfurhud**

Oral and Maxillofacial Surgery and Diagnostic Sciences Department, College of Dentistry, Jouf University, King Khalid Road, Sakaka 72388, Saudi Arabia; dr.aalfurhud@jodent.org or aalfarhood@ju.edu.sa; Tel.: +966-501738443

**Abstract: Background and Clinical Significance:** Sodium hypochlorite (NaOCl) is widely used in root canal treatment for its potent antiseptic and antibacterial effects. However, its cytotoxicity—particularly at higher concentrations and in patients with low immune status—has been associated with serious postoperative complications. This case report describes the risks associated with NaOCl exposure in a medically compromised patient and reviews the relevant literature on NaOCl-related injuries, offering insights into potential current management strategies. **Case Presentation:** This case report describes a challenging scenario of a 25-year-old male with a history of Hodgkin's lymphoma who developed a non-healing bone in the lower right first molar (LR6) region after NaOCl exposure. Several months after undergoing root canal treatment and an extraction of the LR6, the patient presented with exposed necrotic bone in the region. The case's complexity was heightened by the patient's medical and dental history, which included chemotherapy and NaOCl exposure. Following a detailed clinical, radiographic examination and biopsy, the patient was diagnosed with bone necrosis due to NaOCl exposure. The treatment involved the extraction of the LR6, the debridement of the necrotic bone, and long-term follow-up with antimicrobial therapy. Despite efforts to manage the complication, the healing process was prolonged, potentially due to the patient's immunocompromised state from chemotherapy. The patient's condition remained unresolved after nearly a year, and ongoing management, including regular follow-up, was necessary to monitor healing and prevent further complications. This case highlights the challenges of treating dental complications in immunocompromised patients, particularly those with Hodgkin's lymphoma, where delayed healing is a problem that might occur. **Conclusions**: Given the complexity of this case, different adjunctive treatment options, such as leukocyte–platelet-rich fibrin (L-PRF), pentoxifylline and tocopherol (PENTO), and hyperbaric oxygen therapy (HBOT), were discussed as potential treatments to help manage non-healing sockets in patients with similar conditions.

**Keywords:** delayed healing; hodgkin disease; immunocompromised host; osteonecrosis; sodium hypochlorite; treatment outcome

## 1. Introduction

Sodium hypochlorite (NaOCl) has been extensively utilized in dentistry for many years. Its use is critical for achieving successful root canal treatment, functioning as an effective antiseptic and antibacterial irrigating solution to significantly eliminate bacterial populations within the canal system [1]. The clinical technique centers on thorough cleaning and debridement, ensuring the removal of bacteria, necrotic tissue, and residual organic material, which is essential for optimizing treatment outcomes [1]. Nevertheless, concerns have been raised regarding the cytotoxicity of NaOCl, particularly at higher concentrations, with occasional reports of postoperative complications. Several studies have reported both temporary and permanent complications associated with the potential toxicity of NaOCl [1]. Serious complications have been documented in the literature, including unilateral facial swelling, persistent paresthesia in the affected region, and partial paralysis of the facial muscles [2]. Moreover, weakness of the buccal branch of the facial nerve has also been observed, leading to the loss of the nasolabial angle and a downward deviation of the right corner of the mouth [3].

The medical history of a patient is a critical factor in assessing the risk of complications. Medically compromised individuals are particularly at risk of experiencing severe adverse effects from NaOCl compared with healthy patients, as pre-existing systemic conditions may enhance its cytotoxicity, impair tissue repair mechanisms, and increase the likelihood of nerve damage and soft-tissue necrosis. Lymphoma is a diverse malignant condition of the lymphatic system, marked by the abnormal growth of lymphoid cells. Hodgkin's lymphoma predominantly affects the lymph nodes, with more than 90% of cases occurring in these areas, while only 1–4% involve extranodal sites, usually presenting as a nodal disease with a preference for the neck and mediastinal nodes [4].

Diagnosing oral lymphomas can be difficult, as their symptoms often mimic those of other conditions like periodontal disease, osteomyelitis, and other cancers, which may result in delayed treatment and a poorer prognosis [4]. The current case presents significant diagnostic challenges due to the complexity of the patient's medical history. Pre-existing conditions and underlying health factors complicate the identification of symptoms, making it difficult to distinguish between the primary disease, other potential comorbidities, and local complications, thereby complicating the diagnostic process.

## 2. Case Presentation

A 25-year-old male was referred to the Oral and Maxillofacial Surgery Department (OMFS) at the Royal London Dental Hospital (RLDH) with exposed necrotic bone in the lower right first molar (LR6) region. The patient had previously undergone root canal treatment on the LR6 in Romania several months ago. He later presented to a general dental practice in the United Kingdom with exposed bone in the LR6 area, reporting no pain but experiencing an unpleasant taste. Concerned about the exposed necrotic bone in the LR6 socket and the patient's complex medical history, the general dentist referred him to the OMFS Department for further evaluation and management. The patient's medical history included a diagnosis of Hodgkin's lymphoma (stage 2), for which he underwent a six-month course of chemotherapy, completed in September 2020. Additionally, he experienced an endodontic irrigation material-related incident in the LR6 region, which may have contributed to the development of complications in the area.

### 2.1. Clinical Examination

Intraorally, a preoperative photograph (Figure 1), provided by the general dentist who initially examined the patient, revealed a temporary restoration on the LR6. Additionally, there was an area of exposed, non-healing bone on the buccal aspect, extending from the mesial surface of the LR6 to the distal surface of the lower right second molar. A relative blood clot was observed on the mesial surface of the LR6, with no identifiable cause.

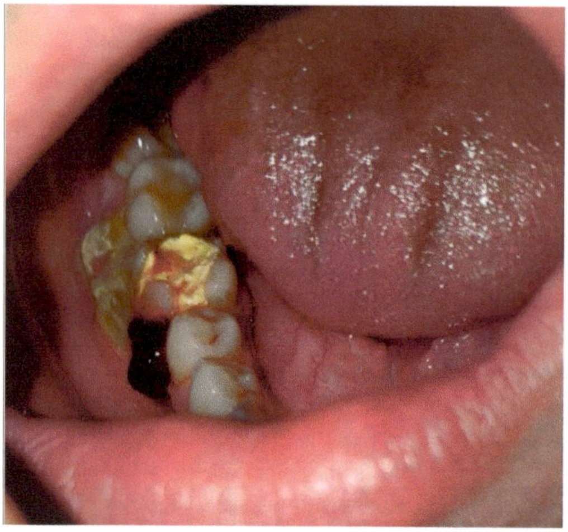

**Figure 1.** A preoperative photograph of the LR6.

A few weeks later, the patient was evaluated by a specialist at the OMFS Department at the RLDS. A clinical examination revealed non-healing exposed necrotic bone in the LR6 region, as illustrated in Figure 2. Additionally, signs of infection were evident, including pain, purulent discharge at the LR6 site, and mild extraoral swelling on the lower right side of the face.

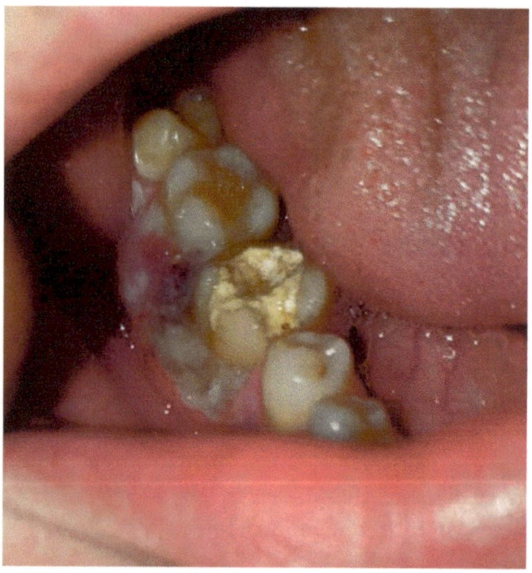

**Figure 2.** A preoperative photograph of the LR6 during the first follow-up visit.

### 2.2. Differential Diagnosis

The clinical findings were suggestive of a differential diagnosis, as follows: the most likely diagnosis in this case was bone necrosis due to a sodium hypochlorite incident, as the patient had a history of an endodontic irrigation-related incident in the LR6 region. Sodium hypochlorite is known for its cytotoxic effects, and accidental extrusion beyond the root canal system can lead to severe tissue damage, necrosis, and delayed healing, which aligns with the patient's clinical presentation of exposed necrotic bone.

However, other differential diagnoses could not be excluded at this stage. Chronic osteomyelitis remains a possibility, as persistent infection in the LR6 area may lead to necrotic bone, purulent discharge, and localized swelling. Additionally, primary or secondary malignancy, such as lymphoma or metastatic carcinoma, should be considered. Lastly, traumatic bone sequestration could also be a contributing factor, particularly if prior dental procedures caused localized trauma, leading to devitalized bone fragments and subsequent exposure.

### 2.3. Management and Intervention

The patient was advised on improving oral hygiene practices to help prevent the progression of bone necrosis, which included proper brushing techniques, antimicrobial mouth rinses, and regular dental check-ups to maintain oral health and minimize the risk of further complications. Given the clinical evidence of infection, a 14-day course of oral 500 mg of amoxicillin, three times a day, was prescribed to control the infection and reduce the bacterial load in the affected area. As the LR6 was deemed non-restorable due to its fragility after the root canal treatment and the presence of a large, mobile, fractured fragment, a simple extraction was performed under local anesthesia to eliminate the source of infection and promote healing, with careful attention to minimizing trauma. A biopsy of the necrotic bone and surrounding mucosa was undertaken to exclude malignancy. Additionally, an ostectomy of the buccal plate of bone (buccal cortex) was performed, followed by curettage of the necrotic bone. The patient was placed on a long-term follow-up protocol to monitor their healing, assess for any recurrence of necrotic bone, and ensure no signs of persistent infection or malignancy, with regular clinical and radiographic evaluations scheduled to track progress and intervene if necessary.

### 2.4. Microscopic Description

Gross examination of the biopsy specimen revealed both hard and soft tissues, with irregular, discolored, and friable bone and mucosa. Histopathological analysis showed acellular necrotic bone, characterized by empty lacunae and loss of osteocytes, surrounded by bacterial aggregates and a mixed inflammatory infiltrate. The bacteria were interspersed with neutrophilic infiltrates and fragments of granulation tissue, with collections of multinucleated osteoclast-type giant cells also observed. The adjacent mucosal biopsy consisted of tissue fragments covered by hyper-parakeratinized epithelium, exhibiting variable hyperplasia, fibrin deposits, and chronic inflammatory cell infiltration. The epithelium demonstrated neutrophilic trafficking and spongiosis, with no significant cytological atypia. Dense infiltrates of neutrophils, lymphoplasmacytic cells, and histiocytes were present, along with scattered hemosiderin deposits. No evidence of epithelial dysplasia or malignancy was identified. The findings are consistent with chemically induced necrosis due to sodium hypochlorite exposure.

### 2.5. Follow-Up and Outcomes

The initial radiographic assessment was conducted a few weeks after the surgery. As shown in Figure 3, the orthopantomograph (OPG) revealed a non-healing bony defect within the extraction socket. This defect extended inferiorly, encroaching upon the inferior alveolar canal, which may suggest the potential involvement of the nerve. Notably, there was an increase in the bony density adjacent to the socket, consistent with sclerosing osteitis.

These findings necessitate further radiographic evaluation and monitoring to assess the progression of healing and any potential complications.

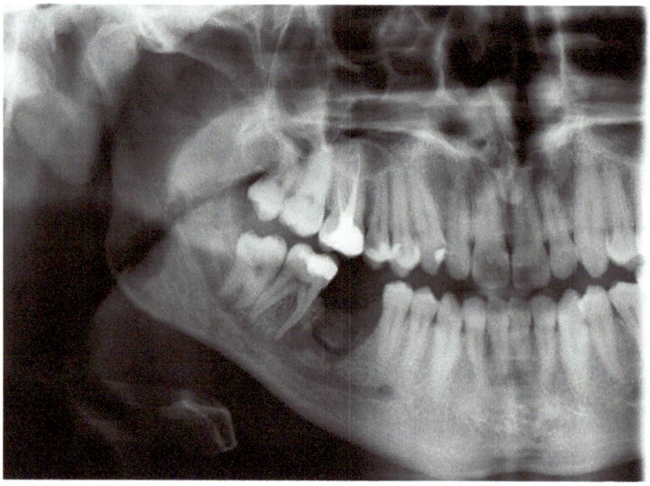

**Figure 3.** A postoperative radiograph of the LR6 during the follow-up visit.

A cone-beam computed tomography (CBCT) scan of the posterior mandible revealed a bony sequestrum in the region of the missing LR6 socket, as shown in Figure 4. There was a subtle periosteal bone reaction on both the buccal and lingual aspects of the socket, along with a marked increase in the adjacent bony density. The bony defect extended inferiorly to involve the inferior alveolar canal, with a small dehiscence of its superior cortex. Additionally, the defect extended mesially to the root of the LR7, with apical periodontal ligament space widening at both LR7 apices. The inferior alveolar canal was in contact with the buccal aspect of the radiolucency associated with the distal apex of the LR7, and there was partial loss of the canal's cortical outline in this region.

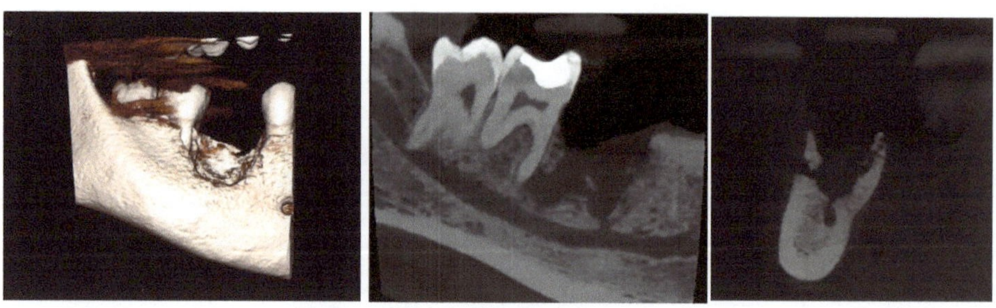

**Figure 4.** A postoperative CBCT of the LR6 during the follow-up visit.

Although the definitive diagnosis, confirmed by the histopathological examination, was necrosis due to sodium hypochlorite exposure, the patient required ongoing regular follow-up to monitor the healing process. Given the patient's complex medical history, including prior chemotherapy, there was an increased risk of delayed healing, secondary infection, and potential complications, such as osteomyelitis. Regular clinical and radiographic assessments are essential to evaluate bone regeneration, soft-tissue healing, and any signs of persistent inflammation or further necrosis.

The primary objective in this case was to achieve primary closure to minimize the risk of infection at the surgical site. However, this was not possible due to the compromised healing process, likely resulting from the patient's history of chemotherapy. Chemotherapy can impair wound healing by affecting cellular regeneration, reducing vascular supply, and compromising immune response, increasing the risk of delayed epithelialization and secondary infection. As a result, the open wound remained vulnerable to bacterial colonization and further necrosis.

As can be seen in Figure 5, the healing process in this case was prolonged and complex. During follow-up, the surgical site showed minimal progress, with no complete healing observed. Despite nearly a year of monitoring, primary closure was not achieved, likely due to impaired tissue regeneration and delayed healing associated with the patient's medical history. This necessitated continued follow-up and potential adjunctive interventions to support tissue repair and minimize the risk of further complications.

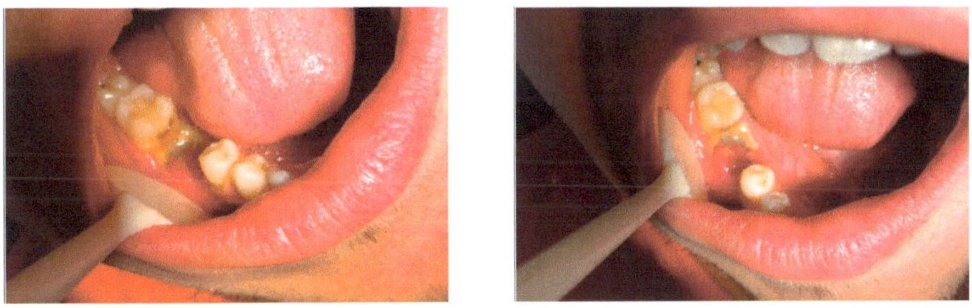

**Figure 5.** A postoperative clinical photograph of the LR6 area, taken one year after the surgery, showing the healing status of the site.

The clinical findings, as shown in Figure 5, were recorded during the patient's last attended appointment, one year after the surgery. Unfortunately, the patient did not return for the remaining follow-up appointments for unknown reasons, making it challenging to assess the long-term healing progress and any potential complications.

### 2.6. *Review of the Literature*

Several case reports identified in the literature review, summarized in Table 1, describe a wide range of complications associated with NaOCl exposure. Most of these complications are typically uncomplicated and resolve within a few days to weeks; however, some complications may persist for a prolonged period or even become permanent. Accidental exposure to NaOCl during endodontic procedures typically results in mild to moderate complications, including pain and swelling, which generally resolve within a period ranging from several days to weeks. However, some severe symptoms, such as skin discoloration, chemical burns, and mucosal or bone necrosis, may require a prolonged healing period, with full recovery potentially taking up to months. Accidental NaOCl exposure can result in severe, long-lasting, or permanent complications, such as sensory impairment, paresthesia, facial nerve dysfunction and facial muscle weakness potentially persisting for years or even becoming permanent. Therefore, most NaOCl-related injuries are self-limiting, with the majority healing completely within a few weeks. However, in severe cases involving extensive nerve tissue damage, the healing period may extend for a long time. A summary of the included case reports is provided in Table 1.

**Table 1.** A summary of the case reports discussed in this paper.

| Reference | Signs and Symptoms | Duration | Managements | Outcomes |
|---|---|---|---|---|
| [2] | Pain and swelling, paresthesia in the infraorbital nerve area and weakness in the buccal branch of the facial nerve, leading to loss of upper lip and cheek function. | Pain and swelling lasted for about 1 week. Paresthesia persisted for 3 years with no signs of improvement in the facial nerve weakness. | Local anesthesia, cold compress, antibiotics, and analgesics. The patient was later referred to a neurologist for further assessment of the persistent sensory and motor deficits. The patient underwent prosthetic rehabilitation to replace the upper front teeth. | The patient experienced permanent facial nerve weakness and reduced sensitivity in the infraorbital region. No significant improvement occurred even after 3 years, despite daily attempts to train the mimic musculature. Permanent paresthesia and weakness of the mimic musculature, causing difficulty with facial movements like smiling and uncontrolled salivation. |
| [3] | Pain and swelling, weakness of the buccal branch of the facial nerve, leading to loss of upper lip and cheek function, with the mouth corner being pulled down by unopposed lower lip muscles. Infra-orbital ecchymosis and altered sensation in the right infra-orbital nerve area. | One month later: Swelling had almost resolved, mouth opening was improved, and the patient was pain-free. However, there was no improvement in facial nerve weakness after one month. | The patient was treated with intravenous dexamethasone (8 mg, three times a day) and co-amoxiclav (1.2 g, three times a day), along with regular analgesia. | Outcome after one month: The patient was free from pain, with significant improvement in mouth opening. However, the weakness of the facial nerve persisted, and there was minimal improvement in infra-orbital nerve paresthesia. |
| [5] | Burning sensation around the rubber dam during sodium hypochlorite irrigation. A rash developed around the patient's chin, which later formed scabs. | Burning sensation ceased after 3 days, and the scab began to fall off after 7 days. The skin discoloration from the burn disappeared after 3 months, and the patient fully recovered. | The patient was treated with topical Hamamelis virginiana extract (Hametan) twice a day for 2 weeks. | The patient fully recovered with no long-term effects. The burning sensation and skin discoloration were alleviated, and there were no further complications after 3 months. |
| [6] | Pain and massive edema on the right cheek and upper lip. The swelling extended to the right orbit, and the patient experienced right eye pain, blurred vision, and corneal discoloration. A necrotic area appeared on the upper lip mucosa. | The symptoms developed rapidly within minutes to hours, with the swelling extending over two weeks. | The patient received intravenous hydrocortisone and penicillin G for swelling and pain control. Surgical debridement was performed to excise the necrotic mucosa and clean the affected area. The area was irrigated daily with saline to remove necrotic tissue, and intravenous antibiotics were administered to treat the infection. | After two weeks, the wound healed, but the patient experienced long-term scarring, dimples, and right infraorbital nerve anesthesia. |

**Table 1.** *Cont.*

| Reference | Signs and Symptoms | Duration | Managements | Outcomes |
| --- | --- | --- | --- | --- |
| [7] | The patient reported burning, stinging, and sharp pain during the injection of 1% sodium hypochlorite. Edema, difficulty swallowing, redness on the cheek, and loss of sensation were noted in the mental nerve area. | The patient underwent regular debridement of necrotic tissue, and re-epithelialization was observed by the third month. All symptoms resolved by the sixth month. | The patient was administered pheniramine maleate, dexamethasone, and intraoral antibiotics (1000 mg of amoxicillin, twice a day, for two weeks), along with alpha-lipoic acid (300 mg, daily, for one month). Regular clinical follow-up was performed, and necrotic tissue was debrided every 3 days for 4 weeks. The patient was advised to avoid smoking and consuming hot food and alcohol. | Re-epithelialization of necrotic tissue was observed after one month. The paresthesia of the mental nerve decreased after three months, and all symptoms completely disappeared by the sixth month. |
| [8] | Severe chemical burn on the right infraorbital area and partial necrosis of the hard palate. Erythematous, tender skin on the right cheek, numbness, and blackish discharge from the nose. | Mucosal damage healed completely after six weeks, but facial scar discoloration remained. | The patient was treated with creams and ointments for chemical burns. The symptoms were managed conservatively without surgical intervention. The patient was monitored for two weeks and did not require further surgical treatment. | The facial scar remained, but the mucosal damage healed nearly completely. The patient recovered without significant long-term complications, though facial discoloration remained. |
| [9] | Case 1: Gross left facial swelling extending from the mandible to the zygomatic arch with diffuse subcutaneous ecchymosis, mouth-opening limited to 20 mm, and intra-oral necrosis, ulceration, and ecchymosis.<br>Case 2: Severe pain and swelling in the left cheek, extending from the mandible to the left eye, with no intra-oral tissue damage. | The swelling and pain reduced significantly within a few days. In Case 1, mouth opening and facial swelling improved by the 7th day, and by the 3rd week, and the face and mouth were normal. In Case 2, the symptoms improved significantly within 4 weeks. | Case 1: The oral cavity was irrigated with normal saline, and ice packs were applied for 1 day, followed by warm saline rinses. Prednisone was prescribed to control inflammation, and co-amoxiclav and analgesics were given. Regular monitoring was undertaken over the next few days.<br>Case 2: Cold and warm compresses, saline rinses, acetaminophen-based narcotic analgesics, prophylactic antibiotics, and corticosteroids were prescribed. | Case 1: Complete resolution of symptoms, normal mouth opening, and absence of pain by 3 weeks.<br>Case 2: All symptoms resolved satisfactorily after 4 weeks. The root canal treatment was successfully completed with alternative irrigants (hydrogen peroxide and chlorhexidine gluconate). |
| [10] | Severe burning pain, swelling of the surrounding tissue, and redness observed at the tissues beyond the root apex. Profuse bleeding, severe tissue necrosis, and potential nerve involvement. | Symptoms improved appropriately, but full resolution may take several weeks, and nerve recovery could take several months. | Immediate irrigation with normal saline to flush out the NaOCl, followed by ice packs to reduce swelling. Steroids like prednisone were administered to control inflammation. Antibiotics to prevent secondary infections were prescribed, along with warm compresses to stimulate healing and improve circulation after the initial 24 h period. | The patient showed significant improvement over several weeks, with the swelling and ecchymosis reducing. In some cases, tissue necrosis was resolved after several weeks with non-surgical interventions, but facial nerve damage (e.g., numbness or weakness) could persist for a few months. |

**Table 1.** *Cont.*

| Reference | Signs and Symptoms | Duration | Managements | Outcomes |
|---|---|---|---|---|
| [11] | Sudden onset of pain in the left hemimandible and numbness in the left lower lip. Persistent pain in the left lower molar region and the left lower lip remained numb after the initial procedure. | Pain and numbness persisted for 15 days. After the gutta-percha point was removed surgically, pain subsided within 15 days, but numbness in the lower lip persisted for about a month before resolving completely. | A surgical procedure was performed to remove the gutta-percha point that had overfilled the root canal and entered the mandibular canal. The patient underwent an outpatient surgical procedure to remove the gutta-percha point, with the lesion being addressed by raising a mucoperiosteal flap for ostectomy and careful curettage. | The pain was resolved after the surgical removal of the gutta-percha, although the paresthesia (numbness) persisted for a while. The numbness in the lower lip was fully recovered within a month after the surgery. |
| [12] | Severe pain at the injection site, which began immediately after the sodium hypochlorite was injected instead of the anesthetic solution. Rapid development of local edema and tissue necrosis, labial ptosis (drooping), paresthesia in the upper lip, and visual blurring. | The severe pain and edema appeared immediately. The visual discomfort resolved after 8 days. The mucosal injury healed with scarring after 60 days. The labial ptosis resolved after 3 months, but the lip paresthesia persisted for 3 years. | The patient was given Arcoxia (anti-inflammatory), amoxicillin (antibiotic), and dexamethasone with B-complex vitamins for inflammation control. The patient received a combination of antibiotics and anti-inflammatory medications to manage the necrosis and prevent infection. Regular follow-up ensured proper tissue healing and symptom management. | The edema and necrosis resolved with scarring. Lip ptosis improved within 3 months, but paresthesia in the lip persisted for 3 years despite treatment. |
| [13] | Severe pain upon injection, which was followed by tissue necrosis in the palatal mucosa. Swelling and discoloration (purple) around the necrotic area, with the center being yellow-white. The area was painless during palpation. | Pain persisted for 2 days after the injection, after which it subsided. Swelling and tissue necrosis were visible for the next 15 days. | The patient was monitored conservatively as the mucosa showed signs of healing. No surgical intervention was needed since the tissue was healing naturally. Regular monitoring was carried out for 30 days, ensuring that no further complications arose. | Complete healing without scarring was achieved within 30 days. No long-term complications were reported, and the mucosal tissue healed effectively. |
| [14] | Severe pain occurred immediately after the accidental injection of NaOCl instead of the intended anesthetic solution. Swelling of the gingiva and surrounding tissues, followed by the formation of necrotic tissue and bone sequestration. | Pain persisted for 3 days after the injection. Swelling and tissue necrosis were present for the following 2 months. | The patient was treated with anti-inflammatory medication (diclofenac) and antibiotics (amoxicillin) to manage pain, inflammation, and prevent infection. After 2 months, surgical coverage with a laterally positioned flap was performed to address the necrotic tissue and bone sequestration. | The area affected by chemical necrosis healed after 3 weeks, with no further tissue damage or complications. The root canal treatment of the adjacent tooth was completed 30 days after the surgical procedure. |

**Table 1.** *Cont.*

| Reference | Signs and Symptoms | Duration | Managements | Outcomes |
|---|---|---|---|---|
| [15] | Severe pain upon injection, swelling, and hyperemia in the right half of the face, along with black necrotic areas on the right buccal mucosa. No facial paralysis, but the patient exhibited significant tissue damage and edema in the affected area. | Severe swelling, pain, and necrosis developed within 4–5 h of the accidental injection. After 24 h of treatment, the patient's symptoms regressed. Full recovery occurred within 4 weeks, with no residual effects. | The patient was hospitalized and treated with IV antibiotics (ceftriaxone and metronidazole), anti-inflammatory medication (dexketoprofen), and analgesics (paracetamol). Cold compresses and bed rest were recommended. The patient was monitored for 4 weeks, after which they showed complete recovery with no complications. | The patient recovered fully without any long-term effects, and the necrotic tissue healed completely within a month. There were no additional issues reported after the treatment. |
| [16] | Report A: Swelling and ecchymosis on the right side of the face, particularly around the mouth and periorbital region. Ulcerative lesions on the internal lip mucosa. Report B: Mild edema and ecchymosis on the right commissure lip with no mucosal lesions. Report C: Swelling and ecchymosis on the left side of the face, particularly near the mouth and periorbital region. Report D: Severe pain and bleeding from the root canal, followed by mild edema and swelling on the face. | Report A: Swelling and bruising peaked within 24 h, which improved significantly after 3–5 days. Report B: Swelling and ecchymosis persisted for 5 days but resolved with minimal symptoms remaining. Report C: Symptoms like swelling and ecchymosis reduced after 5 days. Report D: Swelling persisted for several days, but pain and symptoms resolved within 6 days. | Report A: Cold compress, antibiotic (amoxicillin with clavulanic acid), pain control (paracetamol and ibuprofen), and corticosteroids (prednisone). Report B: Saline solution flush, cold compress, and prescribed medications (ciprofloxacin, paracetamol, ibuprofen, and betamethasone). Report C: Saline flush, cold compress, and medications (amoxicillin, prednisone, and ibuprofen). Report D: Saline flush, cold compress, and prescribed medications (amoxicillin, prednisone, and ibuprofen). | Report A: Significant improvement in 3–5 days, with the continuation of root canal treatment using chlorhexidine. Report B: Symptoms reduced significantly after 5 days; root canal treatment continued with chlorhexidine. Report C: Recovery within 5 days, root canal treatment continued with a side-vented needle after CBCT revealed apical fenestration. Report D: Significant reduction in symptoms after 6 days, treatment completed with no legal actions taken. |

## 3. Discussion

Identifying the risk factors that predispose individuals to prolonged bone necrosis following NaOCl exposure is essential for both prevention and effective management. The presented case led to bone necrosis and a non-healing extraction socket, with the complication persisting for a much longer period than expected. This extended healing time exceeded the typical duration described in the literature, indicating that there may be additional factors influencing wound healing and tissue repair, which likely contributed to the prolonged nature of the complication. Individuals with impaired immune function or those undergoing immunosuppressive treatment are at a significantly higher risk of developing severe complications following NaOCl injuries [17]. In immunocompromised patients, such as those with Hodgkin's lymphoma, a usually localized area of tissue necrosis may progress more rapidly or show delayed healing.

The clinical outcome of a NaOCl accident is largely influenced by patient-related factors, such as medical history. This factor determines whether the injury remains a self-limiting or transient event in otherwise healthy patients or progresses into more severe complications, such as persistent osteonecrosis, as demonstrated in the presented case.

In patients with a healthy immune status, NaOCl injuries typically present with acute pain and swelling, which generally resolve with conservative management [5,7,9–11,13–16]. In contrast, the presence of a high-risk factor, particularly immunocompromised states, such as in patients with Hodgkin's lymphoma, can dramatically alter the clinical trajectory. In such individuals, a compromised inflammatory response and impaired ability to contain secondary infection may lead to more extensive soft-tissue destruction and involvement of the alveolar bone [17], even when procedural guidelines are followed and predisposing conditions and risk factors are carefully considered [18]. These complex cases often require surgical intervention, such as debridement of the necrotic bone, along with prolonged wound care and monitoring to aid healing, as was performed in the presented case. However, despite these efforts, the desired outcomes were not achieved.

Notably, no clinical cases documenting NaOCl injuries in patients with Hodgkin's lymphoma have been identified in the existing literature. Consequently, there is no specific management protocol designed for this patient group. This poses a clinical challenge, as extended monitoring in such an individual may increase the risk of secondary infection over time, while early surgical intervention, such as debridement of the necrotic bone, could potentially worsen the condition by causing further bone damage.

Therefore, as the conventional management approach failed, this patient should be managed according to the most up-to-date treatment strategies, as suggested in situations similar to those involving Hodgkin's lymphoma patients, where individuals exhibit a low immune status.

One of the recently established therapies for managing non-healing sockets, particularly in the context of medication-related osteonecrosis of the jaw (MRONJ) [19], is leukocyte–platelet-rich fibrin (L-PRF). This treatment has demonstrated promising outcomes in addressing non-healing sockets in non-malignant conditions, such as osteoporosis, and oncology patients, offering a potential solution for enhancing healing and improving clinical outcomes.

A retrospective observational study [19] was conducted to evaluate the effectiveness of L-PRF as an adjunct to surgical intervention in the treatment of patients at risk of MRONJ development. The study included 22 participants, who were allocated into two groups: Group A, which received surgery alone, and Group B, which received both surgery and L-PRF. Treatment success was determined based on complete soft-tissue healing and the absence of infection, inflammation, fistula formation, or exposed bone. The results demonstrated that 100% of patients in Group B achieved complete healing, in contrast with 54.5% of patients in Group A. The study concluded that L-PRF is a promising adjunct to the surgical management of MRONJ, providing favorable treatment outcomes and enhanced healing potential. A similar study [20] found that none of the patients in the L-PRF group developed established MRONJ, while five high-risk patients in the control group presented with MRONJ during follow-up. The study concluded that L-PRF may be effective in preventing MRONJ following dental extractions and also introduced a management protocol for these individuals.

Another group of bone necrosis and non-healing sockets is observed in osteoradionecrosis of the jaws (ORNJ), a severe and complex complication that arises following head and neck radiation therapy. In the management of ORNJ, one promising therapeutic option is the combination of pentoxifylline and tocopherol (PENTO). A systematic review [21] was conducted to assess the efficacy of PENTO in the treatment of ORNJ. The review revealed that PENTO treatment resulted in complete mucosal coverage with no exposed bone in patients, with success rates ranging from 16.6% to 100%, depending on the study. Additionally, clinical improvement or disease stabilization was reported in 7.6% to 66.6% of patients, while disease progression occurred in 7.6% to 32% of cases across five studies. The findings of the review suggest that PENTO may effectively achieve complete disease control in a significant proportion of patients.

Another treatment approach for ORNJ involves addressing radiation tissue injury. Hyperbaric oxygen therapy (HBOT) has been proposed as a potential treatment for such complications, owing to its ability to enhance blood flow to irradiated tissues. A Cochrane systematic review [22] was conducted to evaluate the effectiveness and risks of HBOT in treating or preventing late radiation tissue injury. The review found that HBOT is associated with improved outcomes in managing osteonecrosis. Additionally, it appears to reduce the risk of osteoradionecrosis following tooth extraction, indicating its potential benefit as an adjunctive therapy for patients with radiation-induced complications.

These adjunctive management strategies have been utilized in the treatment of various medical conditions, such as MRONJ and ORNJ, which share similar underlying pathophysiologies of NaOCl injury. Additionally, these conditions exhibit notable parallels to the present case, particularly in the manifestation of bone necrosis and delayed wound healing in immunocompromised patients.

The pathophysiology of NaOCl injury is predominantly attributed to its potent cytotoxic effects on living tissues. When NaOCl is accidentally extruded beyond the confines of the root canal during endodontic procedures, it comes into direct contact with surrounding vital tissues, leading to a cascade of harmful biological responses. NaOCl induces hemolysis by disrupting the integrity of red blood cells and releasing their intracellular contents into the surrounding tissues, thereby contributing to the disruption of the local tissue environment [14]. Additionally, NaOCl causes the ulceration of the affected tissue, leading to a compromised mucosal barrier [14]. The resultant disruption of the mucosal integrity creates a vulnerable site where microorganisms can more easily penetrate the exposed underlying bone, potentially leading to secondary infection. One of the key mechanisms of injury is the inhibition of neutrophil migration, which diminishes the immune response and compromises the body's ability to combat infection and initiate the healing process [14]. Furthermore, NaOCl inflicts damage to endothelial cells, disrupting vascular integrity, and fibroblast cells, hindering tissue repair and collagen synthesis [14].

As outlined in the 2022 update of the Position Paper by the American Association of Oral and Maxillofacial Surgeons on MRONJ, the pathophysiology of MRONJ is supported by several evidence-based theories. The pathophysiology of MRONJ is multifactorial, involving several interrelated mechanisms. One major factor is the inhibition of bone remodeling due to antiresorptive medications, which directly affect osteoclast formation, differentiation, and function, particularly following bone injury. Additionally, pre-existing inflammation or infection contributes significantly, with elevated levels of pro-inflammatory cytokines—especially at MRONJ lesion sites—supporting the pivotal role of inflammation in disease progression. Inhibition of angiogenesis also plays a key role, characterized by osteocyte death, secondary to reduced blood flow, and a notable decrease in the microvessel density during the early stages of bone healing. Immune dysfunction, such as that caused by chemotherapy, further exacerbates the condition by altering the number and distribution of T-cell populations. Lastly, genetic predisposition has been implicated, with specific single-nucleotide polymorphisms identified as being associated with an increased risk of developing MRONJ [23].

The pathogenesis of ORNJ is primarily driven by the progressive changes induced by radiation therapy. A key mechanism involves the development of hypovascularity, hypocellularity [24], and hypoxia [21] in the irradiated bone. These changes compromise the tissue's ability to regenerate and resist injury, initiating a chronic fibro-atrophic process characterized by fibrosis, reduced tissue elasticity, and impaired wound healing [24]. This leads to the bone and surrounding soft tissues becoming fragile and highly susceptible to necrosis, particularly following trauma, such as tooth extractions [24]. While microorganisms do play a role in exacerbating the condition, their contribution is relatively minor compared with the primary causes of hypovascularity and hypocellularity. Infection can worsen the clinical manifestation of ORNJ [25].

Therefore, the management strategies for MRONJ and ORNJ may be considered applicable in the present case, given the shared elements in their underlying pathophysiological mechanisms. L-PRF [26,27], one of the proposed strategies in the present case, is an autologous platelet concentrate, and regenerative biomaterial composed of a dense fibrin matrix containing high concentrations of platelets and leukocytes. It demonstrates considerable potential in promoting tissue repair through the gradual release of key growth factors, such as platelet-derived growth factor (PDGF), transforming growth factor (TGF), vascular endothelial growth factor (VEGF), and epithelial growth factor (EGF). These molecules collectively enhance angiogenesis, bone regeneration, and soft-tissue healing while also supporting hemostasis and tissue maturation without eliciting an inflammatory response. The fibrin matrix of L-PRF, with its tetra-molecular structure, serves as a biodegradable scaffold containing cytokines and stem cells, facilitating microvascularization and directing epithelial cell migration during the healing process.

Pentoxifylline, a methylxanthine derivative, exerts its antifibrotic effect through multiple mechanisms, including the inhibition of tumor necrosis factor-alpha (TNF-$\alpha$), promotion of vasodilation, enhancement of erythrocyte deformability, and suppression of fibroblast proliferation [21]. Additionally, it increases the activity of collagenase enzymes, thereby facilitating extracellular matrix degradation [21]. Tocopherol (vitamin E), a potent antioxidant, complements these effects by inhibiting oxidative stress and downregulating the expression of procollagen genes, which contributes to the reduction in fibrotic tissue formation [21]. Together, pentoxifylline and tocopherol (PENTO) demonstrate a synergistic interaction, enhancing their overall antifibrotic efficacy.

HBOT has been proposed as a modality to enhance tissue quality, facilitate wound healing, and prevent the breakdown of irradiated tissues. It is defined as the medical use of 100% oxygen delivered at pressures exceeding 1 atmosphere absolute. The procedure involves placing the patient within a sealed hyperbaric chamber, where the ambient pressure is elevated while the patient breathes pure oxygen [22]. This results in a substantial increase in the partial pressure of oxygen in the lungs, bloodstream, and tissues. One of the key therapeutic outcomes of HBOT is the stimulation of angiogenesis, thereby promoting neovascularization within previously irradiated and hypoxic tissues [22].

Although no studies to date have directly investigated the use of these adjunctive management strategies in the context of NaOCl injuries, their therapeutic objectives—particularly the promotion of mucosal coverage over exposed bone—suggest potential applicability in such cases, especially when the patient is immunocompromised due to underlying medical conditions or ongoing treatment, as demonstrated in the presented case.

The dental management of patients with compromised immune systems presents unique challenges. These challenges arise not from the procedures themselves but from the complexities of managing complications in these patients. The current case emphasizes the necessity of careful consideration and expertise in treating such patients. Inexperienced clinicians should exercise caution when managing these cases, as complications could lead to long-term issues without effective management solutions. Hodgkin's lymphoma, in particular, requires specialized attention due to the significant immune compromise associated with the condition. Therefore, a comprehensive and well-coordinated approach is crucial for the successful management of dental complications in this patient group. In this context, it may be advisable to consider the adjunctive management strategies discussed, as they could potentially aid in resolving the complications and promoting optimal healing. However, further well-designed research is required to evaluate the effectiveness of the proposed adjunctive management approaches and determine their suitability for use in such cases as Hodgkin's Lymphoma.

## 4. Conclusions

This case report highlights a challenging clinical scenario commonly encountered in dental practice. While many dental procedures are straightforward, the medical history, particularly in immunocompromised patients, can present significant challenges. It is recommended that such patients be referred to specialists rather than managed by less-experienced clinicians in order to avoid potential long-term complications. The management approaches employed in other conditions, such as MRONJ, may offer valuable insights for managing similar cases to the presented case. Furthermore, a standardized management protocol should be established for handling such cases to ensure optimal patient outcomes.

**Funding:** This study received no external funding.

**Institutional Review Board Statement:** Not applicable.

**Informed Consent Statement:** Verbal and written informed consent were obtained from the patient for the publication of these data.

**Data Availability Statement:** The data concerning this article may be requested from the corresponding author for reasonable purposes.

**Conflicts of Interest:** The author declares no conflicts of interest.

## List of Abbreviations

| | |
|---|---|
| LR6 | Lower right first molar |
| NaOCl | Sodium hypochlorite |
| L-PRF | Leukocyte–platelet-rich fibrin |
| PENTO | Pentoxifylline and tocopherol |
| HBOT | Hyperbaric oxygen therapy |
| OMFS | Oral and maxillofacial surgery department |
| RLDH | Royal London Dental Hospital |
| OPG | Orthopantomograph |
| CBCT | Cone-beam computed tomography |
| MRONJ | Medication-related osteonecrosis of the jaw |
| ORNJ | Osteoradionecrosis of the jaws |

## References


1. Fedorowicz, Z.; Nasser, M.; Sequeira-Byron, P.; de Souza, R.F.; Carter, B.; Heft, M. Irrigants for non-surgical root canal treatment in mature permanent teeth. *Cochrane Database Syst. Rev.* **2012**, *2012*, CD008948. [CrossRef] [PubMed]
2. Pelka, M.; Petschelt, A. Permanent mimic musculature and nerve damage caused by sodium hypochlorite: A case report. *Oral. Surg. Oral. Med. Oral. Pathol. Oral. Radiol. Endod.* **2008**, *106*, e80–e83. [CrossRef] [PubMed]
3. Witton, R.; Brennan, P.A. Severe tissue damage and neurological deficit following extravasation of sodium hypochlorite solution during routine endodontic treatment. *Br. Dent. J.* **2005**, *198*, 749–750. [CrossRef] [PubMed]
4. Silva, T.D.B.; Ferreira, C.B.T.; Leite, G.B.; Pontes, J.R.M.; Antunes, H.S. Oral manifestations of lymphoma: A systematic review. *Ecancermedicalscience* **2016**, *10*, 665. [CrossRef]
5. Serper, A.; Özbek, M.; Çalt, S. Accidental sodium hypochlorite-induced skin injury during endodontic treatment. *J. Endod.* **2004**, *30*, 180–181. [CrossRef]
6. Gatot, A.; Arbelle, J.; Leiberman, A.; Yanai-Inbar, I. Effects of sodium hypochlorite on soft tissues after its inadvertent injection beyond the root apex. *J. Endod.* **1991**, *17*, 573–574. [CrossRef]
7. Akay, N.; Şimşek, G.; Taş, B.M.; Kılıç, R. Inadvertent injection of sodium hypochlorite to oral mucosa. *Eur. J. Rhinol. Allergy* **2019**, *2*, 32–34. [CrossRef]
8. Faras, F.; Abo-Alhassan, F.; Sadeq, A.; Burezq, H. Complication of improper management of sodium hypochlorite accident during root canal treatment. *J. Int. Soc. Prev. Community Dent.* **2016**, *6*, 493–496. [CrossRef]
9. Goswami, M.; Chhabra, N.; Kumar, G.; Verma, M.; Chhabra, A. Sodium hypochlorite dental accidents. *Paediatr. Int. Child. Health.* **2013**, *34*, 66–69. [CrossRef]
10. Gernhardt, C.R.; Eppendorf, K.; Kozlowski, A.; Brandt, M. Toxicity of sodium hypochlorite used as an endodontic irrigant. *Int. Endod. J.* **2004**, *37*, 272–280. [CrossRef]
11. Gallas-Torreira, M.M.; Reboiras-López, M.D.; García-García, A.; Gándara-Rey, J. Mandibular nerve paresthesia caused by endodontic treatment. *Med. Oral.* **2003**, *8*, 299–303. [PubMed]
12. Motta, M.V.; Chaves-Mendonca, M.A.L.; Stirton, C.G.; Cardozo, H.F. Accidental injection with sodium hypochlorite: Report of a case. *Int. Endod. J.* **2009**, *42*, 175–182. [CrossRef] [PubMed]
13. Gursoy, U.K.; Bostancı, V.; Kosger, H.H. Palatal mucosa necrosis because of accidental sodium hypochlorite injection instead of anaesthetic solution. *Int. Endod. J.* **2006**, *39*, 157–161. [CrossRef] [PubMed]
14. Pontes, F.; Pontes, H.; Adachi, P.; Rodini, C.; Almeida, D.; Pinto, D., Jr. Gingival and bone necrosis caused by accidental sodium hypochlorite injection instead of anaesthetic solution. *Int. Endod. J.* **2008**, *41*, 267–270. [CrossRef]
15. Aslan, M.; Özcan, M. Accidental injection of sodium hypochlorite into buccal mucosa before endodontic treatment: Case report. *Essent. Dent.* **2023**, *2*, 66–69. [CrossRef]
16. Salvadori, M.; Venturi, G.; Bertoletti, P.; Francinelli, J.; Tonini, R.; Garo, M.L.; Salgarello, S. Sodium hypochlorite accident during canal treatment: Report of four cases documented according to new standards. *Appl. Sci.* **2022**, *12*, 8525. [CrossRef]
17. da Fonseca Wastner, B.; de Souza Lessa, M.; Sassi, L.M.; Pianovski, M.A. Life-threatening reaction of a pediatric cancer patient to sodium hypochlorite. *Res. Soc. Dev.* **2021**, *10*, e282101320446.
18. Coaguila-Llerena, H.; Denegri-Hacking, A.; Lucano-Tinoco, L.; Aquino, C.E. Accidental extrusion of sodium hypochlorite in a patient taking alendronate: A case report with an 8-year follow-up. *J. Endod.* **2021**, *47*, 1983–1989. [CrossRef]

19. Aslam, R.D.; Pitros, P.; Liew, J.; Besi, E. The adjunctive use of Leukocyte-Platelet Rich Fibrin (L-PRF) in the management of Medication Related Osteonecrosis of the Jaw (MRONJ): A retrospective observational study. *Oral. Maxillofac. Surg.* **2024**, *28*, 1605–1615. [CrossRef] [PubMed]
20. Besi, E.; Pitros, P. The role of leukocyte and platelet-rich fibrin in the prevention of medication-related osteonecrosis of the jaw, in patients requiring dental extractions: An observational study. *Oral. Maxillofac. Surg.* **2024**, *28*, 785–793. [CrossRef] [PubMed]
21. Arqueros-Lemus, M.; Mariño-Recabarren, D.; Niklander, S.; Martínez-Flores, R.; Moraga, V. Pentoxifylline and tocopherol for the treatment of osteoradionecrosis of the jaws. A systematic review. *Med. Oral. Patol. Oral. Cir. Bucal.* **2023**, *28*, e293–e300. [CrossRef] [PubMed] [PubMed Central]
22. Bennett, M.H.; Feldmeier, J.; Hampson, N.B.; Smee, R.; Milross, C. Hyperbaric oxygen therapy for late radiation tissue injury. *Cochrane Database Syst. Rev.* **2016**, *4*, CD005005, Update in: *Cochrane Database Syst. Rev.* **2023**, *8*, CD005005. [CrossRef] [PubMed] [PubMed Central]
23. Ruggiero, S.L.; Dodson, T.B.; Aghaloo, T.; Carlson, E.R.; Ward, B.B.; Kademani, D. American Association of Oral and Maxillofacial Surgeons' position paper on medication-related osteonecrosis of the jaw—2022 update. *J. Oral. Maxillofac. Surg.* **2022**, *80*, 920–943. [CrossRef] [PubMed]
24. Lajolo, C.; Rupe, C.; Gioco, G.; Troiano, G.; Patini, R.; Petruzzi, M.; Micciché, F.; Giuliani, M. Osteoradionecrosis of the jaws due to teeth extractions during and after radiotherapy: A systematic review. *Cancers* **2021**, *13*, 5798. [CrossRef] [PubMed]
25. Marx, R.E. Osteoradionecrosis: A new concept of its pathophysiology. *J. Oral. Maxillofac. Surg.* **1983**, *41*, 283–288. [CrossRef] [PubMed]
26. Cortese, A.; Casarella, A.; Howard, C.M.; Claudio, P.P. Epi-mucosa fixation and autologous platelet-rich fibrin treatment in medication-related osteonecrosis of the jaw. *Dent. J.* **2021**, *9*, 50. [CrossRef]
27. Zelinka, J.; Blahak, J.; Perina, V.; Pacasova, R.; Treglerova, J.; Bulik, O. The use of platelet-rich fibrin in the surgical treatment of medication-related osteonecrosis of the jaw: 40 patients prospective study. *Biomed. Pap. Med. Fac. Univ. Palacky. Olomouc Czech Repub.* **2021**, *165*, 322–327. [CrossRef]

*diagnostics*

MDPI

*Systematic Review*

# Metabolomics Applications for Diagnosing Peri-Implantitis: A Systematic Review of In Vivo Studies

Ana-Maria Condor [1,2,3,†], Andreea Kui [3,*], Daniela Cornelia Condor [4,†], Marius Negucioiu [3], Smaranda Dana Buduru [3] and Patricia Ondine Lucaciu [1]

1 Oral Health Discipline, Department 3—Oral Rehabilitation, Faculty of Dental Medicine, "Iuliu Hațieganu" University of Medicine and Pharmacy, 400012 Cluj-Napoca, Romania; ana.mari.condor@elearn.umfcluj.ro (A.-M.C.)
2 Cluj County Emergency Clinical Hospital, 400006 Cluj-Napoca, Romania
3 Prosthodontics Discipline, Department 4—Prosthodontics and Dental Materials, Faculty of Dental Medicine, "Iuliu Hațieganu" University of Medicine and Pharmacy, 400012 Cluj-Napoca, Romania
4 Periodontology Discipline, Department 3—Oral Rehabilitation, Faculty of Dental Medicine, "Iuliu Hațieganu" University of Medicine and Pharmacy, 400012 Cluj-Napoca, Romania
* Correspondence: gulie.andreea@umfcluj.ro
† These authors contributed equally to this work.

**Abstract: Background/Objectives**: Peri-implantitis is a prevalent inflammatory condition affecting dental implants, leading to increased treatment costs, patient dissatisfaction, and potential implant failure. Novel biomarker-based approaches may contribute to early detection, thereby decreasing the burden of the disease. The aim of this review was to assess in vivo studies using metabolomics to identify the metabolic profiles and potential biomarkers of peri-implantitis. **Methods**: The protocol for this study was registered with PROSPERO (CRD42025634865). Five databases and grey literature sources (PubMed, Scopus, Web of Science, ProQuest, and Google Scholar) were searched using keywords related to metabolomics and peri-implantitis. Studies were selected by independent, intercalibrated researchers. Data were extracted using predefined, custom forms. The risk of bias was assessed using the ROBINS-I tool. **Results**: An electronic literature search retrieved 543 articles, of which five were selected. All studies were published within the last five years of the search. All but one study used untargeted metabolomics, and all studies identified metabolites associated with peri-implantitis or distinct metabolomic profiles of peri-implantitis. SCFAs and lysine metabolites were recurring in the results, confirming the findings of previous metabolomic studies on periodontal disease. **Conclusions**: Metabolomics has not been widely used to study peri-implantitis. Evidence from existing studies confirms the findings of metabolomics studies on periodontitis. Several metabolites related to PI are associated with immune response, tissue degradation, and cellular energy pathways. Integrating -omics technologies into peri-implantitis diagnosis may facilitate biomarker discovery and improve early detection strategies.

**Keywords:** peri-implantitis; peri-implant crevicular fluid; metabolomics; diagnosis

## 1. Introduction

Dental implant therapy is one of the most frequent approaches in dentistry and is used to treat partial or complete edentation cases. As life expectancy continues to grow, so do the challenges of maintaining the health and integrity of oral structures; hence, the number of cases treated with implants is increasing [1,2]. Peri-implantitis is a significant clinical challenge in dental implantology. Dental implant therapy is widely used to address edentulism and maintain oral function; however, the increasing prevalence of complications such as peri-implantitis compromises implant longevity and oral tissue integrity [1,2]. However, managing complications such as peri-implantitis remains a significant challenge [3,4]. Implant complications are common and may impose high financial burdens on patients, leading to dissatisfaction and negative treatment perceptions [5,6]. This is particularly relevant when considering patients' elevated expectations of implant therapy as a permanent solution for oral or dental issues [7].

Implant complications and deficiencies in the surrounding tissues may be a consequence of mechanical, biological, systemic, traumatic, or iatrogenic factors [8]. Peri-implant diseases (mucositis—PIM and peri-implantitis—PI) are the most relevant biological complications, with PI occurring in 19.5% of patients and 12.5% of implants [9]. A systematic review estimated the prevalence of peri-implantitis at 43% and peri-implant mucositis at 22% across Europe, North America, and South America, with an increasing incidence over time [10]. If left untreated, peri-implantitis may lead to implant loss as early as 2 months after the initial diagnosis [4,11–13]. This inflammatory condition is characterised by accelerated bone loss and soft tissue destruction, often leading to implant failure if left untreated [4,11–13]. The biological and mechanical factors contributing to peri-implantitis are multifactorial, including microbial dysbiosis, patient-related risk factors, and the complex interplay of host immune responses, which collectively increase the risk of achieving long-term treatment success [3,8]. However, PI treatment is associated with considerable challenges. A primary concern is patient compliance with oral hygiene practices and implant maintenance. Furthermore, surgical treatment of PI may lead to major aesthetic deficiencies due to subsequent soft tissue retraction [14]. Most importantly, PI treatment is only moderately successful in the short term. A large number of cases (75%) recur or remain unresolved after five years [15]. A recent systematic review reported that fewer than 50% of implants affected by PI achieve disease resolution [16]. PI is triggered and maintained by numerous factors, some of which are difficult to manage. Therefore, due to the unpredictability of treatment success, rigorous prevention measures should be taken to avoid PI whenever possible [17].

Beyond its direct clinical implications, peri-implantitis significantly affects the overall well-being of patients. Affected individuals frequently experience chronic discomfort, reduced masticatory efficiency, and aesthetic deficiencies, which can ultimately diminish the oral health-related quality of life [5,6]. The potential for rapid progression to implant loss and the ensuing need for extensive, costly re-treatment not only intensifies physical discomfort but also contributes to psychological stress and increased financial burden [7,14]. By highlighting these patient-centered consequences, the urgency for early, non-invasive diagnostic methods, such as metabolomic profiling, is underscored, promising improved personalised management strategies that address both clinical and quality-of-life outcomes.

The current PI diagnostic criteria are based on clinical and radiological measurements compared to the baseline values. These include inflammation, bleeding, and/or suppuration upon probing, increased probing depth (PD), and bone loss (BL) [11]. Unfortunately, PI follows a non-linear and accelerating pattern and can occur early during post-surgical follow-up. Therefore, permanent damage to the supporting tissues is frequently observed at the time of diagnosis. This emphasises the need for novel, non-invasive early detection methods for peri-implantitis [14,18,19]. The application of emerging omics technologies in the diagnostic process is essential due to the significant challenges posed by PI therapy and its increasing burden on patients. Integrating -omics technologies into dental practice contributes to the development of precision oral healthcare and personalised treatment [19].

Metabolomics is a powerful tool since it best reflects the molecular phenotype of a sample at the time of analysis [20]. Various molecules (such as cytokines and enzymes) have been previously validated as markers for peri-implantitis [21–23], but no metabolic biomarkers have been identified to date.

Metabolomics could facilitate the early diagnosis, prognosis, and monitoring of PI by non-invasively sampling peri-implant crevicular/sulcular fluid (PICF/PISF). It can detect and quantify metabolites associated with bacterial dysbiosis or incipient disease states, thus preventing large-scale irreversible tissue damage. Integrating metabolic data with other omics or microbiological approaches could contribute to a better understanding of this pathological entity. This could provide opportunities for new preventive strategies and treatment options [24–26]. The objective of this review was twofold: firstly, to assess existing in vivo studies on metabolomics applied in the diagnosis, prognosis, or treatment of peri-implantitis, and secondly, to identify metabolites mentioned in two or more studies, which could represent the subject of future research.

## 2. Materials and Methods

### *2.1. Registration and Validation of Study Protocol*

This review was developed using the Preferred Reporting Items for Systematic Reviews and Meta-Analyses (PRISMA) 2020 reporting guidelines and PRISMA for abstracts [27]. The study protocol was registered with the International Prospective Register of Systematic Reviews (PROSPERO CRD42025634865).

### *2.2. Question of Study*

How can metabolomics technology (metabolic profiling) be applied to the diagnosis, prognosis, or treatment of peri-implantitis in human patients suffering from peri-implantitis?

### *2.3. Eligibility Criteria*

a. Inclusion criteria

P (population) = patients treated with dental implants;
E (exposure) = clinically diagnosed peri-implantitis;
C (control) = implants in a state of clinically determined peri-implant health
O (type of outcome measures) = differences in detectable metabolites from saliva of peri-implant crevicular fluid samples, assessed by both targeted or untargeted metabolomics approaches, marginal bone loss, bleeding on probing, and probing depth.
S (type of studies) = original studies on humans, RCT, NRCT, prospective, retrospective, or cross-sectional studies, case reports and case series, and cohort studies

b. Exclusion criteria

- Study designs: literature reviews and/or meta-analyses, letters to editors, conference abstracts, and commentaries.
- In vitro, animal study designs, and ex vivo studies.
- Studies without full-text articles.
- Studies that presented missing or incomplete data regarding outcome measures or the technologies and pathologies involved.
- Studies published in languages other than English.

### *2.4. Search Strategy*

The existing literature was electronically searched using the following databases and registries: PubMed, Scopus, Web of Science, ProQuest, and Google Scholar. The electronic literature search was designed and conducted by two independent researchers (AMC and CDC), starting from 21 January 2025 until the final date of 30 January 2024. The search strategy included the terms 'peri-implantitis' and 'metabolomics', applied using Boolean operators (AND/OR) in title, abstract, and full-text searches. When available, MeSH terms were included in the search. No date restrictions or language restrictions were applied during the search. This strategy was applied with minor necessary modifications to the queries to accommodate the search particularities and controlled vocabularies of each database. The exact search terminologies are available in Appendix A—Search strategy.

### *2.5. Study Selection Process*

Search results were downloaded in library form from each database (when possible) and centralised using a reference manager (Zotero version 7.0.6.). Duplicates were identified manually and electronically using the same software. The remaining studies were screened for titles and abstracts by 2 researchers and selected based on the inclusion and exclusion criteria. Studies considered relevant were retrieved in full-text form and selected by 2 independent researchers. For databases that had no option of downloading results, the articles were manually selected based on title/abstract and then retrieved in full-text form by the same 2 researchers. Conflicts were resolved by a third researcher. Prior to the selection process, the researchers inter-calibrated and trained for selection on a batch of 100 random results. The inter-researcher's agreement level was calculated by the Kappa coefficient (k = 9.1)

### *2.6. Data Extraction*

The following data were extracted from the included studies using custom, predefined forms:

- General data about the studies (title, main authors, geographical area, DOI, year of publication, study design)
- Population (number of subjects/number of implants, age/gender distribution, personal potential confounding factors)
- Exposure and controls (marginal bone loss, probing depth, bleeding on probing, other periodontal or peri-implant indexes)
- Outcome (metabolomics approaches used, technologies involved, sample types, identified metabolites)

### *2.7. Risk of Bias/Quality Assessment*

ROBINS-I ("Risk Of Bias In Non-randomised Studies—of Interventions") scale was used to assess the risk of bias. This scale assesses the risk of bias in 7 domains: bias due to confounding, study participants' selection, classification of interventions, deviations from intended interventions, missing data, measurements of outcomes, and reporting. Each domain was assessed using the tool guidelines and summarised under the labels proposed by the tool. To generate a visual summary of the assessment, we used the robvis tool to generate a traffic-lights graph [28,29].

## 3. Results

### *3.1. Study Selection*

The search retrieved 543 results. After duplicate removal, 413 articles remained. The screening and study selection processes are summarised in the following PRISMA 2020 flowchart (Figure 1). A total of five studies were included in this review.

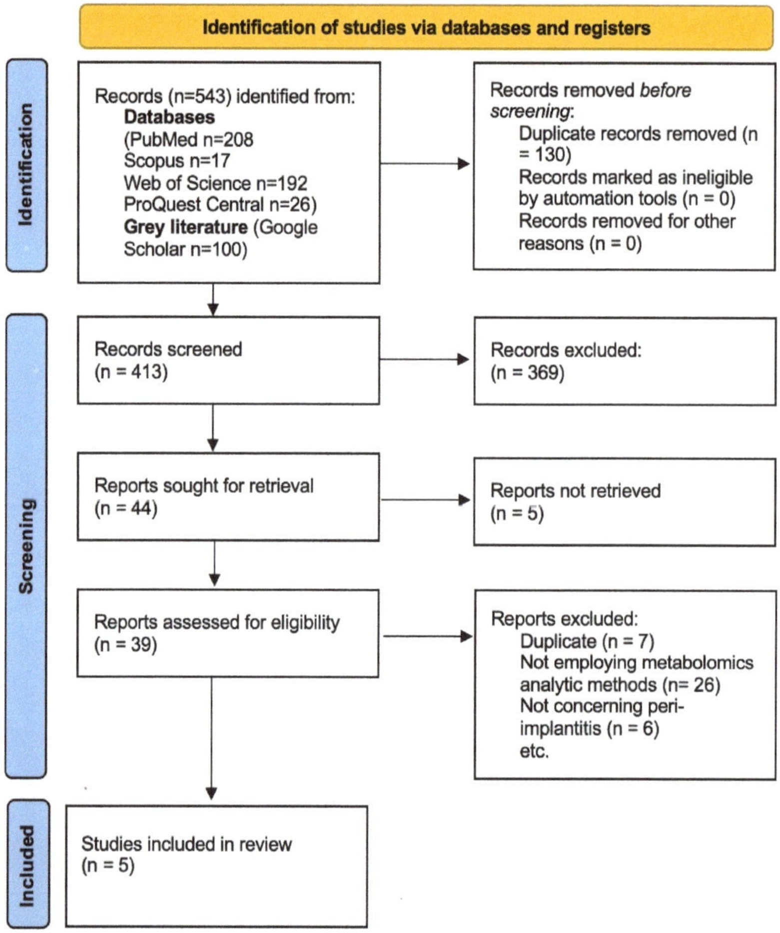


**Figure 1.** PRISMA 2020 flowchart of the study selection process.

### *3.2. Description of Included Studies*

Two of the included studies were theses published in 2020 [30] and 2021 [31]. Two studies were published in 2024 [32,33] and one study was published in 2023 [34]. 2 studies employed H-NMR [30,31], one study SERS [34] and two studies LC and GC [32,33]. All studies analysed peri-implant crevicular (sulcular fluid) samples. All studies clinically diagnosed PI. Excepting for one study [32] based on targeted metabolomics, all studies used untargeted metabolomics. A detailed description of included studies is available in Table 1.

**Table 1.** Description of the included studies.

| Main Author | Year | Analytic Platform | Approach | Study Type | Sample Type | Sample Size | Inclusion Criteria | Metabolites Identified (nr) | Significant Metabolites | Notes | Conclusions |
|---|---|---|---|---|---|---|---|---|---|---|---|
| Song et al. [33] | 2024 | UHPLC-MS, GC-MS | Targeted and untargeted | Cross-sectional | PICF | 56 patients (56 implants) | >18 years old; minimum 12 months functional loading, clinical diagnosis of PI/IH | 179 | succinic acid, fructose-6-phosphate, glucose-6-phosphate (correlated to PI and periodontal parameters); Isobutyric acid, 3-phenylpropionic acid (correlated with periodontal parameters); L-phenylalanine, benzamide, and L-valine (correlated to PD); Photoline, chlorphenguanidine, pyrrolidine, and hypoxanthine (correlated to BOP) | Some participants in the peri-implantitis group also had periodontitis. | A distinct metabolite profile between healthy implants and implants affected by peri-implantitis exists, and it correlates with existing bacterial flora. |
| Alassy [31] | 2021 | H-NMR | Untargeted | Longitudinal | PICF; saliva | 71 patients (130 implants) | Good general health, clinical diagnosis of PI/IH | 36 | Cadaverine/lysine (correlated to PI); alpha-ketoglutarate (correlated to healthy implants); Proline and 1-3-diamino propane (predictors for bone loss >1 mm); arginine (associated with non-progressive PI) | Study included smoking patients; | PI PICF samples demonstrate a distinct metabolic profile compared to healthy implants. |
| Fornasaro et al. [34] | 2023 | SERS | Untargeted | Cross-sectional | PICF | 118 patients (305 implants) | >18 years old; minimum 12 months functional loading, good general health, clinical diagnosis of PI/HI | NR | glutathione, ergothioneine, and hypoxanthine | Study included patients diagnosed with peri-mucositis | SERS could be a non-invasive tool to monitor implant health and PI development |
| Hamilton [30] | 2020 | H-NMR | Untargeted | Longitudinal | PICF | 59 patients (128 implants) | Good general health with controlled systemic diseases, clinical diagnosis of PI/HI | 35 | Cadaverine/lysine, propionate, alanine/lysine, putrescine/lysine, valine, tyramine, and threonine (correlated to PI); a-ketoglutarate, isoleucine, proline, and uracil (correlated to implant health) | Study included patients diagnosed with peri-mucositis | Specific metabolites were significantly correlated with PI or HI but showed insufficient sensitivity/specificity to diagnose PI. |
| Liu et al. [32] | 2024 | GC-MS, HPLC | Targeted | Cross-sectional | PICF | 48 patients (86 implants) | >18 years of age; minimum 5 years since implant placemen; no mechanical complications of implants; clinically diagnosed PI, PIM or PH | NA | Formic acid, acetic, propionic, and isovaleric acids (correlated to PIM); butyric, isobutyric, and isovaleric acids (correlated to PI) | Study searched specifically for SCFAs | Short-chain fatty acids were significantly correlated with PI clinical parameters. Elevated specific SCFAs are correlated with peri-implant disease. |

Abbreviations (in order of appearance): UHPLC-MS = ultra high-performance liquid chromatography coupled with mass spectrometry; GC-MS = gas chromatography coupled with mass spectrometry; PICF = peri-implant crevicular fluid; H-NMR = proton nuclear magnetic resonance; PI = peri-implantitis; HI = healthy implants; SERS = surface-enhanced Raman spectroscopy; HPLC = high-performance liquid chromatography; PIM = peri-implant mucositis; SCFAs = short-chain fatty acids.

### 3.3. Identified Metabolites

The most commonly identified metabolites were consistently associated with peri-implant inflammation and tissue degradation. The following metabolites were reported in studies: isobutyric acid [32,33] and propionic acid [30,32] (short-chain fatty acids or SCFAs), valine [30,33], proline, and cadaverine/lysine [30,31] (amino acids), hypoxanthine [33,34] (a purine), and alpha-ketoglutarate [30,31] (an intermediate in the Krebs cycle).

PI was correlated with SCFAs (propionate, butyric acid, isobutyric acid, isovaleric acid, and succinic acid), carbohydrate derivatives (fructose-6-phosphate and glucose-6-phosphate), amino acids (lysine, alanine, threonine, and valine), polyamines (cadaverine and putrescine), antioxidants (glutathione and ergothioneine), purines (hypoxanthine), and monoamines (tyramine). SCFAs were also correlated with increased periodontal parameters (isobutyric and propionic acids) and PIM (formic, acetic, propionic, and isovaleric acids). Amino acids were also correlated with increased probing depth (phenylalanine, valine), accelerated bone loss (proline), and stabilised PI (arginine).

### 3.4. Risk of Bias/Quality Assessment of the Studies

The risk of bias assessment revealed two studies with a low risk of bias [32,33] and three studies with a moderate risk of bias [30,31,34]. The results are displayed in Figure 2.

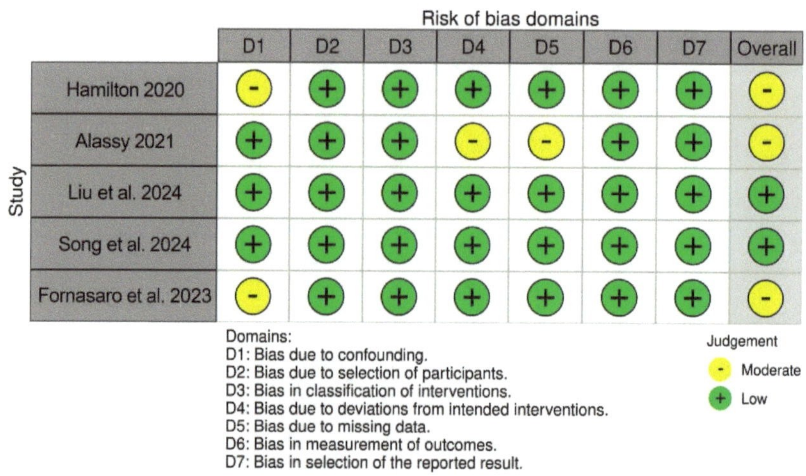


**Figure 2.** Results of risk of bias/quality assessment [30–34].

## 4. Discussion

### 4.1. Main Findings and Interpretation in the Context of Available Literature

Omics-based technologies provide insights into the molecular mechanisms and shifts between healthy and diseased states. Despite limited research, preliminary findings suggest that metabolomics can distinguish the metabolic profiles of healthy and diseased implants, offering the potential for early diagnosis. Current applications of metabolomics in dental research are focused on oral cancer [35–37], periodontitis [38–40], and caries detection [41–43], with little available research focused on PI or PIM. The most common sample types include saliva, gingival crevicular fluid (GCF), microbial plaque, and oral tissues. Metabolites are low-molecular-weight molecules which represent the end-products of metabolic processes and, in contrast to other -omics approaches, directly reflect the biochemical activity and state of tissues in their profile and concentrations. They can be endogenous (produced by the host organism and its microbiota) or exogenous (from diet, environment, and lifestyle) [44–46]. Metabolomics analysis can be conducted in two main directions: targeted and untargeted. Targeted metabolomics measures a defined set of previously characterised metabolites, while untargeted metabolomics comprehensively analyses all detectable metabolites in a sample, including unknown metabolites [47]. Lipidomics is a branch of targeted metabolomics that studies the interactions of lipids in disease processes. Two main analytical platforms are used in metabolomics: mass spectrometry (MS), frequently combined with liquid or gas chromatography (LC or GC), and nuclear magnetic resonance (NMR) spectroscopy [45]. Surface-enhanced Raman spectroscopy (SERS) is a rapid and accurate emerging method for metabolite detection [48,49].

Peri-implant diseases present shared characteristics with periodontal diseases. Both involve dysbiotic biofilms, which trigger host defence immune pathways and lead to chronic inflammation [50]. Studies have reported differences in the bacteriomes of PI and periodontitis, although a distinct microbial profile of peri-implantitis has not yet been established [51]. However, periodontitis is a risk factor for peri-implantitis development. Bacterial colonisation from periodontitis sites to peri-implant sites is frequent [51–54]. Consequently, comparing the results of periodontitis and peri-implantitis metabolomics studies may help validate the initial findings.

No metabolites recurred in more than two studies, probably due to the small number of included studies. The studies by Hamilton [30] and Alassy [31] had three metabolites in common, likely because both studies used H-NMR and similar protocols. The recurrent metabolites identified in all the included studies are discussed further in this section.

Isobutyric acid and propionic acid belong to the group of short-chain fatty acids (SCFAs). SCFAs are produced by gut and oral bacteria. In the oral cavity, they are produced primarily in periodontal pockets by periodontal pathogens like *P. gingivalis* and *Fusobacterium Nucleatum* [55]. Isobutyric acid is an isomer of butyrate. Butyrate has been frequently associated with periodontitis in various metabolomics studies [39,56–58]. It maintains bacterial metabolism and promotes bacterial growth by increasing haeme production. Furthermore, it has destructive effects on the periodontal tissues. In human gingival epithelial cells (HGECs), it promotes cell apoptosis and has a destructive effect on intercellular junctions. In human gingival fibroblasts (HGFs), it promotes cell death and the release of pro-inflammatory cytokines. These cytokines include interleukin-1 beta, interleukin-6, and tumour necrosis factor alpha, which are established biomarkers for periodontal diseases. Therefore, butyrate contributes to promoting and maintaining chronic inflammation [55,59,60]. This validates the findings of Song et al. [33] and Liu et al. [32].

Cadaverine is a metabolite of lysine. Lysine is an essential amino acid whose levels are depleted by pathogenic bacteria during periodontal destruction. Cadaverine has been previously associated with increased periodontal inflamed surface areas (PISA) and periodontitis [61–66]. The association of cadaverine with PI could be linked to both bacterial metabolism and tissue degradation. Both Alassy [31] and Hamilton [30] identified cadaverine in association with PI.

Valine is an essential proteinogenic amino acid involved in stress, energy, and muscle metabolism. Previous studies have associated it with periodontitis, with fluctuating levels [56]. Under experimental conditions, certain concentrations of valine inhibited *P. gingivalis* biofilm formation and affected bacterial polysaccharide production [67]. While Hamilton [30] identified valine as a marker for PI, Song et al. [33] correlated it with increased probing depths.

Hypoxanthine is a purine derivative. It is a chemical intermediate in the production of nucleic acids and the metabolism of adenosine. Purine degradation and reactive oxygen species production are accelerated in disease contexts, suggesting that higher levels of hypoxanthine may be linked to periodontal destruction [68–70]. Hypoxanthine has been associated with PI in the study by Fornasaro et al. [34] and was significantly correlated with bleeding on probing in the study by Song et al. [33].

Proline is a proteogenic amino acid and a component of collagen. Collagen can be found in the extracellular matrix, connective tissues, and bone. Proline molecules can be rapidly released during inflammation by the sequential action of matrix metalloproteinases, peptidases, and prolidase [71]. Extracellular proline increases the rate of collagen production, suggesting a possible connection between proline and healthy implants [72–74]. However, proline is also a marker of tissue degradation. It can be used as a precursor for superoxide radicals, which initiate the process of cellular and extracellular apoptosis [69]. This could potentially explain the correlation between increased levels of proline and periodontitis [40,61,75].

Alpha-ketoglutarate is an intermediate metabolite of the Krebs cycle, which regulates ATP production and contributes to oxidative stress defence. It is indispensable for amino acid and protein synthesis [76,77]. Furthermore, it has a proven anabolic effect on bone metabolism and is associated with bone homeostasis, improving osseointegration of dental implants [77–79]. This confirms the findings of Alassy and Hamilton [30,31], who concluded that alpha-ketoglutarate is associated with healthy implants.

### *4.2. Study Limitations and Strengths*

This review was conducted according to a pre-registered protocol submitted to PROSPERO. It adhered to the PRISMA-2020 guidelines for systematic reviews, ensuring accuracy, transparency, and methodological rigour. To the best of our knowledge, this is the first review of metabolomics applied to the diagnosis of peri-implant disease. An electronic literature search was conducted in numerous databases, including grey literature. This ensured an elaborate and comprehensive approach to identify relevant studies and provide a broad overview. Metabolomics is a novel approach in peri-implantitis research, and there is a scarcity of studies on this subject. Because of the small number of included studies and the variety of approaches used, a meta-analysis could not be conducted. However, the risk of bias assessment results suggest a high degree of study quality. In addition, the findings of the included studies confirmed the results of previous studies on periodontitis. This review provides an initial evaluation of the literature and a starting point for developing new research on metabolomic approaches in peri-implantitis, contributing to periodontics and dentistry.

### *4.3. Clinical Implications*

Based on our research, the integration of metabolomics into clinical practice has significant potential to improve the management of peri-implantitis. By facilitating non-invasive early detection through specific metabolic biomarkers, clinicians can identify peri-implant inflammation at subclinical stages, allowing for timely intervention and potentially preventing irreversible tissue damage. This early diagnostic capability is in line with the principles of personalised dentistry, allowing tailored preventive strategies based on an individual's unique metabolic profile, thus reducing both treatment complexity and associated costs.

In addition, metabolomics could serve as a practical tool for the prognosis and monitoring of therapeutic outcomes, guiding personalised treatment decisions. Regular monitoring of peri-implant crevicular fluid metabolites could provide clinicians with objective, real-time insights into the progression or resolution of peri-implant disease, thereby enabling more precise and effective therapeutic interventions. Eventually, incorporating metabolomic analysis into peri-implant care could lead to improved patient outcomes, reduce treatment burden, and increase patient satisfaction through personalised, targeted preventive strategies.

## 5. Conclusions

Although current evidence is limited, metabolomics shows promise for the diagnosis of peri-implantitis. This technology is increasingly used to study periodontitis, helping to understand its development, biological mechanisms, and progression. In particular, small molecules (metabolites), such as short-chain fatty acids and amino acids, have been frequently identified in relation to disease characteristics, such as periodontal inflammation and tissue degradation. Consequently, metabolomics could provide insights into the differences and similarities between periodontal and peri-implant diseases. Combining metabolomics with other approaches from the -omics spectrum (such as genomics, transcriptomics, and proteomics) is desirable and could provide a deeper understanding of these pathologies. Future research should focus on standardising study protocols, integrating multi-omics platform data, and validating identified metabolites and key findings in larger clinical trials.

**Author Contributions:** Conceptualisation, A.-M.C., D.C.C. and P.O.L.; Methodology, S.D.B. and A.K.; Validation, A.-M.C., A.K., D.C.C., M.N., S.D.B. and P.O.L.; Formal Analysis, S.D.B. and M.N.; Investigation, A.-M.C., D.C.C. and A.K.; Resources, P.O.L.; Writing—Original Draft Preparation, A.-M.C. and D.C.C.; Writing—Review and Editing, A.K.; Visualisation, M.N.; Supervision, P.O.L.; Project Administration, A.K.; Funding Acquisition, A.-M.C. All authors have read and agreed to the published version of the manuscript.

**Funding:** This study was partially funded by the "Iuliu Hațieganu" University of Medicine and Pharmacy, 400012 Cluj-Napoca, Romania (grant number PCD 771/14/11.01.2023).

**Institutional Review Board Statement:** Not applicable.

**Conflicts of Interest:** The authors declare no conflicts of interest.

## Appendix A Search Strategy

| Database/Registry | Query | No. of Results | Date |
|---|---|---|---|
| PubMed | ("peri implantitis"[MeSH Terms] OR "peri implantitis"[All Fields] OR "periimplantitis"[All Fields] OR ("dental implants"[MeSH Terms] OR ("dental"[All Fields] AND "implants"[All Fields]) OR "dental implants"[All Fields] OR ("dental"[All Fields] AND "implant"[All Fields]) OR "dental implant"[All Fields]) OR ("periimplant"[All Fields] AND ("disease"[MeSH Terms] OR "disease"[All Fields] OR "diseases"[All Fields] OR "disease s"[All Fields] OR "diseased"[All Fields])) OR ("peri-implant"[All Fields] AND "crevicular"[All Fields] AND ("fluid"[All Fields] OR "fluid s"[All Fields] OR "fluids"[All Fields])) OR "PICF"[All Fields]) AND ("high-performance liquid chromatography"[Text Word] OR "mass spectrometry"[Text Word] OR "nuclear magnetic resonance spectroscopy"[Text Word] OR "liquid chromatography"[All Fields] OR "gas chromatography"[All Fields] OR ("metabolome"[MeSH Terms] OR "metabolomics"[MeSH Terms]) OR "metabolom*"[All Fields] OR "lipidomic*"[All Fields]) | 208 | 21 January 2025 |

| Database/Registry | Query | No. of Results | Date |
| --- | --- | --- | --- |
| Scopus | TITLE-ABS-KEY (peri-implantitis OR periimplantitis OR "dental implant*" OR peri-implant AND disease OR peri-implant AND crevicular AND fluid OR "PICF") AND TITLE-ABS-KEY (metabolom* OR metabolomics OR metabolome OR lipidom* OR metabolite* OR "high-performance liquid chromatography" OR "mass spectrometry" OR "nuclear magnetic resonance spectroscopy" OR "liquid chromatography" OR "gas chromatography") | 17 | 21 January 2025 |
| Web of Science | ALL=(peri-implantitis OR periimplantitis OR "dental implant*" OR peri-implant AND disease OR peri-implant AND crevicular AND fluid OR "PICF") AND ALL=(metabolom* OR metabolomics OR metabolome OR lipidom* OR metabolite* OR "high-performance liquid chromatography" OR "mass spectrometry" OR "nuclear magnetic resonance spectroscopy" OR "liquid chromatography" OR "gas chromatography") | 192 | 21 January 2025 |
| ProQuest Central | summary((peri-implantitis OR periimplantitis OR ("dental implant" OR "dental implantology" OR "dental implants") OR peri-implant AND disease OR peri-implant AND crevicular AND fluid OR "PICF") AND (metabolom* OR metabolomics OR metabolome OR lipidom* OR metabolite*)) | 26 | 21 January 2025 |
| Google Scholar | peri-implantitis periimplantitis "dental implant*" peri-implant disease peri-implant crevicular fluid PICF metabolom* metabolomics metabolome lipidom* metabolite* high-performance liquid chromatography "mass spectrometry" "nuclear magnetic resonance spectroscopy" 1H NMR "liquid chromatography" "gas chromatography"Results were sorted "by relevance" and the first 10 pages of results were considered | 100 | 21 January 2025 |
| Total | | 543 | |

## References


1. Misch, C.E. Rationale for dental implants. In *Dental Implant Prosthetics*, 2nd ed.; Elsevier Mosby: Maryland Heights, MO, USA, 2014; pp. 1–25.
2. Srinivasan, M.; Meyer, S.; Mombelli, A.; Müller, F. Dental implants in the elderly population: A systematic review and meta-analysis. *Clin. Oral Implant. Res.* **2017**, *28*, 920–930. [CrossRef] [PubMed]
3. Mauer, R.G.; Shadrav, A.; Dashti, M. Predictability of Dental Implants. In *Innovative Perspectives in Oral and Maxillofacial Surgery*; Springer International Publishing: Cham, Switzerland, 2021; pp. 35–45.
4. Berglundh, T.; Jepsen, S.; Stadlinger, B.; Terheyden, H. Peri-implantitis and its prevention. *Clin. Oral Implants Res.* **2019**, *30*, 150–155. [CrossRef] [PubMed]
5. Wang, Y.; Bäumer, D.; Ozga, A.K.; Körner, G.; Bäumer, A. Patient satisfaction and oral health-related quality of life 10 years after implant placement. *BMC Oral Health* **2021**, *21*, 1–14. [CrossRef]
6. Pradyachaipimol, N.; Tangsathian, T.; Supanimitkul, K.; Sophon, N.; Suwanwichit, T.; Manopattanasoontorn, S.; Arunyanak, S.P.; Kungsadalpipob, K. Patient satisfaction following dental implant treatment: A survey. *Clin. Implant. Dent. Relat. Res.* **2023**, *25*, 613–623. [CrossRef]
7. Abrahamsson, K.H.; Wennström, J.L.; Berglundh, T.; Abrahamsson, I. Altered expectations on dental implant therapy; views of patients referred for treatment of peri-implantitis. *Clin. Oral Implants Res.* **2017**, *28*, 437–442. [CrossRef]
8. Hämmerle, C.H.F.; Tarnow, D. The etiology of hard- and soft-tissue deficiencies at dental implants: A narrative review. *J. Clin. Periodontol.* **2018**, *45*, S267–S277. [CrossRef]
9. Diaz, P.; Gonzalo, E.; Villagra, L.J.G.; Miegimolle, B.; Suarez, M.J. What is the prevalence of peri-implantitis? A systematic review and meta-analysis. *BMC Oral Health* **2022**, *22*, 1–13. [CrossRef]
10. Derks, J.; Tomasi, C. Peri-implant health and disease. A systematic review of current epidemiology. *J. Clin. Periodontol.* **2015**, *42* (Suppl. 16), S158–S171. [CrossRef]
11. Renvert, S.; Persson, G.R.; Pirih, F.Q.; Camargo, P.M. Peri-implant health, peri-implant mucositis, and peri-implantitis: Case definitions and diagnostic considerations. *J. Clin. Periodontol.* **2018**, *45*, S278–S285. [CrossRef]
12. Polymeri, A.; Loos, B.G.; Aronovich, S.; Steigmann, L.; Inglehart, M.R. Risk factors, diagnosis, and treatment of peri-implantitis: A cross-cultural comparison of U.S. and European periodontists' considerations. *J. Periodontol.* **2022**, *93*, 481–492. [CrossRef]

13. Saleh, M.H.A.; Dias, D.R.; Kumar, P. The economic and societal impact of periodontal and peri-implant diseases. *Periodontol. 2000* **2024**. *online ahead of print*. [CrossRef] [PubMed]
14. Schwarz, F.; Alcoforado, G.; Guerrero, A.; Jönsson, D.; Klinge, B.; Lang, N.; Mattheos, N.; Mertens, B.; Pitta, J.; Ramanauskaite, A.; et al. Peri-implantitis: Summary and consensus statements of group 3. The 6th EAO Consensus Conference 2021. *Clin. Oral. Implants. Res.* **2021**, *32* (Suppl. 21), 245–253. [CrossRef] [PubMed]
15. Heitz-Mayfield, L.J.; Aaboe, M.; Araujo, M.; Carrión, J.B.; Cavalcanti, R.; Cionca, N.; Cochran, D.; Darby, I.; Funakoshi, E.; Gierthmuehlen, P.C.; et al. Group 4 ITI Consensus Report: Risks and biologic complications associated with implant dentistry. *Clin. Oral Implants Res.* **2018**, *29*, 351–358. [CrossRef] [PubMed]
16. Garaicoa-Pazmino, C.; Couso-Queiruga, E.; Monje, A.; Avila-Ortiz, G.; Castilho, R.; Amo, F. Disease Resolution Following the Treatment of Peri-implant Diseases: A Systematic Review. *Int. J. Periodontics Restor. Dent.* **2025**, *45*, 115–133. [CrossRef]
17. Fu, J.H.; Wang, H.L. Breaking the wave of peri-implantitis. *Periodontol. 2000* **2020**, *84*, 145–160. [CrossRef]
18. Alassy, H.; Parachuru, P.; Wolff, L. Peri-implantitis diagnosis and prognosis using biomarkers in peri-implant crevicular fluid: A narrative review. *Diagnostics* **2019**, *9*, 214. [CrossRef]
19. Bornes, R.; Montero, J.; Correia, A.; Marques, T.; Rosa, N. Peri-implant diseases diagnosis, prognosis and dental implant monitoring: A narrative review of novel strategies and clinical impact. *BMC Oral Health* **2023**, *23*, 183. [CrossRef]
20. Kabbashi, S.; Roomaney, I.A.; Chetty, M. Bridging the gap between omics research and dental practice. *BDJ Open* **2024**, *10*, 1–9. [CrossRef]
21. Sorsa, T.; Gursoy, U.K.; Nwhator, S.; Hernandez, M.; Tervahartiala, T.; Leppilahti, J.; Gürsoy, M.; Könönen, E.; Emingil, G.; Pussinen, P.J.; et al. Analysis of matrix metalloproteinases, especially MMP-8, in gingival creviclular fluid, mouthrinse and saliva for monitoring periodontal diseases. *Periodontol. 2000* **2016**, *70*, 142–163. [CrossRef]
22. Duarte, P.M.; Serrão, C.R.; Miranda, T.S.; Zanatta, L.C.S.; Bastos, M.F.; Faveri, M.; Figueiredo, L.C.; Feres, M. Could cytokine levels in the peri-implant crevicular fluid be used to distinguish between healthy implants and implants with peri-implantitis? A systematic review. *J. Periodontal Res.* **2016**, *51*, 689–698. [CrossRef]
23. Carinci, F.; Romanos, G.E.; Scapoli, L. Molecular tools for preventing and improving diagnosis of peri-implant diseases. *Periodontol. 2000* **2019**, *81*, 41–47. [CrossRef] [PubMed]
24. Clish, C.B. Metabolomics: An emerging but powerful tool for precision medicine. *Mol. Case Stud.* **2015**, *1*, a000588. [CrossRef] [PubMed]
25. Gardner, A.; Carpenter, G.; So, P.W. Salivary Metabolomics: From Diagnostic Biomarker Discovery to Investigating Biological Function. *Metabolites* **2020**, *10*, 47. [CrossRef] [PubMed]
26. Hyvärinen, E.; Savolainen, M.; Mikkonen, J.J.W.; Kullaa, A.M. Salivary Metabolomics for Diagnosis and Monitoring Diseases: Challenges and Possibilities. *Metabolites* **2021**, *11*, 587. [CrossRef] [PubMed]
27. Page, M.J.; McKenzie, J.E.; Bossuyt, P.M.; Boutron, I.; Hoffmann, T.C.; Mulrow, C.D.; Shamseer, L.; Tetzlaff, J.M.; Akl, E.A.; Brennan, S.E.; et al. The PRISMA 2020 statement: An updated guideline for reporting systematic reviews. *Syst. Rev.* **2021**, *10*, n71. [CrossRef]
28. Sterne, J.A.; Hernán, M.A.; Reeves, B.C.; Savović, J.; Berkman, N.D.; Viswanathan, M.; Henry, D.; Altman, D.G.; Ansari, M.T.; Boutron, I.; et al. ROBINS-I: A tool for assessing risk of bias in non-randomised studies of interventions. *BMJ* **2016**, *355*, i4919. [CrossRef]
29. McGuinness, L.A.; Higgins, J.P.T. Risk-of-bias VISualization (robvis): An R package and Shiny web app for visualizing risk-of-bias assessments. *Res. Synth. Methods* **2021**, *12*, 55–61. [CrossRef]
30. Hamilton, J. Investigation of Diagnostic and Prognostic Testing for Peri-Implantitis Using Quantitative Metabolomics. Master's Thesis, University of Minnesota, Minneapolis, MN, USA, 2020.
31. Alassy, H. Peri-Implantitis Prognosis Using Metabolomic Biomarkers in Peri-Implant Crevicular Fluid: A Longitudinal Study. Ph.D. Thesis, University of Minnesota, Minneapolis, MN, USA, 2021.
32. Liu, Y.; Yang, H.; Wang, P.; Shi, Y.; Shi, R.; Zhang, S.; Zhao, Y.; Lan, J.; Ge, S. Correlation between short-chain fatty acids and peri-implant disease: A cross-sectional study. *J. Periodontol.* **2024**, *96*, 21–29. [CrossRef]
33. Song, L.; Lu, H.; Jiang, J.; Xu, A.; Huang, Y.; Huang, J.P.; Ding, P.H.; He, F. Metabolic profiling of peri-implant crevicular fluid in peri-implantitis. *Clin. Oral Implants Res.* **2024**, *35*, 719–728. [CrossRef]
34. Fornasaro, S.; Rapani, A.; Farina, F.; Ibishi, M.; Pisnoli, G.; Stacchi, C.; Sergo, V.; Bonifacio, A.; Di Lenarda, R.; Berton, F. Spectroscopic insights into peri-implant mucositis and peri-implantitis: Unveiling peri-implant crevicular fluid profiles using surface enhanced Raman scattering. *Analyst* **2023**, *149*, 885–894. [CrossRef]
35. Mikkonen, J.J.W.; Singh, S.P.; Herrala, M.; Lappalainen, R.; Myllymaa, S.; Kullaa, A.M. Salivary metabolomics in the diagnosis of oral cancer and periodontal diseases. *J. Periodontal Res.* **2016**, *51*, 431–437. [CrossRef] [PubMed]

36. Kouznetsova, V.L.; Li, J.; Romm, E.; Tsigelny, I.F. Finding distinctions between oral cancer and periodontitis using saliva metabolites and machine learning. *Oral Dis.* **2021**, *27*, 484–493. [CrossRef] [PubMed]
37. Papale, F.; Santonocito, S.; Polizzi, A.; Giudice, A.L.; Capodiferro, S.; Favia, G.; Isola, G. The New Era of Salivaomics in Dentistry: Frontiers and Facts in the Early Diagnosis and Prevention of Oral Diseases and Cancer. *Metabolites* **2022**, *12*, 638. [CrossRef] [PubMed]
38. Baima, G.; Corana, M.; Iaderosa, G.; Romano, F.; Citterio, F.; Meoni, G.; Tenori, L.; Aimetti, M. Metabolomics of gingival crevicular fluid to identify biomarkers for periodontitis: A systematic review with meta-analysis. *J. Periodontal Res.* **2021**, *56*, 633–645. [CrossRef]
39. Alamri, M.M.; Williams, B.; Le Guennec, A.; Mainas, G.; Santamaria, P.; Moyes, D.L.; Nibali, L. Metabolomics analysis in saliva from periodontally healthy, gingivitis and periodontitis patients. *J. Periodontal Res.* **2023**, *58*, 1272–1280. [CrossRef]
40. Romano, F.; Meoni, G.; Manavella, V.; Baima, G.; Tenori, L.; Cacciatore, S.; Aimetti, M. Analysis of salivary phenotypes of generalized aggressive and chronic periodontitis through nuclear magnetic resonance-based metabolomics. *J. Periodontol.* **2018**, *89*, 1452–1460. [CrossRef]
41. Heimisdottir, L.H.; Lin, B.M.; Cho, H.; Orlenko, A.; Ribeiro, A.A.; Simon-Soro, A.; Roach, J.; Shungin, D.; Ginnis, J.; Simancas-Pallares, M.; et al. Metabolomics Insights in Early Childhood Caries. *J. Dent. Res.* **2021**, *100*, 615–622. [CrossRef]
42. Li, K.; Wang, J.; Du, N.; Sun, Y.; Sun, Q.; Yin, W.; Li, H.; Meng, L.; Liu, X. Salivary microbiome and metabolome analysis of severe early childhood caries. *BMC Oral Health* **2023**, *23*, 30. [CrossRef]
43. Schulz, A.; Lang, R.; Behr, J.; Hertel, S.; Reich, M.; Kümmerer, K.; Hannig, M.; Hannig, C.; Hofmann, T. Targeted metabolomics of pellicle and saliva in children with different caries activity. *Sci. Rep.* **2020**, *10*, 1–11. [CrossRef]
44. Turi, K.N.; Romick-Rosendale, L.; Ryckman, K.K.; Hartert, T.V. A review of metabolomics approaches and their application in identifying causal pathways of childhood asthma. *J. Allergy Clin. Immunol.* **2018**, *141*, 1191–1201. [CrossRef]
45. Chen, Y.; Li, E.M.; Xu, L.Y. Guide to Metabolomics Analysis: A Bioinformatics Workflow. *Metabolites* **2022**, *12*, 357. [CrossRef] [PubMed]
46. Zhang, Y.; Chen, R.; Zhang, D.D.; Qi, S.; Liu, Y. Metabolite interactions between host and microbiota during health and disease: Which feeds the other? *Biomed. Pharmacother.* **2023**, *160*, 114295. [CrossRef] [PubMed]
47. Roberts, L.D.; Souza, A.L.; Gerszten, R.E.; Clish, C.B. Targeted metabolomics. *Curr. Protoc. Mol. Biol.* **2012**, *98*. [CrossRef] [PubMed]
48. Lu, Y.; Lin, L.; Ye, J. Human metabolite detection by surface-enhanced Raman spectroscopy. *Mater. Today Bio.* **2022**, *13*, 100205. [CrossRef]
49. Premasiri, W.R.; Lee, J.C.; Sauer-Budge, A.; Théberge, R.; Costello, C.E.; Ziegler, L.D. The biochemical origins of the surface-enhanced Raman spectra of bacteria: A metabolomics profiling by SERS. *Anal. Bioanal. Chem.* **2016**, *408*, 4631–4647. [CrossRef]
50. Robitaille, N.; Reed, D.N.; Walters, J.D.; Kumar, P.S. Periodontal and peri-implant diseases: Identical or fraternal infections? *Mol. Oral Microbiol.* **2016**, *31*, 285–301. [CrossRef]
51. Sahrmann, P.; Gilli, F.; Wiedemeier, D.B.; Attin, T.; Schmidlin, P.R.; Karygianni, L. The Microbiome of Peri-Implantitis: A Systematic Review and Meta-Analysis. *Microorganisms* **2020**, *8*, 661. [CrossRef]
52. Ferreira, S.D.; Martins, C.C.; Amaral, S.A.; Vieira, T.R.; Albuquerque, B.N.; Cota, L.O.M.; Lima, R.P.E.; Costa, F.O. Periodontitis as a risk factor for peri-implantitis: Systematic review and meta-analysis of observational studies. *J. Dent.* **2018**, *79*, 1–10. [CrossRef]
53. Darby, I. Risk factors for periodontitis & peri-implantitis. *Periodontol. 2000* **2022**, *90*, 9–12.
54. Dalago, H.R.; Schuldt Filho, G.; Rodrigues, M.A.P.; Renvert, S.; Bianchini, M.A. Risk indicators for Peri-implantitis. A cross-sectional study with 916 implants. *Clin. Oral Implants Res.* **2017**, *28*, 144–150. [CrossRef]
55. Guan, X.; Li, W.; Meng, H. A double-edged sword: Role of butyrate in the oral cavity and the gut. *Mol. Oral Microbiol.* **2021**, *36*, 121–131. [CrossRef] [PubMed]
56. Brito, F.; Curcio, H.F.Q.; da Silva Fidalgo, T.K. Periodontal disease metabolomics signatures from different biofluids: A systematic review. *Metabolomics* **2022**, *18*, 83. [CrossRef] [PubMed]
57. Na, H.S.; Kim, S.; Yu, Y.; Kim, S.Y.; Kim, H.J.; Lee, J.Y.; Lee, J.H.; Chung, J. Molecular subgroup of periodontitis revealed by integrated analysis of the microbiome and metabolome in a cross-sectional observational study. *J. Oral Microbiol.* **2021**, *13*, 1902707. [CrossRef]
58. Kim, S.; Kim, H.J.; Song, Y.; Lee, H.A.; Kim, S.; Chung, J. Metabolic phenotyping of saliva to identify possible biomarkers of periodontitis using proton nuclear magnetic resonance. *J. Clin. Periodontol.* **2021**, *48*, 1240–1249. [CrossRef]
59. Leonov, G.E.; Varaeva, Y.R.; Livantsova, E.N.; Starodubova, A.V. The Complicated Relationship of Short-Chain Fatty Acids and Oral Microbiome: A Narrative Review. *Biomedicines* **2023**, *11*, 2749. [CrossRef]
60. Basic, A.; Dahlén, G. Microbial metabolites in the pathogenesis of periodontal diseases: A narrative review. *Front. Oral Health* **2023**, *4*, 1210200. [CrossRef]

61. Kuboniwa, M.; Sakanaka, A.; Hashino, E.; Bamba, T.; Fukusaki, E.; Amano, A. Prediction of Periodontal Inflammation via Metabolic Profiling of Saliva. *J. Dent. Res.* **2016**, *95*, 1381–1386. [CrossRef]
62. Sakanaka, A.; Kuboniwa, M.; Katakami, N.; Furuno, M.; Nishizawa, H.; Omori, K.; Taya, N.; Ishikawa, A.; Mayumi, S.; Isomura, E.T.; et al. Saliva and Plasma Reflect Metabolism Altered by Diabetes and Periodontitis. *Front. Mol. Biosci.* **2021**, *8*, 742002. [CrossRef]
63. Sakanaka, A.; Kuboniwa, M.; Hashino, E.; Bamba, T.; Fukusaki, E.; Amano, A. Distinct signatures of dental plaque metabolic byproducts dictated by periodontal inflammatory status. *Sci. Rep.* **2017**, *7*, 42818. [CrossRef]
64. Rashid, M.H.; Yellarthi, S.P.K.; Yellarthi, P.K.; Didugu, B.G.L.; Mamillapalli, A. Combined assessment of lysine and N-acetyl cadaverine levels assist as a potential biomarker of the smoker periodontitis. *Amino Acids* **2024**, *56*, 41. [CrossRef]
65. Andörfer, L.; Holtfreter, B.; Weiss, S.; Matthes, R.; Pitchika, V.; Schmidt, C.O.; Samietz, S.; Kastenmüller, G.; Nauck, M.; Völker, U.; et al. Salivary metabolites associated with a 5-year tooth loss identified in apopulation-based setting. *BMC Med.* **2021**, *19*, 161. [CrossRef] [PubMed]
66. Barnes, V.M.; Ciancio, S.G.; Shibly, O.; Xu, T.; Devizio, W.; Trivedi, H.M.; Guo, L.; Jonsson, T.J. Metabolomics Reveals Elevated Macromolecular Degradation in Periodontal Disease. *J. Dent. Res.* **2011**, *90*, 1293–1297. [CrossRef] [PubMed]
67. Qi, H.; Li, B.; Wang, H.; Cai, Q.; Quan, X.; Cui, Y.; Meng, W. Effects of d-valine on periodontal or peri-implant pathogens: Porphyromonas gingivalis biofilm. *J. Periodontol.* **2018**, *89*, 303–314. [CrossRef]
68. Liebsch, C.; Pitchika, V.; Pink, C.; Samietz, S.; Kastenmüller, G.; Artati, A.; Suhre, K.; Adamski, J.; Nauck, M.; Völzke, H.; et al. The Saliva Metabolome in Association to Oral Health Status. *J. Dent. Res.* **2019**, *98*, 642–651. [CrossRef]
69. Citterio, F.; Romano, F.; Meoni, G.; Iaderosa, G.; Grossi, S.; Sobrero, A.; Dego, F.; Corana, M.; Berta, G.N.; Tenori, L.; et al. Changes in the salivary metabolic profile of generalized periodontitis patients after non-surgical periodontal therapy: A metabolomic analysis using nuclear magnetic resonance spectroscopy. *J. Clin. Med.* **2020**, *9*, 1–12. [CrossRef]
70. Barnes, V.M.; Teles, R.; Trivedi, H.M.; Devizio, W.; Xu, T.; Mitchell, M.W.; Milburn, M.V.; Guo, L. Acceleration of purine degradation by periodontal diseases. *J. Dent. Res.* **2009**, *88*, 851–855. [CrossRef]
71. Phang, J.M.; Pandhare, J.; Liu, Y. The Metabolism of Proline as Microenvironmental Stress Substrate. *J. Nutr.* **2008**, *138*, 2008S. [CrossRef]
72. Karna, E.; Szoka, L.; Huynh, T.Y.L.; Palka, J.A. Proline-dependent regulation of collagen metabolism. *Cell Mol. Life Sci.* **2019**, *70*, 1911. [CrossRef]
73. Fouillen, A.; Mary, C.; Ponce, K.J.; Moffatt, P.; Nanci, A. A proline rich protein from the gingival seal around teeth exhibits antimicrobial properties against Porphyromonas gingivalis. *Sci. Rep.* **2021**, *11*, 2353. [CrossRef]
74. Jayasinghe, T.N.; Harrass, S.; Erdrich, S.; King, S.; Eberhard, J. Protein Intake and Oral Health in Older Adults-A Narrative Review. *Nutrients* **2022**, *2022*, 4478. [CrossRef]
75. García-Villaescusa, A.; Morales-Tatay, J.M.; Monleón-Salvadó, D.; González-Darder, J.M.; Bellot-Arcis, C.; Montiel-Company, J.M.; Almerich-Silla, J.M. Using NMR in saliva to identify possible biomarkers of glioblastoma andchronic periodontitis. *PLoS ONE* **2018**, *13*, e0188710. [CrossRef] [PubMed]
76. Wang, Y.; Deng, P.; Liu, Y.; Wu, Y.; Chen, Y.; Guo, Y.; Zhang, S.; Zheng, X.; Zhou, L.; Liu, W.; et al. Alpha-ketoglutarate ameliorates age-related osteoporosis via regulating histone methylations. *Nat. Commun.* **2020**, *11*, 5596. [CrossRef] [PubMed]
77. Liu, R.; Gao, Y.; Huang, L.; Shi, B.; Yin, X.; Zou, S. Alpha-ketoglutarate up-regulates autophagic activity in peri-implant environment and enhances dental implant osseointegration in osteoporotic mice. *J. Clin. Periodontol.* **2023**, *50*, 671–683. [CrossRef] [PubMed]
78. Chen, L.; Li, Q.; Ma, S.; Wang, B. α-Ketoglutarate promotes autophagic activity under a peri-implant condition to enhance osseointegration of dental implant in rats with osteoporosis. *Connect. Tissue Res.* **2024**, *66*, 1–9. [CrossRef]
79. Li, Y.; Liu, L.; Li, Y.; Song, W.; Shao, B.; Li, H.; Lin, W.; Li, Q.; Shuai, X.; Bai, M.; et al. Alpha-ketoglutarate promotes alveolar bone regeneration by modulating M2 macrophage polarization. *Bone Rep.* **2023**, *18*, 101671. [CrossRef]

*diagnostics*

MDPI

*Interesting Images*

# Extensive Synovial Chondromatosis of the Temporomandibular Joint Extending to the Cranial Base

**Chi-Heon Sung [1], Seo-Young An [1], Hae-Seo Park [1], Wonae Lee [2] and Moon-Young Kim [1,*]**

[1] Department of Oral and Maxillofacial Surgery, College of Dentistry, Dankook University, Cheonan 31116, Republic of Korea; kom4809@gmail.com (C.-H.S.); u8042222@naver.com (S.-Y.A.); haeseopk@dankook.ac.kr (H.-S.P.)

[2] Department of Pathology, College of Medicine, Dankook University, Cheonan 31116, Republic of Korea; walee@dankook.ac.kr

* Correspondence: kmyomfs@dankook.ac.kr

**Abstract:** A 42-year-old male presented to the Department of Oral and Maxillofacial Surgery with the chief complaint of pain and stiffness in the right temporomandibular joint (TMJ). The patient's height was 174 cm and his body weight was 65 kg. The patient's occupation was heavy equipment operator. According to the patient, the pain had initiated a week prior to his first visit and was exacerbated during mastication. Evaluation of the range of motion revealed extensive crepitus along the right TMJ. The active and passive range of motion were measured at 45 mm and 42 mm, respectively, indicating adequate mouth-opening capacity. Occlusion was also favorable, and no other clinical symptoms were shown intraorally.

**Keywords:** head and neck neoplasms; synovial chondromatosis; middle cranial fossa; TMJ

Synovial chondromatosis in the TMJ may occur as either primary idiopathic lesions or secondary lesions related to trauma or degenerative arthritis [1]. Patients often report discomfort within the TMJ that is exacerbated by physical activities such as mouth opening and mastication, thus resulting in TMJ dysfunction. Since the risk of degenerative arthritis resulting from constant mechanical friction increases with delay in the surgical removal of synovial chondromatosis, it is necessary to perform surgical excision as soon as the initial diagnosis is made.

On magnetic resonance imaging (MRI), synovial chondromatosis of the temporomandibular joint (TMJ) is indicated by the presence of cartilaginous nodules with signs of low and isointensity in the joint space, which may present small or localized rounded shapes, with different degrees of calcification, similar to a "ring" [2]. On computed tomography (CT), multiple loose bodies of moderate to increased density can be identified, delimited, and located, with expansion of the intra-articular space and bone changes, such as erosions of the mandibular fossa, joint tubercle, and head of the mandible [2].

Synovial chondromatosis is an uncommon articular disorder characterized by synovial metaplasia with intra-articular proliferation of cartilaginous nodules originating from the synovial membrane [3–5]. This disorder usually affects large joints and is rarely observed in the TMJ. Synovial chondromatosis in the TMJ may occur as either primary idiopathic lesions or secondary lesions related to trauma or degenerative arthritis [6].

Panoramic radiography, CT, and MRI are the typical radiological evaluation tools required for the diagnosis of TMJ bony lesions. However, a histopathological biopsy of the specimen acquired via surgery is crucial for definitive diagnosis. Synovial chondromatosis arising in the TMJ is most commonly reported to be confined within the joint cavity [7]. We herein report a rare extra-articular case of synovial chondromatosis extending to the cranial base. Panoramic radiographs taken upon the patient's first visit revealed multiple calcified particles in the right TMJ area. CT and MRI were consecutively performed for accurate diagnosis. Radiological examinations revealed multiple nodules within the joint capsule of the right TMJ, extending to the middle cranial fossa. The shape of the mandibular condyle appeared to be smooth. The patient was provisionally diagnosed with pigmented villonodular synovitis and subsequently admitted for surgical treatment (Figures 1–3).

Blood tests showed normal results with a white blood cell count of 9560/mm$^3$, C-reactive protein at 0.36 mg/dL, and an erythrocyte sedimentation rate of 3 mm/h. Under general anesthesia, a temporo-preauricular incision was made to access the right temporomandibular joint, and surgical excision of the loose bodies was performed. A total of 25 loose bodies were removed, and histopathological examination was performed. At the 1-month post-surgery follow-up, the patient showed decreased pain, with a measured range of motion (ROM) of 35 mm. At the 6-month post-surgery follow-up, the patient still complained of occasional clicking in the right TMJ but stated that the pain had completely resolved. A follow-up CT scan taken at 6 months post-surgery also revealed no signs of loose body formation.

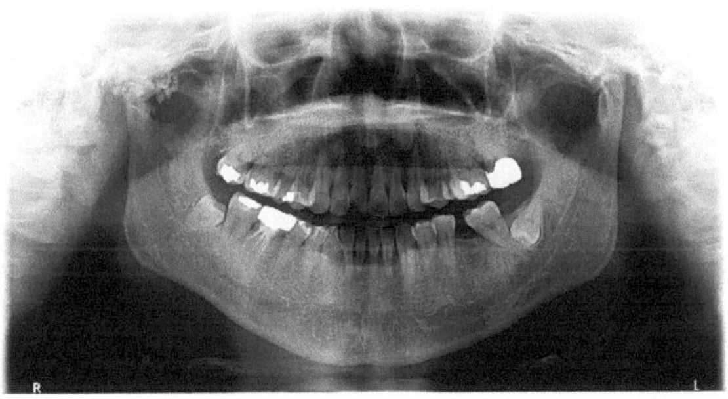


**Figure 1.** Panoramic view: multiple calcified nodules around the right condyle of the mandible, showing cortical disruption and possible erosion of the condyle head. The right condylar process shows a sclerotic appearance with mixed radiopacity and radiolucency. The joint space is reduced because of the lesion.

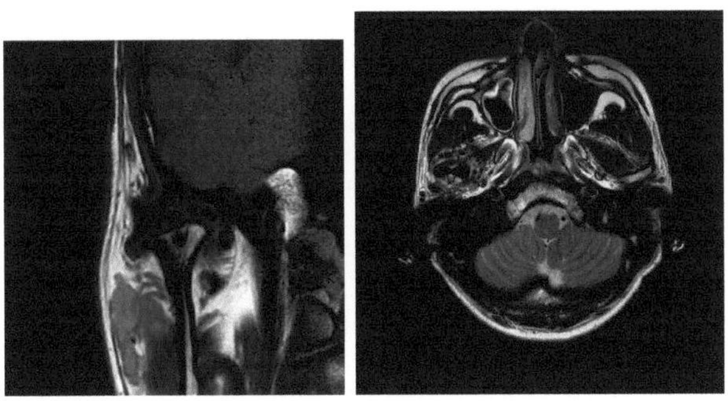

**Figure 2.** Coronal view of magnetic resonance (MR) TMJ T1-weighted image, showing a mass extending to the cranial base. The coronal view shows flattening of the right condylar head with a heterogeneous signal intensity, particularly in the cortical and subcortical areas, which may indicate sclerosis or degeneration. The articular disk of the right TMJ appears to be displaced anteriorly.

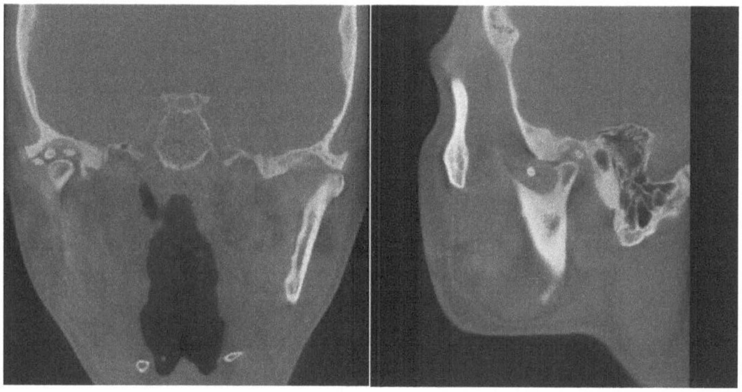

**Figure 3.** Coronal and sagittal view of computed tomography. Right glenoid fossa erosion was present compared to the opposite condyle. The right condylar head shows a loss of the normal smooth cortical margin with evidence of mixed sclerosis and radiolucency which shows cortical irregularity, and possible erosion is noted on the superior aspect of the condyle. The joint space is narrowed, suggesting possible degenerative changes.

Synovial chondromatosis is a rare, benign condition of unknown etiology in which the synovium undergoes metaplasia leading to cartilaginous nodules that ultimately break free, mineralize, and even ossify [8]. This disorder usually affects large joints and is rarely observed in the TMJ [1]. The process of hyaline cartilage degeneration within the TMJ was originally described by Paré in 1558. Although the exact etiology remains yet unclear, it is characterized pathologically by degeneration of the synovial membrane within the articular space that results in the formation of calcified nodules [3]. The mean age of presentation is between the 4th and 5th decade, with a preponderance of female cases and unilateral presentation [8].

The common symptoms of synovial chondromatosis of the TMJ are pain, restricted mandibular range of motion, crepitation, and deviation to the affected site [5]. Typically, synovial chondromatosis occurring in the TMJ is predominantly localized within the joint space. Among the rare cases in which the extra-articular calcified nodules remarkably erode the skull base, neurological manifestations only still occur when the cranial base is perforated. The objective of this paper is to review the risk factors that may cause synovial chondromatosis arising from the TMJ, which previously led to neurological symptoms, by sharing our rare case.

Lieger et al. reviewed 80 cases of TMJ synovial chondromatosis patients to find only 7 cases with lesions extending to the cranial base [9]. They reported no significant differences in the neurological symptoms between this group and other cases with lesions not affecting the cranial base. However, neurological deficits (hearing loss) were identified when the loose body penetrated the temporal bone. It would be natural to assume that the delayed treatment of this condition would be one of the major causes leading to such an extension to the cranial base. However, von Lindern et al. reported contrary findings [10]. In their recent literature review of 60 references with a total of 74 cases, it was revealed that the mean delay to confirmation of diagnosis among patients with intracranial/cranial extension (21 months) was significantly shorter than that of extracranial cases (32 months). Age, gender, and the location of the lesion were similar in both groups. This case demonstrates the possibility of synovial chondromatosis of the TMJ extending to the base of the skull, underscoring the importance of the meticulous examination of the skull base in future diagnosis and treatment planning. In conclusion, we propose that a thorough evaluation of adjacent structures for signs of invasion be essentially accompanied when diagnosing TMJ synovial chondromatosis. Further research is necessary to elucidate the pathological mechanisms and clinical significance of such an invasion.

**Author Contributions:** Conceptualization, M.-Y.K.; methodology, C.-H.S., H.-S.P., W.L. and M.-Y.K.; resources, C.-H.S. and M.-Y.K.; writing—original draft preparation, C.-H.S. and M.-Y.K.; writing—review and editing, C.-H.S., S.-Y.A., W.L. and M.-Y.K.; supervision, M.-Y.K.; funding acquisition, M.-Y.K. All authors have read and agreed to the published version of the manuscript.

**Funding:** M.-Y.K. was supported by a National Research Foundation of Korea (NRF) grant funded by the Ministry of Science and ICT (2021R1C1C1008843).

**Institutional Review Board Statement:** Not applicable.

**Informed Consent Statement:** Informed consent was obtained from all subjects involved in the study. Written informed consent has been obtained from the patient to publish this paper.

**Data Availability Statement:** The original contributions presented in the study are included in the article, further inquiries can be directed to the corresponding author.

**Conflicts of Interest:** The authors declare no conflicts of interest.

## References

1. Oksana, I.; Edvitar, L.; Ülle, V.-O. Synovial chondromatosis in the temporomandibular joint: Case report with review of the literature. *Stomatol. Balt. Dent. Maxillofac. J.* **2015**, *17*, 97–101.
2. Jang, B.G.; Huh, K.H.; Kang, J.H.; Kim, J.E.; Yi, W.J.; Heo, M.S.; Lee, S.S. Imaging features of synovial chondromatosis of the temporomandibular joint: A report of 34 cases. *Clin. Radiol.* **2021**, *76*, 627–e1. [CrossRef]
3. Neumann, J.A.; Garrigues, G.E.; Brigman, B.E.; Eward, W.C. Synovial Chondromatosis. *JBJS Rev.* **2016**, *4*, 1. [CrossRef]
4. Agaram, N.P.; Zhang, L.; Dickson, B.C.; Swanson, D.; Sung, Y.; Panicek, D.M.; Hameed, M.; Healey, J.H.; Antonescu, C.R. A Molecular Study of Synovial Chondromatosis. *Genes Chromosomes Cancer* **2020**, *59*, 144–151. [CrossRef]
5. Moorthy, V.; Tay, K.S.; Koo, K. Arthroscopic Treatment of Primary Synovial Chondromatosis of the Ankle: A Case Report and Review of Literature. *J. Orthop. Case Rep.* **2020**, *10*, 54–59.
6. Paparo, F.; Massarelli, M.; Cordeschi, R.; Sciannameo, V.; Spallaccia, F. Chondromatosis of the Temporomandibular Joint as a Consequence of Persistent Long-Lasting Joint Dysfunction. *J. Craniofacial Surg.* **2016**, *27*, e636–e637. [CrossRef]
7. Sozzi, D.; Bocchialini, G.; Novelli, G.; Valente, M.G.; Moltrasio, F.; Bozzetti, A. A rare case of synovial chondromatosis of the inferior TMJ compartment: Diagnosis and treatment aspect. *Ann. Stomatol.* **2016**, *6*, 91–95. [CrossRef]
8. Morales, R.J.; Cabrales, R.A. Cabrales: Synovial chondromatosis affecting the temporomandibular joint: A case report and literature review. *Oral. Maxillofac. Surg. Cases* **2020**, *6*, 100144. [CrossRef]
9. Lieger, O.; Zix, J.; Stauffer-Brauch, E.J.; Iizuka, T. Synovial Chondromatosis of the Temporomandibular Joint With Cranial Extension: A Case Report and Literature Review. *J. Oral Maxillofac. Surg.* **2007**, *65*, 2073–2080. [CrossRef]
10. von Lindern, J.J.; Theuerkauf, I.; Niederhagen, B.; Bergé, S.; Appel, T.; Reich, R.H. Synovial chondromatosis of the temporomandibular joint: Clinical, diagnostic, and histomorphologic findings. *Oral. Surg. Oral. Med. Oral. Pathol. Oral. Radiol. Endod.* **2002**, *94*, 31. [CrossRef]

MDPI AG
Grosspeteranlage 5
4052 Basel
Switzerland
Tel.: +41 61 683 77 34

*Diagnostics* Editorial Office
E-mail: diagnostics@mdpi.com
www.mdpi.com/journal/diagnostics

www.ingramcontent.com/pod-product-compliance
Lightning Source LLC
Chambersburg PA
CBHW041354210926
51850CB00013B/3080
* 9 7 8 3 7 2 5 8 4 5 0 1 9 *